Endorsements

Anyone in my field knows that if you want to get healthy and stay healthy, it's all about body composition. *Sustainable Weight Loss* is a must have book for anyone, including physicians like myself, who want to go above and beyond the limits of just diet and exercise. *In the war against aging, the bigger your arsenal, the better the outcome.* This book has expanded my arsenal considerably.

**Michael Reilly, MD - Holistic Practitioner &
Board Certified in Anti-Aging Medicine**

In my nearly 70 years of health and fitness, I have never seen a collection of health and weight management information as comprehensive, complete and well researched as *Sustainable Weight Loss*. My only regret is that it wasn't available years earlier.

**Bill Pearl - Mr. America, five-time Mr. Universe and author of the
best selling books, *Beyond the Universe* and *Getting Stronger***

In our society people are always looking for a quick fix to anything and everything. In *Sustainable Weight Loss* the thing that really resonates with me, as an athlete is to set goals that you can really achieve and let people encourage you and help you reach those goals. It's exactly the same way in sports. This book is full of important facts about why we all need to be fit and healthy. After reading it even I need to make some changes to live a healthier life. Thank you Lee, now I'm heading off the gym!

Shannon Bahrke - two-time Olympic Medalist (Freestyle Skiing)

Dr. Waller's book on weight management offers a unique and interesting perspective on a subject that has no dearth of information in the popular media. Dr. Waller examines the psychological dynamics as well as giving sound nutritional advice for success in achieving weight goals and overall balance.

Carla Edwards, MS, PhD, LAc, Dipl OM

Obesity, diabetes and cancer could bankrupt our country. *Sustainable Weight Loss* leaves no stone unturned in its search for helpful suggestions to these problems, while at the same time allowing its readers an array of choices in line with their health, lifestyle, age, mental well being, etc. I think that Primary Care Physicians might want to keep this book handy as a valuable desk reference.

Bob Quesnel - 1977 Mr. Arizona Over Age 35

Sustainable Weight Loss

The Definitive Guide to Maintaining a Healthy Body Weight

D. Lee Waller, JD, ND

iUniverse, Inc.
Bloomington

Sustainable Weight Loss
The Definitive Guide to Maintaining a Healthy Body Weight

iUniverse books may be ordered through booksellers or by contacting:

iUniverse
1663 Liberty Drive
Bloomington, IN 47403
www.iuniverse.com
1-800-Authors (1-800-288-4677)

ISBN: 978-1-4620-0160-6 (pbk)
ISBN: 978-1-4620-0161-3 (ebk)

Printed in the United States of America

iUniverse rev. date: 04/27/2011

Dedication

This book is dedicated to military men and women worldwide, who have throughout the history of mankind, been called upon to give of themselves for the cause of freedom. Especially the freedom to:

- Read, write, speak and think what we want to,
- Elect those that govern our political institutions,
- Live our lives without undue interference from government.

Frequently we disagree with the conflict, venue or engagement but we should never lose sight of what is at stake. It should be obvious to all of us in the free world that many people don't enjoy the same freedoms we do. We must also realize without the commitment from the men and women who protect our freedom, there are those who would take it away from us.

My deepest thanks go out to all of them. Without their efforts it is possible this book could not have been written.

Acknowledgements

An undertaking like the writing and publication of this book can only be fully appreciated by a first-time author, as the task progresses. From the beginning, I was prepared for a sizable task; however, I had no idea how much I would come to rely on the skills and talent of other people. Although the group of contributors was fairly small, the magnitude and significance of their contributions cannot be overstated. I offer each and every one my deepest gratitude and most heartfelt thanks. Following is what each individual did to help me move my idea from an embryonic stage to a fully developed and functional finished product.

Research

- **Lillian Hardison** - is a Graduate Secretary in the history department at Chicago's Loyola University, who through the course of this project helped me locate my research assistants from the Loyola student body.

- **Kirsten DeVries, PhD** - was my first research assistant and even though juggling her time between teaching and finishing her doctoral thesis, she found time to research two thirds of the material used in this book, before she moved on to take a full-time teaching position in Virginia.

- **Andrew Altepeter** - picked up where Kirsten left off, and while working part-time and conducting his own graduate study work, he found time to collect the remainder of the research needed to complete this project.

- **Barbara Wilensky** – is my personal assistant and the person responsible for locating and initiating conversations with all of the individuals who endorsed this book.

Presentation Review

- **Jayne Kurschner** - is a close friend and fellow natural health devotee who offered to review my work because of her: (1) interest in the subject, (2) outstanding grammatical skills, and (3) voracious appetite for reading. Thanks Jayne for your input.

- **Bruce Braker** - is a long-time business associate and wise old sage who I welcomed as a reviewer because of his common sense, superior writing skills and previous reviewer experience. I am very grateful to Bruce for the depth of his review.

Technical Content Review

- **Michael Reilly, MD** - is board-certified in the use of anti-aging treatments. His extensive background in the effective use of hormone protocols, his understanding of the genetic contribution to weight loss, coupled with his personal exercise and nutrition experience made his review invaluable.

- **John Funovits, DC** - is a long time friend, natural healing counselor and fellow natural health devotee, who brought a broad knowledge of biomechanics, exercise physiology and nutrition to the review process, making his contribution to this work priceless.

- **Joseph Harbosky, DC** - is a long time friend and natural health care professional and confidant, whose broad array of skills in nutrition, kinesiology, biofeedback, herbology and homeopathy gave his review exceptional credibility.

Publishing and Marketing

- **Helen Gallagher** - is my Publishing Consultant who brought knowledge and experience that only comes with having been immersed in this field for years. Although I have read several books on the topic of publishing, Helen was able to distill that looming cloud into simple, easy to follow steps that moved this project forward expeditiously. Without her help the lengthy transitionary period from writing to publishing would have been all but impossible.

It has been both an honor and a privilege for me to be able to rely on the expertise of these people during the life of this project, and I will always regard them as personal friends.

About the Author

I was born November 4, 1942 in Saginaw, Michigan and spent most of my life in Michigan. I have been driven by an interest in personal health and physical fitness for over fifty years. While I have never suffered from any of the maladies that have driven many people to seek improved health practices, I have been moved by the burning notion we all can improve our current health status, if we just apply a little knowledge, patience, energy and will power. Although I didn't initially choose a career in healthcare, my interest, curiosity and propensity towards personal health improvement and preservation has increasingly moved me from my business roots to a very well rounded and knowledgeable devotee of natural health practices.

I have worked in a number of businesses over the years while at the same time formally pursuing my passion for natural health and weight control. In 1991 I founded Genesis 1 Technology, Ltd., a Chicago based consulting firm, which also serves as a platform for my healthcare ventures.

I have achieved an extensive and diversified educational background, which includes:

- Doctor of Naturopathy - Trinity College of Natural Health,
- Certified Personal Trainer - American Council on Exercise,
- Certified Lifestyle and Weight Management Coach - American Council on Exercise,
- Juris Doctor - Thomas M. Cooley Law School,
- MA Business Management - Central Michigan University,
- MA Personnel Administration - Central Michigan University,
- BS Mechanical Engineering - General Motors Institute.

I want you to understand in writing this book I have no competing interests. I am not selling any products, services or anything else that might bias me in terms of what I tell you and I have tried to keep my personal opinions in check, basing this work on solid, factual research. My interpretation of the research was done with an open mind and an honest heart.

It is my deepest hope you will be able to tap into all that is offered within these pages, for the benefit of your own successful and *Sustainable Weight Loss*, coupled with outrageous health improvement.

To learn more and obtain the companion workbook, visit www.sustainableweightloss.net

Contents

Dedication v

Acknowledgements vii

About the Author ix

Foreword xvii

Preface xix
- Why I Wrote This Book xix
- How to Use This Book xxii
- Endnotes xxii

Introduction xxv
- Metabolic Syndrome (MS) xxvii
- Health Risk Factors xxviii
- Endnotes xxxi

Warning / Disclaimer xxxv

Part One	Understanding the Basics	1

  1 An Overview of the Human Body 3

- Understanding Entropy 3
- How Cells Produce Energy 4
- Good Health and Weight Control are Inseparable 5
- The Set Point Theory 6
- Body Type 7
- Body Composition 7
  - o Body Mass Index (BMI) 8
  - o Waist to Hip Ratio (WHR) 8
  - o Waist Circumference (WC) 9
  - o Fat Free Mass (FFM) 9
- Metabolism - Friend or Foe 10
- Endnotes 11

  2 The Role of Genetics 13

- Your Future is Not Completely Controlled by Genetics 15

- ○ The Link Between Genetics and Obesity...15
- • Summary...18
- • Endnotes..19

Part Two   Consider Your Options   23

3   The Importance of Food Choices 25

- • Diets and Dieting...26
  - ○ Reasons for Dieting 27
  - ○ Types of Diets 28
  - ○ Caloric Balance..32
  - ○ Successful Dieters 33
  - ○ The Downside of Dieting 33
- • Nutrition - It's a Bigger Deal Than You Might Think.......................35
  - ○ Fuel the Engine - Healthy Eating 36
  - ○ What to Include in Your Food Plan...37
  - ○ What to Limit in Your Food Plan 44
  - ○ It is Easier Than You Think (The Rule of Thirds)........................50
  - ○ Nutritional Supplements / Meal Replacements / Diet Aids...........53
    - – Nutritional Supplements..54
    - – Meal Replacements...54
    - – Diet Aids 55
  - ○ Read the Labels...57
- • Summary...58
- • Endnotes..61

4   The Power of Exercise...69

- • Why Exercise is Important...71
  - ○ Fat Oxidation 71
  - ○ Reduced Health Risk Factors...71
  - ○ Exercise Can be a Predictor 72
  - ○ Psychological Benefits..73
- • Disease Prevention and Treatment..74
  - ○ Heart Disease...74
  - ○ Cancer 75
  - ○ Diabetes 76
  - ○ Brain Function 78
  - ○ Bone Density 79
  - ○ Inflammation 82
  - ○ Other..83
- • Exercise Specifics 84

       o Exercise Type 85

       o Exercise Duration 88

       o Exercise Frequency 89

       o Exercise Intensity 90

   • Obstacles to Exercise 91

   • Summary 92

   • Endnotes 95

5   Psychological Aspects of Weight Loss 105

   • How the Brain Affects Weight Loss 107

   • Stress 111

   • Depression 114

       o Arguments "In Favor of" a Relationship Between Obesity and Depression 115

       o Arguments "Against" a Relationship Between Obesity and Depression 116

   • Eating Disorders 118

       o Anorexia Nervosa 121

       o Bulimia Nervosa 122

       o Binge-Eating Disorder 123

       o Night Eating Syndrome 125

   • Self Esteem 126

   • Behavior Changes 129

   • Summary 135

   • Endnotes 137

6   The Role of Hormones 153

   • What are Hormones 153

   • Hormones and Weight Loss 154

       o Thyroid Hormones 154

       o Testosterone 156

       o Estrogen / Progesterone 157

       o Growth Hormone 158

       o Ghrelin 160

       o Leptin 160

       o Adiponectin 162

       o Cortisol 163

       o Dehydroepiandrosterone (DHEA) 163

       o Melatonin 163

       o Parathyroid Hormone (PTH) 164

       o Corticotropin-Releasing Hormone 164

        o   Prolactin 164

        o   Lesser Known Gut Hormones and Peptides 165

    • Determining Your Hormone Levels 165

    • Synthetic Vs Bio-Identical Hormones 166

    • Summary 167

    • Endnotes 168

Part Three   How to Make a Difference   175

7   The Driving Force Within 177

    • Motivation 178

    • Self-Discipline 182

    • Goal Setting 186

    • Building a Support System 198

    • Summary 203

    • Endnotes 207

8   Lesser-Known Weight Loss Considerations 219

    • Special Needs Groups 219

        o   The Chronically Ill 220

        o   Children 221

        o   The Elderly 225

        o   Pregnant Women 226

    • The Relationship Between Sleep and Weight Loss 231

    • Acupuncture 235

    • Massage Therapy 236

    • Sauna / Steam Room 236

    • Mind Machines 237

    • Summary 237

    • Endnotes 238

9   The Last Resort - A Hidden Trap Awaits 245

    • Prescription Drugs 245

    • Children's Issues with Prescription Drugs 250

    • Bariatric Surgery 251

    • Children's Issues with Bariatric Surgery 253

    • Liposuction 255

    • Summary 255

    • Endnotes 256

10 Summary - What Action to Take Now 263

- Remember the Basic Rules 264
- Evaluate Your Readiness for Change 265
- Goal Setting 266
- Putting it all Together - Proceeding From Here 269
- The Planning Phase 270
- Endnotes 282

Appendix How to Find Help 285

Index 289

Foreword

Obesity really is the major disease of the 21st Century. For reasons no one fully understands, excess weight and true obesity have doubled in the last 30 to 40 years. There is evidence, of course: (1) the fast food industry is partially responsible, (2) the excess of sugar and fructose in many processed foods is partially responsible, and (3) monosodium glutamate is partially responsible. In addition, there is evidence the widespread use of mood drugs, tranquilizers, and antidepressants are contributors. Whatever the cause, obesity is now the number one recognizable cause of death in the United States. Interestingly, only 3 percent of Americans have the four essentials for optimal health:

- Body mass index between 18 and 24,
- No smoking,
- A minimum of 5 servings a day of fruits and vegetables. (The average American is 2.4),
- Exercise a minimum of 30 minutes 5 days a week.

I have spoken to well over 100 groups of people in the past few years and the best I have found when asking people how many have these four habits is approximately 25 percent. That low percentage even applies to a group of so-called holistic nurses. Personally, I don't think you can be a holistic nurse or holistic physician or a conscious, sane individual if you don't have those four health habits.

Personally, I have tried many approaches to offer individuals opportunities to lose weight in programs that would work if they would do them. In one such program, 12 individuals showed up for an initial two-hour visit. The following week only one of them showed up. In another situation seven smokers and eight obese people showed up for a weekend workshop designed to help them. By Sunday morning, less than half of them were still involved and at the follow up a month later, four showed up.

In other words, as far as I can tell, obesity is no different from drug addiction, alcoholism or smoking. It is a serious psychosocial problem, as well as a public health problem. Theoretically, if everyone in the United States just adopted the four basic health habits, within 10 to 20 years our average age of death would go up to about 100 years of age, instead of the current 78 years of age. Our total expenses for managing disease would probably drop at least 50 percent. That is how simple health is. And, of course, we all know there is a new weight control program at least once a month to make some kind of national news.

Dr. Waller's book is a true encyclopedia of health information for everyone who has the most essential requirement, WILL. This outstanding work offers all the information you need to assist you in making willful choices that will normalize and optimize your weight. The vast majority of people who do lose weight, stop drinking, stop smoking, and stop drug use, do so with willpower. If you have the will to live, *Sustainable Weight Loss* offers you all you need to accomplish your goals. I know of nothing that can actually give you that WILL but for those intelligent individuals who have the WILL and are willing to use it, this is the best guide I know for accomplishing your goals.

C. Norman Shealy, MD, PhD
President, Holos Institutes of Health
Professor Emeritus of Energy Medicine
President Emeritus, Holos University Graduate Seminary

Preface

Why I Wrote This Book

Growing up in the 1940's and 1950's was a time quite unlike it is today. Life was simpler, less stressful, and people seemed to have a greater interest in taking care of themselves, or at least they were more successful at it. As the decades rolled by many changes took place, many not so good. Among the most noticeable changes I have seen are:

- A reduced consciousness about our dietary habits,
- A decline in the quality of the foods we eat,
- A decrease in the amount of physical energy we expend,
- An increase in the size of people,
- An increase in the recognized health risk factors associated with obesity,
- A decrease in the general health of the population. Wow, could there be a relationship between these changes and obesity? We will explore that concept in later chapters.

As the process of growing larger has ratcheted up over time, the data reveals people are growing heavier at a much faster rate than they are growing taller. As far back as 1998 it was reported that the number of adults in the US who were obese had doubled over the previous 30 years.[1] In 2006 the Center for Disease Control reported that 60 percent of the US adult population was overweight and 24 percent was obese.[2] In the early years of my delving into health and weight control there didn't seem to be enough impetus for me to write a book on the subject. However, as time passed the problem continued to grow and with that growth, the engineer/health devotee in me decided to further investigate the causes. After a lot of study on the subject I decided the time was right for this book. After thoroughly evaluating the available information, the book's framework began to take shape.

As I learned more about obesity and its cause, I noticed the vast majority of the solutions offered were focused on a single remedy. Many of the so-called experts are actually nothing more than one-trick ponies. They haven't figured out there is no such thing as the proverbial silver bullet. They suggest if you do the one thing they propose (e.g. diet or exercise) you will easily control your weight and possibly your physical condition. To verify what I am saying is true, turn on the television on Sunday morning and look at the advertising. It goes like this: if you use my one of a kind exercise apparatus or if you follow my diet or if you take my weight loss potion you will soon look like the beautiful person in the ad. These claims generally aren't true and don't offer a healthy, lasting result! Complete and sustainable weight control is a combination of multiple factors and those factors vary amongst individuals, much like hair color or eye color. If you get the combination right and are persistent you will be successful. If you get the combination wrong or are lazy with your approach you will struggle. This book: (1) exposes the factors you need to consider, (2) gives you a game plan for determining which of those will help you the most, and (3) helps you develop a personalized strategy for solving the problem.

Another problem is often the solutions offered by the gurus are so complicated they become unworkable. Some of the diet experts advocate every time you eat you need to count the calories you are about to consume, or the grams of fat or the grams of carbohydrate. This kind of complexity is one of the reasons many people fail with diets. Again these one-size-fits-all approaches are only a small part of the overall reality and as you will see later they need to be integrated into the bigger picture.

The main reasons I wrote this book are:

- People need help with weight loss,
- People need something workable,
- People need something based on sound science,
- People need something affordable,
- I am knowledgeable and experienced in this field, and
- I am a master at taking the complex and boiling it down into something simple, that can be used. As we progress I will show you how easily you can manage your body weight without obsessing over watching your bathroom scale).

There are a few concepts that will be repeated throughout this book. They will be discussed at length and are of vital importance to your weight loss success. They are:

- **Weight Control = Good Health** - Weight control and good health go hand-in-hand. As detailed in the chapter on the functioning of the human body, the affects of modest weight loss on personal health can be enormous; in fact the success of any weight loss program should be evaluated by the overall health improvement achieved.[3]

- **Goal Setting** - The importance of good goal setting and sound implementation of your plan cannot be overstated. As explained further in the chapter on the psychological aspects of weight loss the ability to set good goals and to achieve them is paramount to the success of any weight loss program. If I were working directly with you, I would ensure you never lost sight of your goal(s) and you adjusted them as often as needed.

- **Lifestyle Changes** - Good weight management cannot be accomplished without some basic lifestyle changes. This does not mean you must give up everything you like but it does mean some of the things you like may need to be done in moderation and some additional changes will probably need to be integrated into your daily activities.

- **Caloric Balancing** - The hallmark of good weight management is a balance between calories consumed and calories burned. Obviously to maintain your body weight the number of calories consumed must equal the number of calories burned. In order to lose weight you must burn more calories than you consume.

- **Rarely is it Simple** - Weight-loss approaches touted as overly simple and easy rarely provide the lasting results you want.

- **Have Fun Maintaining Your Weight** - The process of losing weight and improving your health doesn't have to be an onerous task. It can actually be fun. As you will see throughout the chapters to come much of the fun comes from what you feel, what you believe and the successes you experience.

- **Reasonable vs Perfect Body** - We all see people in magazines, on TV, and in the movies with what appears to be the perfect body. We must take an honest look at ourselves, and our own personal traits to determine what body size and shape is reasonable for us. It has recently been proposed we abandon traditional weight-loss goals based on tables, charts and measurements in favor of attaining a reasonable weight. Good health benefits are associated with even a modest weight loss.[4] Don't be fooled into believing anyone who wants to can have the perfect body that is being advertised. I don't say this to discourage you but setting realistic and attainable goals is very important.

This book is not about discovering a great new secret to weight management rather it is about coming to grips with the basic requirements of weight control and being able to apply them in your life. In the real world obese people experience an endless accumulation of problems affecting all aspects of their lives.[5] A lot of people hope to make a major transformation in themselves through weight loss but what they find is frequently their loss of weight produces only subtle changes in them.[6] This book is intended to be a self-help tool that you can use to change your life with minimal outside help. For those who need outside help, you will be able to use this book to determine what help you need, how much help you need, where to find help and to determine the quality of the help you are getting.

How to Use This Book

By looking at the title of this book you are already aware the subject is *weight loss*. If you are a body builder, athlete or any other person who is trying to gain weight, while there may a lot of pertinent information in this book for you, it is not intended to serve your needs. If you want to maintain continuity in your understanding of the subject of weight loss and if you want to fully understand my logic, please read this book from the beginning to the end. If you have a fairly good understanding of anatomy then you will not lose much benefit if you begin with Part Two. Please don't skip both Part One and Part Two.

Part One - Presents an overview of the body. It describes what entropy is, how health and weight control are inseparable, the set point theory of weight loss, body type and composition, how the cells produce energy, what they use for fuel and how metabolism affects weight loss. It also explains the role of genetics in weight loss and how to work with your genetics to achieve desirable results.

Part Two - Discusses the things you need to consider to lose weight and to keep it off the rest of your life. These considerations include the importance of what you eat and drink, what your exercise habits are and what they need to be, what psychological roadblocks can impede your progress, the role hormones can play and a discussion of special needs.

Part Three - Is the *how-to* portion of the book. It goes into detail as to what you need to do to make a difference in your life. The topics discussed are the importance of proper support systems, motivation and discipline and the hidden traps you might want to avoid. Finally you will gain an understanding of how to evaluate your readiness for change, how to determine the right lifestyle for your personal success, how to implement the changes needed, how to monitor your progress and how to maintain your new lifestyle.

This document is not intended to be a treatise that can be used by researchers to further build the body of supporting evidence for their work but rather was written to be used by everyday folks, who are struggling with reducing their weight. Finally, as you read on you will see I took the liberty of translating the complexity of a lot of technical jargon into plain and simple English.

It is my sincere hope you can use this book to begin an exciting new chapter in your life leading you on a rewarding journey to improved weight control, health and self-esteem.

Endnotes

1.   K.M. Flegal, M.D. Carroll, R.J. Kuczmarski, C.L. Johnson, "Overweight and obesity in the United States prevalence and trends, 1960-1964," *Int'l J Obes Relat Metab Disord* 22 (1998) 39-47.
2.   Centers for Disease Control and Prevention, "State specific prevalence of obesity among adults - U.S. 2005," *MMWR* 55 (2006) 985-988.

3. World Health Organization, "Obesity: preventing and managing the global epidemic. Report of a WHO consultation on obesity, Geneva, 3-5 June 1997," (World Health Organization, Geneva, 1998).

4. M.J. Devlin, S.Z. Yanovski, G.T. Wilson, "Obesity: what mental health professionals need to know," *Am J Psychiatry* 157 (2000) 854-866.

5. M.E.J. Lean. "Pathophysiology of Obesity, 1st plenary session on obesity," *Proceeding of the Nutr Soc,* 59 (2000) 331-336.

6. E. Granberg, "Is that all there is? Possible selves, self change and weight loss," *Soc Psych Qtrly* 69 (2006) 109-126.

Introduction

Throughout the world, obesity is a condition affecting a large and growing number of adults and children.[1] Obesity is a complex phenomenon influenced by a variety of genetic, physiological, psychological and social factors,[2] and to make matters worse there is a major disconnect between what the general public considers a healthy bodyweight and what the World Health Organization thinks it is.[3] This book is based on a broader set of contributors, namely:

- Genetic,
- Hormonal,
- Behavioral,
- Diet and exercise,
- Cultural and socioeconomic.[4]

Although in some cases obesity may be attributable to certain genetic predispositions and metabolic abnormalities, the huge increase in obesity in the past 20 years has been caused by behavioral and social ecological factors.[5] In 2006 there were over one billion overweight people in the world and more than 300 million of them were obese.[6] In 2010 annual US obesity health related costs were $147 billion.[7] In countries like the "USA, Britain, Canada and Australia as many as one in four children and adolescents, and more than half of the adult population

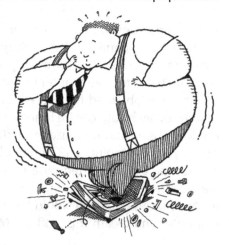

carry excess body fat that puts them at increased risk for a range of chronic conditions."[8] Parents of children who are transitioning from adolescence to adulthood need to be aware these kids are in a particularly high-risk period for the development of obesity,[9] since about "50%-70% of obese children become obese adults."[10] Obesity beginning at a young age frequently sets the stage for a lifetime of difficult to overcome, obesity related health problems.

Here's an indication of why I think the study data might be accurate. In June of 2008, I went on the website of a major US underwear manufacturer, to make a purchase. I was quite surprised to find the manufacturer not only stocked the popular sizes of S, M, L, XL but they found it advantageous to also stock 2XL, 3XL, 4XL, 5XL and 6XL shorts and T-shirts, in several styles. 6XL shorts are a 60-62 inch waist size, and 6XL T-shirts are a 66-68 inch chest size. This prompted me to make a phone call to the manufacturer to convince myself I fully understood what I had just read. I was blown away to find they routinely take special orders for larger sizes. Wow! Just think of the possible implications.

The procurement of food and water is one of the most important behaviors for all living creatures. From the beginning of evolution until the present time a major part of the nervous system has been dedicated to all aspects of survival, one of the most prevalent of them being that of acquiring food; therefore, it is not surprising the human brain has developed an extraordinary ability to deal with the procurement of food.[11]

Some researchers suggest there might be two basic causes of obesity. They focus primarily on two aspects of the body's control system. First is the claim of a defective sensing of ingested nutrients. When the signals to the brain cannot accurately convey the availability of nutrients, individuals lose their ability to properly control their energy balance resulting in either starvation or obesity. Second is an over stimulated reward mechanism. The downside of a diet that tastes extremely good (e.g. a fast food diet) is it tends to over stimulate appetite and food consumption.[12]

There is a stigma to being overweight or obese. Overweight people are oftentimes the target of a bias against them, because of their body weight. A body weight bias has been documented among employers, educators, healthcare providers and family members, with the result being a significant blow to the individual's emotional and physical well being.[13] In addition, as the percentage of overweight children has increased over the years, their stigmatization has become worse as well.[14] For example, it has been found overweight children are only half as likely to be named as a friend by another child.[15] It seems obvious people in the developed world need to acquire some specialized skills, honed to perfection, if prompt, effective remedial action is to be taken.

The material used in this book came from a variety of sources. A small amount was taken from my personal experience and an ongoing dialog with other people of similar interest. A much larger amount was derived from my reading and study in the field of natural health. As you can see from the extensive chapter Endnotes, the vast majority of the material included in this body of work was obtained from research data that was collected through an exhaustive search. I realize research data can be found to support almost any view. After reviewing the data for this book, it was initially organized into three different categories: (1) in favor of a specific point, (2) opposed to that point, or (3) some other middle ground opinion. I've tried to promote research points that are supported by a preponderance of the research without excluding opposing views. If the research took a neutral position I presented that as well. I took great pains to ensure in reading this book you would be comfortable with the fact that I didn't just sit in front of my computer and dream this stuff up. My goal has always been to present you with information you can understand and will help you achieve your weight loss goal. This material was prepared, digested and cataloged in a way I hope you will find to be interesting, understandable and most importantly, usable.

To set the stage for what follows you need to understand some basic concepts that are both frequently discussed among western healthcare practitioners and are often referred to in the research data cited.

Metabolic Syndrome (MS)

One such concept is that of the metabolic syndrome, which is a medically recognized combination of multiple risk factors that primarily increase the risk of cardiovascular disease[16] and type 2 diabetes. "Metabolic syndrome is more common among socio-economically disadvantaged individuals, and is associated with certain risky lifestyle practices."[17] Metabolic syndrome "appears to be triggered by adverse social circumstances and chronic stress."[18] Although there is frequent disagreement as to exactly what metabolic syndrome is comprised of and how it is precisely identified it has been referred to by a variety of titles, such as "syndrome X, insulin resistance syndrome, dysmetabolic syndrome, deadly quartet and plurimetabolic syndrome."[19] According to one study metabolic syndrome is diagnosed when the patient has more than three of the following conditions:

- Abdominal obesity,
- High triglycerides,
- Low HDL (good) cholesterol,
- High fasting glucose,
- High blood pressure.[20]

Metabolic syndrome may include a number of additional conditions:

- Osteoporosis,
- Sleep apnea,
- Sarcopenia (i.e. age related decline in muscle mass),
- Type 2 diabetes,
- Cardiovascular disease,
- Erectile dysfunction, and
- Cognitive decline (e.g. Alzheimer's Disease).

Obese subjects with psychiatric conditions ranging from mild depression to more advanced anxieties, with the perception of uncontrollable stress, frequently have stress-induced abdominal obesity and metabolic syndrome.[21] Now for the bad news! 2000 census data estimated 47 million US residents have metabolic syndrome.[22] The real downside is stress-induced abdominal obesity and related cardiovascular dysfunction increase the risk of mortality of affected subjects, two to three fold and shortens their life expectancy by several years.[23]

One researcher has attempted to put a numerical scoring on the metabolic syndrome risk factors:

- High fasting glucose greater than 100 mg/dl,
- Low HDL (good) cholesterol less than 40 mg/dl for men and less than 50 mg/dl for women,
- High LDL (bad) cholesterol greater than 150 mg/dl,
- High systolic blood pressure greater than 130 mmHg,
- High diastolic blood pressure greater than 85 mmHg,
- Abdominal obesity defined as a waist circumference greater than 40 inches for men and greater than 35 inches for women.[24]

A grouping of risk factors is referred as a *clustering* of risk factors. Abdominal obesity is one risk factor that has been shown to correlate strongly with the other metabolic syndrome conditions, especially insulin resistance.[25] It has been demonstrated to be a key element in the group of risk factors linked to an increased risk of cardiovascular disease and type 2 diabetes.[26] One of the most alarming aspects of metabolic syndrome is that it is a growing epidemic among children. This might be expected since it parallels the growing epidemic in childhood obesity, where a large percentage of obese children become obese adults. As in adults "the major benefit of identifying metabolic syndrome in children is to draw attention to the risk factor clustering associated with obesity and insulin resistance."[27] Here's a surprise! "One promising type of therapy might be weight reduction…and increased physical activity."[28] This approach, reported in the Diabetes Prevention Program, was found to be successful in reducing the incidence of diabetes and metabolic syndrome.[29] Viner & Cole followed adolescents into adulthood and concluded it was important to reduce sedentary behavior and unhealthy eating patterns if the obesity link between childhood and adulthood was to be broken.[30] They also found fast food consumption contributed to the largest gains in BMI.[31]

Health Risk Factors

Another important concept is that of health risk factors. As discussed later in this book the endocrine system is the hormonal control system of the body. Interestingly, fat tissue is the body's largest endocrine gland.[32] It has been well documented obesity is directly associated with the increased health risk factors of many common chronic diseases, including coronary heart disease, stroke, cancer, diabetes, hypertension and dyslipidemia.[33] There is also evidence-linking obesity with osteoarthritis, gallstones, asthma, depression and sleep disorders.[34] Women suffer from obesity related health conditions more than men.[35] The prevention and control of obesity is the result of a variety of factors that contribute to energy balance.[36] Risk factors include: (1) high calorie diets, (2) poor eating habits, (3) high levels of sedentary behavior, and (4) inadequate exercise. There is strong evidence that multiple behavioral factors tend to occur in combination, in most people.[37]

Coronary heart disease, stroke, high blood pressure and high cholesterol are the most highly publicized of the health risk factors. "Obesity…is an independent risk factor for arteriosclerosis, stroke and cardiovascular disease."[38] Visceral adipose tissue (VAT) (i.e. fat located around the internal organs especially the abdomen) is associated with carotid atherosclerosis and there seems to be a VAT threshold that is reached in men at an earlier age than in women. It seems the accumulation of VAT precedes the development of atherosclerosis.[39] Furthermore, studies have found "obese children are at increased risk of coronary artery calcification and cardiovascular disease in adulthood."[40] There is support for the idea that although being overweight is a risk factor for mortality, "it is a moderate risk factor for severe morbidity."[41] Finally, "a 10% weight loss is sufficient to see significant improvement in risk factors."[42] There is obvious value in modifying health behaviors to reduce coronary risk factors in patients with coronary heart disease. Reducing dietary fat intake, increasing the level of exercise and employing stress management techniques can lower the risk of coronary heart disease.[43] On the surface this finding makes sense but it must be applied with care, because the idea of arbitrarily reducing dietary fat intake could be problematic. As discussed later attempting to reduce dietary fat intake without understanding the individual's needs and current consumption level, can be downright dangerous.

"Overweight and obesity increase the risk of developing several types of cancer."[44] The majority of research on obesity related cancer focuses primarily on breast, prostate and colon cancer. Additionally, obese people have an increased risk of cancer recurrence and poorer survival rates, than lean people.[45] "Compounding this is the fact that weight gain after a diagnosis is common in some cancer patients, this is especially true among breast cancer patients receiving…therapy."[46] Study data indicates weight gain influences the characteristics of breast tumors among adult women who are not using postmenopausal hormone therapy and "the risk of breast cancer increased with increasing weight gain regardless of tumor stage, grade or…type."[47] Women with the highest weight gain are three times more likely to have cancer than women who gained less than 20 pounds in adulthood.[48] Here is the good news. An American Cancer Society study found women aged 40-64 who intentionally lost weight had a reduction in mortality of 20-25 percent.[49]

"Obesity is a major risk factor for developing type 2 diabetes mellitus, and an estimated 60-90% of patients are overweight or obese prior to diagnosis."[50] In a recent study of 44,000 patients with type 2 diabetes 80 percent were overweight and 37 percent were obese.[51] The location of body fat is equally important. Abdominal fat can cause a worsening of glucose tolerance in patients with type 2 diabetes.[52] Losing "about 5% of body weight can significantly reduce the risk of developing type 2 diabetes in high risk individuals."[53] In addition to diabetes, "being overweight increases the risk of coronary heart disease (CHD) in healthy individuals, and this association may be even more important in people with diabetes, as CHD is responsible for >75% of deaths in these individuals."[54] Because of the relationship between cardiac risk factors and the risk factors associated with diabetes, "it is essential that medical providers treat modifiable risk factors in patients with diabetes aggressively, with lifestyle modifications and pharmacotherapy."[55]

Obesity increases the risk of dementia and brain atrophy,[56] and "those with metabolic syndrome are also more likely to have a greater cognitive decline."[57] More specifically obesity has been associated with a 25 percent increase in: (1) common mood and anxiety disorders, and (2) increased risk of substance use disorder.[58] As discussed abdominal fat is a risk factor for developing cardiovascular disease and diabetes and recent findings suggest it has the same effect on risk for dementia.[59]

What about something as remote as infertility? It has been demonstrated overweight men experience increased infertility.[60]

Health risk factors aren't often the main motivator for people deciding to lose weight instead their goal is generally an increased sense of self-esteem. These people typically find it difficult to sustain a radical approach to weight loss for more than a limited amount of time,[61] so to help them achieve their objective simplicity is a key factor. Social support, regular monitoring and an effective, well-executed exercise regime appear to be beneficial.

Obesity results from a variety of social, behavioral, cultural, environmental and physiological factors.[62] "Addressing nutrition and physical activity jointly is essential to the prevention and treatment of obesity…because of its complex etiology, no single approach to weight management is adequate."[63]

Studies have suggested obese people suffer substantial hardships. Here is how researchers say they are discriminated against:

- The obese are less likely to receive financial aid for college,[64]
- When their qualifications are the same or similar to non-obese people, the obese are less frequently hired for a job,[65]
- The obese earn lower wages than non-obese people performing the same work,[66]
- The obese are less likely to be rented apartments,[67]
- The obese are less sought after as mates,[68]
- The obese are less likely to marry economically upward,[69]
- The obese are waited on more slowly by salespeople,[70]
- Health care professionals frequently hold negative attitudes towards the obese.[71]

"One of the greatest challenges in the clinical management of obese patients is addressing the significant disparity between actual and expected weight losses."[72] There are certain biological and physiological limitations on what it takes for each of us to lose weight and to maintain a reasonable body weight. "Not everyone who eats the same and exercises the same weighs the same."[73] Because long-term weight loss results are so disappointing, some weight-loss experts are suggesting stringent weight-loss recommendations be abandoned and more healthy weight loss goals be adopted.[74] The Institute of Medicine claims the goal of obesity treatment should move away from weight loss alone and while weight loss is often aimed at appearance it would be better if weight management systems aimed to achieve a reasonable body weight within a framework of overall good health.[75] The health benefit of losing only ten percent of body weight is used to justify this modest goal.[76] This type of goal focuses on behavioral changes intended to result in health benefits even if weight loss is minimal.[77] Lifestyle changes (e.g. reducing caloric intake and increasing exercise levels) should be used to motivate people towards good health regardless of weight loss.[78]

A "reality of life with obesity is steady accumulation of problems affecting every aspect of life and almost every system of the body."[79] If you are substantially overweight or obese and want to enjoy life more fully, improve your overall health, experience the possibility of reversing or avoiding chronic illness and avoid a premature death, you need to get your weight under control, and this book is designed to help you do just that. **Obesity is one of the leading causes of preventable death.**"[80]

Endnotes

1. P.T. James, R. Leach, E. Kalamara, M. Shayeghi, "The worldwide obesity epidemic," *Obes Res* 9 (2001) 228S-233S.
2. K.D. Brownell, T.A. Wadden, " Etiology and treatment of obesity: understanding a serious, prevalent and refractory disorder," *J Consult Clin Psych* 60 (1992) 505-517.
3. G. Heading, "Rural obesity, healthy weight and perceptions of risk: struggles, strategies and motivation for change," *Aust J Rural Health* 16 (2008) 86-91.
4. K.M. Flegal, R.P. Troiano, R. Ballard-Barbash, "Aim for a healthy weight: what is the target?" *J Nutr* 131 (2001) 440S-450S.
5. T. Baranowski, K.W. Cullen, T. Nicklas, D. Thompson, J. Baranowski, "Are current health behavioral change models helpful in guiding prevention of weight gain efforts," *Obes Res* 11 (2003) 23S-43S.
6. S. Gazdzinski, J. Kornak, M.W. Weiner, D.J. Meyerhoff, R. Nat, "Body mass index and magnetic resonance markers of brain integrity in adults," *Ann Neurol* 63 (2008) 652-657.
7. Dr. Julian Whitaker's, "*Health & Healing: your definitive guide to wellnes medicine,*" 20 (2010) 5.
8. D. Crawford, K. Ball, "What help young women want in their efforts to control their weight? implications for program development," *Nutr Diet* 64 (2007) 99-104.
9. M.C. Nelson, P. Gordon-Larsen, K.E. North, L.S. Adair, "Body mass index gain, fast food, and physical activity: effects of shared environments over time," *Obesity* 14 (2006) 701-709.
10. R.M. Viner, T.J. Cole, "Who changes body mass between adolescence and adulthood? Factors predicting change in BMI between 16 year and 30 years in the 1970 British birth cohort," *Intl J Obes* 30 (2006) 1368-1374.
11. H.R. Berthoud, C. Morrison, "The brain, appetite and obesity," *Annual Rev Psych* 59 (2008) 55-92.
12. Ibid.

13. R.M. Puhl, C.A. Moss-Racusin, M.B. Schwartz, "Internalization of weight bias: implications for binge eating and emotional well-being," *Obesity* 15 (2007) 19-23.

14. J.D. Latner, A.J. Stunkard, "Getting worse: the stigmatization of obese children," *Obes Res* 11 (2003) 452-456.

15. R.S. Strauss, H.A. Pollack, "Social marginalization of overweight children," *Arch Pediatr Adolesc Med* 2 (1994) 38-43.

16. T. Yasuda, M. Matsuhisa, N. Fujiki, F. Sakamoto, M. Tsuji, N. Fujisawa, M. Kimura, R. Ishibashi, H. Kaneto, Y. Yamasaki, T. Watari, E. Imano, "Is central obesity a good predictor of carotid atherosclerosis in Japanese type 2 diabetes with metabolic syndrome," *J Endcrinol* 54 (2007) 695-702.

17. B.J. Stewart-Knox, "Psychological underpinnings of metabolic syndrome," *Proceedings of the nutrition society,*" 64 (2005) 363-369.

18. Ibid.

19. Ibid.

20. T. Yasuda, M. Matsuhisa, N. Fujiki, F. Sakamoto, M. Tsuji, N. Fujisawa, M. Kimura, R. Ishibashi, H. Kaneto, Y. Yamasaki, T. Watari, E. Imano, "Is central obesity a good predictor of carotid atherosclerosis in Japanese type 2 diabetes with metabolic syndrome," *J Endcrinol* 54 (2007) 695-702.

21. G.P. Chrousos, "The role of stress and the hypothalamic - pituitary - adrenal axis in the pathogenesis of the metabolic syndrome: neuro - endocrine and target tissue related causes," *Int'l J Obes* 24 (2000) S50-S55.

22. S.G. Aldana, "*The Culprit & the Cure,*" (Mapleton, UT: *Maple Mountain Press,* 2005) 60.

23. G.P. Chrousos, "The role of stress and the hypothalamic - pituitary - adrenal axis in the pathogenesis of the metabolic syndrome: neuro - endocrine and target tissue related causes," *Int'l J Obes* 24 (2000) S50-S55.

24. B.J. Stewart-Knox, "Psychological underpinnings of metabolic syndrome," *Proceedings of the nutrition society,*" 64 (2005) 363-369.

25. B. Carr, K. Utzschneider, R. Hull, K. Kodama, B. Retzlaff, J. Brunzell, J. Shofer, B. Fish, R. Knopp, S. Kahn, "Intra-abdominal fat is a major risk determinant of the National Cholesterol Education program Adult Treatment Panel III criteria for the metabolic syndrome," 53 *Diabetes* (2004) 2087-2094.

26. D.H. Ryan, "The relationship among risk factor clustering, abdominal obesity and residual risk for cardiovascular events," *Rev Cardio Med* 8 (2007) 9-15.

27. S. Dhuper, H.W. Cohen, J. Daniel, P. Gumidyala, V. Agarwalla, R. St Victor, S. Dhuper, "Utility of the modified ATP III defined metabolic syndrome and severe obesity as predictors of insulin resistance in overweight children and adolescents: a cross-sectional study," *Cardio Diabet* 6 (2007) 1-9.

28. S.M. Haffner, "Unmet needs in controlling metabolic disease," *Cardio Med* 8 (2007) S17-S24.

29. Ibid.

30. R.M. Viner, T.J. Cole, "Who changes in body mass between adolescence and adulthood? Factors predicting change in BMI between 16 year and 30 years in the 1970 British birth cohort," *Int'l J Obese* 30 (2006) 1368-1374.

31. Ibid.

32. R.A. Whitmer, " The epidemiology of adiposity and dementia," Cur *Alzheimer Res* 4 (2007) 117-122.

33. National Task Force on the Prevention and Treatment of Obesity, "Overweight, obesity and health risk," *Arch Intern Med* 160 (2000) 898-904.

34. R.E. Patterson, L.L. Frank, A.R. Kristal, E. White, "A comprehensive examination of health conditions associated with obesity in older adults," *Am J Prev Med* 27 (2004) 385-390.

35. Ibid.

36. National Institutes of Health, "Strategic plan for NIH obesity research: a report of the NIH obesity research task force," (2004) http://obesityresearch.nih.gov.

37. A. Sanchez, G.J. Norman, J.F. Sallis, K.J. Calfas, C. Rock, K. Patrick, "Patterns and correlates of multiple risk behaviors in overweight women," *Prev Med* 46 (2008) 196-202.

38. S.A. Lear, K.H. Humphries, S. Kohli, J.J. Frohlich, C.L. Birmingham, G.B.J. Mancini, "Visceral adipose tissue, a potential risk factor for carotid atherosclerosis," *Stroke* 38 (2007) 2422-2429.

39. Ibid.

40. D.S. Freedman, D.A. Patel, S.R. Srinivasan, W. Chen, R. Tang, M.G. Bond, G.S. Berenson, "The contribution of childhood obesity to adult carotid intima-media thickness: the Bogalusa Heart Study," *Int'l J Obes* 32 (2008) 749-756.

41. G.R. Weitoft, M. Eliasson, M. Rosen, "Underweight, overweight and obesity as risk factors for mortality and hospitalization," *Scan J Pub Health* 36 (2008) 169-176.

42. G.A. Bray, "Medical consequences of obesity," *J Clin Endocrinol & Metab* 89 (2004) 2583-2589.

43. J.J. Daubenmier, G. Weidner, M.D. Sumner, N. Mendell, T. Merritt-Worden, J. Studley, D. Ornish, "The contribution of changes in diet, exercise and stress management to changes in coronary risk in women and men in the multisite cardiac lifestyle intervention program," *Ann Behav Med* 33 (2007) 57-68.

44. A. McTiernan, "Obesity and cancer: the risks, science and potential management strategies," *Oncology* (2005) 871-881.

45. Ibid.

46. Ibid.

47. H. Spencer-Feigelson, A.V. Patel, L.R. Teras, T. Gansler, M.J. Thun, E.E. Calle, "Adult weight gain and histopathologic characteristics of breast cancer among postmenopausal women," American Cancer Society (2006) www.interscience.wiley.com.

48. Ibid.

49. G.A. Bray, "Medical consequences of obesity," *J Clin Endocrinol & Metab* 89 (2004) 2583-2589.

50. K. Hermansen, L.S. Mortensen, "Bodyweight changes associated with antihyperglycaemic agents in type 2 diabetes mellitus," *Drug Safety* 30 (2007) 1127-1142.

51. Ibid

52. Ibid.

53. G.A. Bray, "Medical consequences of obesity," *J Clin Endocrinol & Metab* 89 (2004) 2583-2589.

54. K. Hermansen, L.S. Mortensen, "Bodyweight changes associated with antihyperglycaemic agents in type 2 diabetes mellitus," *Drug Safety* 30 (2007) 1127-1142.

55. M. McCollum, S.L. Ellis, E.H. Morrato, P.W. Sullivan, "Prevalence of multiple cardiac risk factors in US adults with diabetes," *Cur Med Res & Opin* 22 (2006) 1031-1034.

56. S. Gazdzinski, J. Kornak, M.W. Weiner, D.J. Meyerhoff, R. Nat, "Body mass index and magnetic resonance markers of brain integrity in adults," *Ann Neurol* 63 (2008) 652-657

57. R.A. Whitmer, " The epidemiology of adiposity and dementia," Cur *Alzheimer Res* 4 (2007) 117-122.

58. G.E. Simon, M. Von Korff, K. Saunders, D.L. Miglioretti, P.K. Crane, G. Van Belle, R.C. Kessler, "Association between obesity and psychiatric disorders in the US population," *Arch Gen Psych* 63 (2006) 824-830.

59. Ibid.

60. R.H.N. Nguyen, A.J. Wilcox, R. Skjaerven, D.D. Baird, "Men's body mass index and infertility," *Human Repro* 22 (2007) 2488-2493.

61. A.M. Herriot, D.E. Thomas, K.H. Hart, J. Warren, H. Truby, " A qualitative investigation of individuals' experiences and expectations before and after completing a trial of commercial weight-loss programs," *J Hum Nutr Diet* 21 (2007) 72-80.

62. N.S. Wellman, B. Friedberg, "Causes and consequences of adult obesity: health, social and economic impacts in the United States," *Asia Pac J Clin Nutr* 11 (2002) S705-S709.

63. Ibid.

64. C. Crandall, "Do heavy weight students have more difficulty paying for college," *Pers & Soc Psych Bull* 17 (1991) 606-612.

65. E.D. Rothblum, P.A. Brand, C.T. Miller, H.A. Oetjen, "The relationship between obesity, employment discrimination and employment related victimization," *J Voc Behav* 37 (1990) 251-266.

66. C.A. Register, D.R. Williams, "Wage effects of obesity among young workers," *Soc Sci Quart* 70 (1990) 130-141.

67. L. Karris, "Prejudice against obese renters," *J Soc Psych* 101 (1977) 159-160.

68. M.B. Harris, "Is love seen as different for the obese," *J App Soc Psych* 20 (1990) 1209-1224.

69. S. Sonne-Holm, T.I.A. Sorensen, "Prospective study of attainment of social class of severely obese subjects in relation to parental social class, intelligence and education," *BMJ* 292 (1986) 586-589.

70. L.L. Pauley, "Consumer weight as a variable in salespersons response time," *J Soc Psych* 129 (1989) 713-714.

71. B.S. Liese, "Physicians' perceptions of the role of psychology in medicine," *Prof Psych: Res Prac* 17 (1986) 276-277.

72. G.D. Foster, A.P. Makris, B.A. Bailer, "Behavioral treatment of obesity," *Am J Clin Nutr* 82 (2005) 230S-235S.

73. Ibid.

74. G. L. Blackburn, S. Rosofsky, "Making the connection between weight loss, dieting and health: the 10% solution," *Weight Contr Digest* 2 (1990) 121-127.

75. Institute of Medicine, "Weighing the options: criteria for evaluating weight management programs," (Washington, DC: National Academy Press, 1995).

76. G.L. Blackburn, "Effects of weight loss and weight-related risk factors. In K.D. Brownell & C.G. Fairburn (eds), Eating Disorders Obesity: a comprehensive handbook (New York, NY: Guilford, 1995) 406-410.

77. M.S. Faith, K.R. Fontaine, L.J. Cheskin, D.B. Allison, "Behavioral approaches to the problems of obesity," Behav Mod 24 (2000) 459-493.

78. K.D. Brownell, T.A. Wadden, " Etiology and treatment of obesity: understanding a serious, prevalent and refractory disorder," *J Consult Clin Psych* 60 (1992) 505-517.

79. M.E.J. Lean, "1st plenary session on obesity," *Proceeding Nutri Soc* 59 (2000) 331-336.

80. L.A. Barness, J.P. Opitz, E. Gilbert-Barness, "Obesity: genetic, molecular, and environmental aspects," *Am J Med Genet* 143A (2007) 3016-3034.

Warning / Disclaimer

This book was written to provide information on weight loss and life style modification. It is sold with the understanding the publisher and author are not engaged in the practice of medicine, psychology, or any other regulated healthcare professional service. If medical, psychological or other expert healthcare assistance is needed, the services of a competent professional should be obtained.

Every effort has been made to make this book as accurate and complete as possible. If there are mistakes, errors or omissions, they are not intentional. No attempt has been made to deliberately mislead or deceive the reader. This book and its contents should only be used as a guide in the quest for weight loss and improved health. If you have questions or doubts about anything contained in this book, I recommended that you raise them with a competent health care provider.

This book is a compilation of many researched sources of information and should be considered current only up to the date of its printing. The publisher and author shall have no liability or responsibility, to any person or entity, regarding any loss or damage caused or alleged to have been caused, either directly or indirectly, by use of the information contained in this book.

The author has no financial interest in, and is not engaged in the sale or promotion, of any weight loss product or equipment; therefore, specific product names have been mentioned only: (1) because they were cited in a referenced research study, or (2) for informational purposes.

Part One
Understanding the Basics

1   An Overview of the Human Body

The human body is a marvelous creation intended to operate flawlessly for decades, by adapting to its surroundings in order to serve its changing needs. While the plant kingdom is tethered to the earth the animal kingdom is intended to move freely and independently of its surroundings. The existence of physical objects, plants, animals and others, appears at first blush like they should last for long periods, but existence on earth is not quite that simple. There is one rule of the physical universe that interferes with that idea. It is called *entropy*.

Understanding Entropy

Entropy is "the tendency of any system to move toward randomness or disorder."[1] More entropy equates to greater disorder of the system.[2] "In general most systems within the physical universe tend toward increasing positive entropy and towards more disorder over time, (i.e. things tend to fall apart)."[3] If we look at the things around us, for example a car, a refrigerator, a TV, etc., we see entropy at work. Through use all of these items deteriorate over time. Ah, but there is good news for all of us mortals! There is an exception to the entropic rule of the physical universe and it is this.

The plant and animal kingdoms actually experience *negative entropy*. Both plants and animals move toward decreasing disorder of their systems. The bodies of plants and animals continuously try to correct themselves. If the body is damaged or contracts an illness it works tirelessly to heal itself. For example when the human body experiences a laceration, abrasion or bruise or when it contracts a cold or the flu, if left alone it will heal itself. The one and only time negative entropy doesn't work for the human body is when the body is too weak or run down to be able to wage the appropriate fight, at which point the organism experiences a steady decline in health, resulting in death.

By applying this fact to the condition of excess body weight it is easy to understand the body works diligently, around the clock to maintain a stable and homeostatic weight. In reality your body is not only constantly fighting for your survival it is also trying to optimize your weight, what ever that weight might be.

Having identified negative entropy, it must be understood no matter how much the body fights on behalf of us, it is still possible to override its propensity for perfection. In the context of obesity there have arisen two interesting theories that support this idea. The first theory is called the *Absence of Protection Model*, which believes obesity is the result of living in an obese causing or obese promoting environment. The second theory is called the *Central Resistance Model*, which believes under normal circumstances the body's energy balance system provides an effective defense against weight gain and/or weight loss and obesity involves genetic or acquired defects, impairing the function of this system.[4] There will be more as to how this might work in the chapters on genetics and the role of hormones.

How Cells Produce Energy

The science of Cellular Physiology is the study of cells, including their internal structure and function. While it is not the goal of this book to turn you into an expert on this subject, it will be necessary for you to have at least an elementary understanding of a few basic concepts of how a cell produces energy. Let's take a closer look at some aspects of the internal functioning of a cell.

"Cells are the fundamental structural and functional units of living organisms."[5] Cells are the building blocks for tissue, organs and bones within the body. It has been said we live and die at the cellular level.

Cells are comprised of a vast array of component parts. One that is critical to our understanding is the mitochondria (mye-toh-KON-dree-ah). All cells in the human body contain one or more mitochondria. The "mitochondria could be called the power plant of the cell because it is here that energy from nutrients is converted into a form that is usable by the cell."[6] The end product of this nutrient conversion process is adenosine triphosphate (ATP). ATP is the source of energy the cell uses to function.

There are two ways the mitochondria produce ATP. They are:

- Aerobic Metabolism - The word aerobic means in the presence of oxygen. This process occurs when either fatty acids or glucose are taken from the bloodstream into the mitochondria and combined with oxygen to produce ATP, water and carbon dioxide.[7]

- Anaerobic Metabolism - The word anaerobic means in the absence of oxygen. This process occurs when glucose is taken from the bloodstream into the mitochondria and is involved in a fermentation process called lactate fermentation, where it is combined with creatine phosphate, resulting in the production of ATP and lactic acid.[8]

There will be a more detailed discussion of this process in the chapter on exercise.

Good Health and Weight Control are Inseparable

For more than 100 years there has been substantial support for the idea that a homeostatic system exists in the body that adjusts energy intake and energy expenditure to promote the stability of body fat.[9] To support this hypothesis data cited in the chapter on the role of hormones demonstrates there are in fact hormones that perform this task precisely (e.g. ghrelin, leptin). This concept supports the previously mentioned rule of negative entropy. The controversy that remains is that if our bodies are truly homeostatic systems then why has the condition of obesity grown so rapidly in recent years. While this question lingers, research has already proven that our modern lifestyle is causing defects in the homeostatic system. There are also some additional facts that we know relative to health and obesity.

It is virtually impossible for an obese person [usually defined as a person with a Body Mass Index (BMI) greater than 30], to return to a normal body weight (a BMI of 18.5-25), and not experience measurable health improvement. In both Finland,[10] and the United States,[11] it has been shown that a reduction of five percent of body weight can reduce the risk of developing type 2 diabetes, in high-risk individuals. Minimal weight loss can reduce: (1) systolic blood pressure during rest, (2) systolic blood pressure and pulse rate after mental stress, during the recovery period, and (3) the time it takes for the body to reach a resting systolic blood pressure level.[12] A decrease of five to ten, percent of body weight is also known to improve triglycerides and HDL cholesterol, in addition to blood pressure.[13]

I believe there are six critical factors contributing to optimal health. They are shown on the Wheel of Health and will be considered in detail in later chapters. The Wheel of Health suggests the percentage contribution each factor makes to our health and identifies several important considerations, that may help control those factors. The factors are:

- Genetics (10 percent),
- Stress (10 percent),
- Rest (10 percent),
- Environmental considerations (20 percent),
- Exercise (20 percent),
- What we put in our bodies (30 percent).

Wheel of Health

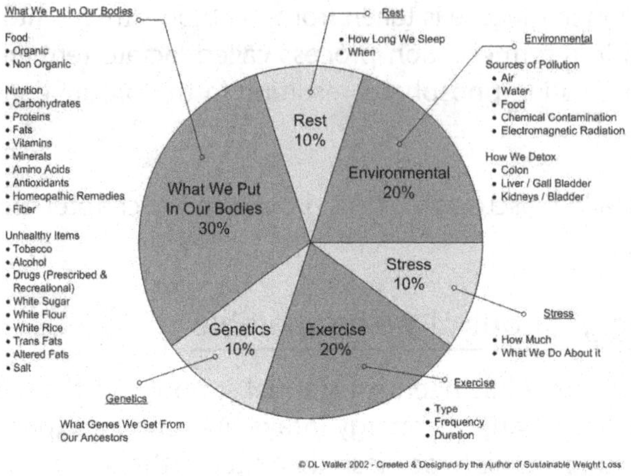
What We Put in Our Bodies
Food
• Organic
• Non Organic
Nutrition
• Carbohydrates
• Proteins
• Fats
• Vitamins
• Minerals
• Amino Acids
• Antioxidants
• Homeopathic Remedies
• Fiber
Unhealthy Items
• Tobacco
• Alcohol
• Drugs (Prescribed & Recreational)
• White Sugar
• White Flour
• White Rice
• Trans Fats
• Altered Fats
• Salt
Rest
• How Long We Sleep
• When
Environmental
Sources of Pollution
• Air
• Water
• Food
• Chemical Contamination
• Electromagnetic Radiation
How We Detox
• Colon
• Liver / Gall Bladder
• Kidneys / Bladder
Rest 10%
Environmental 20%
What We Put In Our Bodies 30%
Stress 10%
Genetics 10%
Exercise 20%
Stress
• How Much
• What We Do About it
Exercise
• Type
• Frequency
• Duration
Genetics
What Genes We Get From Our Ancestors
© DL Waller 2002 - Created & Designed by the Author of Sustainable Weight Loss

The Set Point Theory

In 1982 a couple of researchers named Bennett and Gurin proposed what they called the *Set Point Theory*, where they explained how the human body resists changes in body weight from its own natural state of equilibrium.[14] Their theory holds that, "when body weight is reduced below a given a set point, the body makes a series of internal adjustments to resist weight change and conserve fat stores."[15] The body's main control mechanism is believed to be the brain's hypothalamus, which plays a key role in maintaining the body's homeostasis.[16] When dieting begins the metabolism slows down in order to conserve the calories it already has, and as a result of "this innate biological response, dieting becomes progressively less effective, and...a plateau is reached at which further weight loss seems all but impossible."[17] This situation is especially troubling for people attempting to lose weight by dieting, because as soon as normal eating is resumed the body returns to its previous weight.[18]

A few years later Harris suggested the state of equilibrium characterized by the set point may also regulate a number of other parameters, "including nutrient balance, energy balance, and physical aspects of adipose tissue, such as fat cell number and size."[19] Over the years the set point theory has been extended, and it has been shown the body's set point can be changed.[20] Factors shown to lower the set point are: (1) dietary changes (e.g. lowered fat consumption), (2) exercise levels (e.g. increased aerobic activity), (3) drugs (e.g. fenfluramine),[21] and (4) hormone changes (e.g. ghrelin).[22]

I didn't mentioned the set point theory, to give you something more to think about but if it comes up in conversation with others, you will have heard of it and understand what it's all about. If you proceed forward with the recommendations from other chapters regarding proper dietary practices, exercise programs, hormone evaluation, etc. you will lose the weight you want to and will keep it off, without having to concern yourself about your set point.

Body Type

In the 1940's an American psychologist named William Sheldon while studying the association of body types and human temperaments, proposed that human body types be classified into three somatotypes, which he named, *ectomorphic*, *mesomorphic* and *endomorphic*. Here's how these three body types are characterized:

- **Ectomorphic** - The person with a light bone structure, long, thin muscles and limbs, low fat storage, who tends to be slender (perhaps underweight) and finds gaining weight difficult.

- **Mesomorphic** - The lean athletic person with a medium bone structure, who gains muscle easily with minimal fat gain, and is often described as muscular or well-built.

- **Endomorphic** - The large bone structure person who gains weight easily, with predominately more fat than muscle and often battles a weight problem throughout life.[23]

It is possible for any of us to have characteristics of more than one somatotype. After looking closely at ourselves and at others it should be easy to see how different people tend to fall into one of these body types. Although many experts have attempted to discredit the somatotype criteria as being outdated,[24] I think you will find this to be very useful as you progress forward with weight loss. I have focused on this distinction, not to make you believe your somatotype locks you into a particular body for life, quite the contrary. It is true you cannot change your bone structure, one of the basics of your somatotype, but you certainly can change your body composition. So what is body composition?

Body Composition

The body is composed of five distinct parts. They are fat, muscles, organs, bones and everything else. Since the topic of this book is weight loss and the goal is weight reduction, coupled with weight maintenance, the main thing we want to get rid of is body fat. During weight loss it is important to know where the lost weight is coming from, (e.g. fat, muscle, water), because you certainly don't want the loss to come from lean muscle mass. What is important to know is how much fat your body contains, usually defined as a percentage of total body weight. Below we will look at three of the most popular measurement techniques.

Body Mass Index (BMI)

Body mass index (BMI), became popular in the 1980's, as rates of obesity climbed sharply. BMI is often mistakenly used as a measure of body composition, while it is really a measure of relative heaviness. BMI is referenced extensively in the research data discussed in later chapters. It is noteworthy that BMI tends to increase with age, then plateau or even decline slightly.[25] A person's BMI is the result of a numerical calculation using their height and weight. It is not important to be able to calculate BMI since BMI data tables and calculators have been developed to give you that information. Should you need your exact BMI, go online and Google BMI calculator and follow the directions. What is important to understand is the BMI number is a gauge, often used to determine whether a person is underweight, proper weight, overweight or obese. Once a person's BMI has been determined, the following table is used to identify the body condition.

Body Mass Index Comparison Chart	
Condition	**BMI Number**
Underweight	Less Than 18.5
Proper Weight	18.5 – 24.9
Overweight	25.0 – 29.9
Obesity (Class I)	30.0 – 34.9
Obesity (Class II)	35.0 – 39.9
Obesity (Class III)	Greater Than 40.0

The major problem with the BMI calculation is it uses total body weight rather than estimates of fat and lean body mass separately, therefore it does not discriminate between the overly fat individual and the athletic more muscular body type. Since BMI calculations frequently favor body weight only, while the makeup of the individual is really a combination of genetic and environmental factors, BMI frequently fails to accurately reflect the actual body composition.[26] I feel this is enough of a problem to deem the BMI almost worthless, even though researchers cannot seem to give it up.

Waist to Hip Ratio (WHR)

The waist to hip ratio (WHR) may be the most widely used body composition technique. Since abdominal obesity is known to increase health risks, WHR is one quick means of determining body fat distribution. It is calculated by dividing the waist measurement by the hip measurement. The American College of sports medicine interprets WHR measurements outside the following ranges to indicate a high level of health risk:[27]

Waist to Hip Ratio – Health Risk Indicator Chart		
Age	**Men**	**Women**
Less Than 59	More Than .95	More Than .86
60 - 69	More Than 1.03	More Than .90

Waist Circumference (WC)

The waist circumference (WC) is used frequently because it is a convenient measurement of fat tissue.[28] It is nothing more than a waist measurement or more simply, your current pant size. I believe using the waist of your pants, as a fat monitoring tool, is much simpler than having to take a physical measurement, like you do with WC. Instead of using a tape measure, simply apply my Belt Hole Rule and monitor the belt you normally wear to hold your pants up. Whenever you put your belt on take a close look at which hole you are using. If you are running out of holes you are gaining weight and if you are seeing extra holes you are losing weight. This technique usually works well for men since the waist is the first place weight is gained and the last place it is lost. Since women tend to gain first in the hips and thighs the Belt Hole Rule may work better if combined with a visual observation of those areas.

Fat Free Mass (FFM)

The most reliable body composition technique and a good method of determining an overweight condition or obesity is to determine fat free mass (FFM), which is also frequently referred to as lean body mass or lean muscle mass. FFM is expressed as a percentage of total body weight. There are a number of methods used to determine fat-free mass. Among the most popular are skin fold measurements, bioelectric impedance and hydrostatic weighing. These three techniques require skills and equipment beyond the scope of this book; therefore, they will be left for you to explore with a personal trainer or other health professional, should you wish to do so. Below is a table showing estimated fitness levels as they relate to percent of body fat.[29] If you are serious about measuring your FFM, you can find inexpensive fat loss monitors on the Internet. I personally have a battery operated, Omron model HBF-306F that can be purchased for less than $35.00.

Estimated Fitness Levels - Related to Body Fat		
Classification	Women (% fat)	Men (% fat)
Essential Fat	10% - 13%	2% - 5%
Athletic	14% - 20%	6% - 13%
Fit	21% - 24%	14% - 17%
Average	25% - 31%	18% - 24%
Obese	32% or More	25% or More

Metabolism - Friend or Foe

"Metabolism is the aggregate of all the chemical reactions that take place in the body."[30] Metabolism "involves a complex network of hormones and enzymes that not only convert food into fuel but also affect how efficiently you burn that fuel."[31] The speed and efficiency of our metabolic processes are what is called our metabolic rate. The majority of our metabolic rate is determined by our gender, age, amount of lean muscle mass, and by the amount of exercise we do. Our basal metabolic rate (BMR), which is also known as resting metabolic rate (RMR), "is the amount of energy that is necessary to maintain life and to keep the body functioning at a minimal level,"[32] and about 60 to 75 percent of the our daily energy use is for basal metabolism.[33] The reason this is important for you to know is because the remaining 25 to 40 percent of daily metabolism is something you have control over.

These processes only become detrimental when they slow down or become sluggish and don't burn the calories they're supposed to or don't burn them as efficiently as are supposed to. The key to a successful weight loss program is, to fire up your metabolism and get it burning more calories. Here are a few things you can do to ramp up your metabolism, all of which will be discussed in greater detail, in later chapters:

- Don't skip meals - the minute your body senses you are restricting calories it goes into a starvation mode and the first thing that happens is your metabolism slows.

- Be sure you get enough protein in your diet - I am not suggesting you eat an all meat diet like some popular diet advocates do, but protein consumption helps stabilize blood insulin levels which helps keep your metabolism at the proper level.

- Move around more - park farther from the grocery store, walk more, take the stairs, etc., all of which help keep your metabolism burning.

- <u>Build muscle mass</u> - when you add lean muscle you automatically burn more calories, and you burn them both during daily activity and while at rest.

- <u>Be sure to get adequate sleep</u> - yep, sounds unbelievable but plenty of research studies agree that sleep deprivation appears to contribute to obesity.

Whether your metabolism is your friend or your foe is up to you. It will be your friend as long as you can keep it burning to help you lose weight, but it can quickly become your enemy if you let it get sluggish and lazy.

Endnotes

1. "Entropy," *Dorland's Illustrated Medical Dictionary*, 30th edition: 623.
2. R. Gerber, *Vibrational Medicine*, The #1 Handbook of Subtle Energy Therapies (Rochester, VT: Bear & Company, 2001) 147.
3. Ibid.
4. M.W. Schwartz, K.D. Hiswender, "Adiposity signaling and biological defense against weight gain: absence of protection or central hormone resistance," *J Clin Endrocrinol & Metab* 89 (2004) 5889-5897.
5. "Cell," *Dorland's Illustrated Medical Dictionary*, 30th edition: 315.
6. E.J. Applegate, *The Anatomy & Physiology Learning System*, 2nd Edition (Philadelphia, PA: Saunders, 2000) 43.
7. *"Ace personal trainer manual-American Council on Exercise,"* 3rd ed (San Diego, CA: *American Council on Exercise*, 2003) 8.
8. Ibid.
9. R.O. Neumann, "Experimental contributions to the science of human daily nutritional needs with particular regard to the necessary amount of protein," *Arch Hyg Bacteriol* 45 (1902) 69-78.
10. J. Tuomilehto, J. Lindstrom, J.G. Eriksson, T.T. Valle, H. Hamalainen, P. Ilanne-Parikka, S. Keinanen-Kiukaanniemi, M. Laakso, A. Louheranta, M. Rastas, V. Salminen, M. Uusitupa; Finnish Diabetes Prevention Study Group, "Prevention of type 2 diabetes mellitus by changes in lifestyle among subjects with impaired glucose intolerance," *N Engl J Med* 344 (2001) 1343-1350.
11. Diabetes Prevention Program Research Group, "Reduction in the incidence of type 2 diabetes with lifestyle intervention or metformin," *N Engl J Med* 346 (2002) 393-403.
12. S.J. Torres, C.A. Nowson, "Effect of a weight-loss program on mental stress-induced cardiovascular responses and recovery," *Nutri* 23 (2007) 521-528.
13. C.D. Sjostrom, L. Llissner, L. Sjostrom, "Relationships between changes in body composition and changes in cardiovascular risk factors: the SOS intervention study," *Obes Res* 5 (1997) 519-530.
14. H. Riess, M. Dockray-Miller, *"Set-point theory,"* (The center for health promotion & wellness at MIT Medical) http://web.mit.edu/medical/pdf/set_point_theory.pdf
15. *"Lifestyle and weight management consultant manual-American Council on Exercise,"* (San Diego, CA: *American Council on Exercise*, 2005) 111.

16. E.J. Applegate, *"The Anatomy & Physiology Learning System,"* 2nd ed, (Philadelphia, PA: Saunders, 2000) 167.

17. H. Riess, M. Dockray-Miller, *"Set-point theory,"* (The center for health promotion & wellness at MIT Medical) http://web.mit.edu/medical/pdf/set point theory.pdf

18. S. Knecht, T. Ellger, J.A. Levine, "Obesity in Neurobiology," *Prog Neurobio* 84 (2008) 85-103.

19. R.B.S. Harris, "Role of set-point theory in regulation of body weight," *FASEB J* 4 (1990) 3310-3318.

20. R.E. Keesey, M.D. Hirvonen, "Body weight set-points: determination and adjustment," *J Nutr* 127 (1997) 1875S-1883S.

21. Ibid.

22. H.J. Leidy, J.K. Gardner, B.R. Frye, M.L. Snook, M/K/ Schuchert, E.L. Richard, N.I. Williams, "Circulating ghrelin is sensitive to changes in body weight during a diet and exercise program in normal-weight young women," *J Clin Endocrinol Metab* 89 (2004) 2659-2664.

23. C.M. Colker, *Extreme Muscle Enhancement*, 2nd ed (Manasquan, NJ: ProSource Publications, LLC, 2007) 52.

24. Ibid., 112.

25. L. Strug, L. Sun, M. Corey, "The genetics of cross-sectional and longitudinal body mass index," *BMC Genetics* 4 (2003).

26. Y.-F. Guo, H. Shen, Y.-J. Liu, W. Wang, D.-h. Xiong, P. Xioa, Y.-z. Liu, L.-j. Zhao, R.R. Recker, H-w. Deng, "Assessment of genetic linkage and parent-of-origin effects on obesity," *J. Clin Endocrinol & Metab* 91 (2006) 4001-4005.

27. American College of sports medicine: guidelines for exercise testing and prescription, 7th edition (Baltimore, MD: Lippincott, Williams & Wilkins, (2006).

28. J.P. Despres, I. Lemieux, D. Prud'homme, "Treatment of obesity: need to focus on higher risk abdominally obese patients," *BMJ* 322 (2001) 716-720.

29. *ACE Personal Trainer Manual: The Ultimate Resource for Fitness Professionals*, (San Diego, CA: American Council on Exercise, 3rd edition 2003) 188.

30. E.J. Applegate, *The Anatomy & Physiology Learning System*, 2nd Edition (Philadelphia, PA: Saunders, 2000) 354.

31. C. Bouchez, *"Make the most of your metabolism,"* (WebMD) http://www.webmd.com/fitness-exercise/guide/make-most-your-metabolism

32. E.J. Applegate, *The Anatomy & Physiology Learning System*, 2nd Edition (Philadelphia, PA: Saunders, 2000) 361.

33. *"Lifestyle and weight management consultant manual-American Council on Exercise,"* (San Diego, CA: *American Council on Exercise*, 2005) 157.

2   The Role of Genetics

Through the ages it has become clear the body is genetically programmed for fat accumulation when food is available. This fat accumulation is the source of survival in times of shortage. Some have suggested that, "a *thrifty gene* that helped cavemen survive food shortages appears to be a common underlying trigger of both obesity and diabetes. This gene is advantageous in times of food scarcity."[1] However, Neal suggests that an emphasis on the thrifty gene alone is incorrect and needs to incorporate consideration of muscle conditioning as well.[2]

Throughout history there has been a link between physical exercise and the procurement of food. Today, where starvation seldom occurs and the majority of people live a more sedentary lifestyle than their ancestors did, the thrifty gene hypothesis is the subject of a lot more scrutiny. To further complicate genetic research overweight individuals tend to create circumstances in their lives, by their eating and exercise habits, promoting their overweight condition and making genetic and environmental characteristics largely inseparable.[3]

The topic of genetics, as it relates to obesity, is one gaining a lot of visibility today. There are a number of reasons:

- Worldwide, obesity is growing rapidly,
- The health problems related to obesity are becoming more evident every day,
- Obese people frequently find losing weight to be a struggle they're not prepared for,
- If scientists could find a genetic cause for obesity the road would be paved for a medical solution.
- If genetic manipulation was found to solve the obesity problem, it would:
  - Offer an easy solution,
  - Generate billions of dollars for those who posses the solution.

My review of the genetic research material used as the basis of this chapter makes it apparent to me that "over the last two decades, an increasing effort has been directed toward identifying the genes that influence the risk for the development of such complex conditions as coronary heart disease, type 2 diabetes, and obesity."[4] The objective of most of today's genetic related obesity research is to find a significant, positive correlation, between genetics and obesity, yet in the majority of case studies there is only a modest correlation.

One good example is the search for the so-called *Fat Gene*. Even though its function is still largely unknown, the most popular fat gene candidate today, is the fat mass and obesity-associated gene identified as FTO.[5] The FTO gene has not been implicated in severely obese children and there does not appear to be a difference based on children's gender.[6] Later that year a group of researchers summarized their FTO gene study by claiming they had verified the results of previous studies confirming the role of the FTO gene in the pathogenesis of obesity, even though the precise function of the FTO gene was unknown.[7] Even though some claim a correlation between the FTO gene and obesity, it could be a very long time before its function is understood and a possible therapy for its manipulation made available. What that means to those now struggling with excess body weight is, don't sit back and wait for FTO gene treatment discoveries to become available, because that may not happen for years. Instead grab the bull by the horns and begin to put all of the other currently available knowledge to work immediately.

I frequently hear overweight people comment on the fact they believe they are destined to be overweight because of their genetic makeup. They may say something like, it's a genetic thing that causes me to be overweight, or being overweight is in my genes, or it's my family history causing me to be overweight, implying some sort of genetic control that causes the overweight condition. Some researchers have claimed that, "up to 80% of the tendency to obesity has a genetic basis,"[8] but be careful here.

Since genetic research invariably fails to demonstrate a significant cause-and-effect relationship between genetic expression and obesity, the researchers frequently use words like susceptibility, tendency and predisposition, to hedge their bets. A susceptibility, tendency or predisposition towards obesity is not the same thing as a cause. As you will see later in this chapter, all of these thoughts posses a measure of truth, but only a small measure. We all have certain genetic tendencies but most genes can only express themselves if they are provided with the proper environment.

You're probably asking yourself at this point what are genes anyway? Are they the same as chromosomes? What is DNA? Is there a relationship? Although the whole conversation becomes very technical, here is some fundamental information that may help your understanding.

- **DNA** - "DNA is the genetic material of the cell."[9] It is a chemical hereditary coding, peculiar to each individual, found in the nucleus of every cell except for red blood cells, which don't have a nucleus. DNA is the same in all of the individual's cells. Effectively DNA defines who we are as individuals.

- **Gene** - A gene is "a segment of the DNA molecule that contains all the information required for synthesis of a product ... including both coding and non-coding sequences."[10] Coding sequences determine what the gene does while non-coding sequences determine when the gene is active. "It is the biologic unit of heredity, self reproducing and transmitted from parent to progeny."[11] In plain words genes are subunits of DNA carrying complete instructions for replicating the various cells. Because there are many different kinds of cells in the body (e.g. heart cells, brain cells, liver cells, muscle cells) there are also many different genes. Effectively genes are the instruction manuals, which define what each cell looks like.

- **Chromosome** - A chromosome in animal cells is "a structure in the nucleus containing a linear thread of DNA, which transmits genetic information... Each organism of a species normally has a characteristic number of chromosomes in its somatic cells, 46 being the number normally present in man,"[12] with these 46 chromosomes being arranged in 23 pairs. Chromosomes "contain several hundred genes arranged in a specific linear order."[13] One of the main functions of chromosomes is to facilitate proper cellular division.

Your Future is Not Completely Controlled by Genetics

A review of recent genetic research demonstrates there is a lot of difference of opinion, if not downright disagreement among authorities as to whether or not genetic malfunctions cause obesity. A lot more research needs to be conducted to determine the exact role genetics plays in the obesity problem we see today. The research results fall into one of two broad categories. First are those who appear to believe genetics are the primary cause of obesity. Second are those who believe the connection is much weaker and other factors play an equally important role. Let's explore these views.

The Link Between Genetics and Obesity

Epidemiologic observations of the constancy of body composition over long periods of time give strong support for a biological basis for the regulation of body fat.[14] Both the amount of body fat and the body shape and composition in adults are strongly influenced by genetic factors.[15] Even if family members don't live together, having obese relatives increases a person's risk for obesity.[16] Of course, rather than a genetic problem it may be a learned behavior affecting eating or exercise habits. In fact "first-degree relatives of obese patients have up to a 9-fold increase in disease risk."[17]

There is some genetic regulation of BMI between the ages of 1 and 18, but there are also long-lasting environmental influences.[18] "Persons who matured rapidly in adolescence were generally more obese than were those who matured slowly,"[19] but there is a decreased genetic influence with increased age.[20] What all this means is there are not only genetic and environmental influences impacting our tendency to gain and retain body weight but at different ages those factors affect us differently.

"A number of genes involved in the regulation of energy expenditure, appetite, lipid metabolism and adipogenesis have been reported to affect body weight regulation and the risk of treatment failure in some obese subjects."[21] For example, as discussed above "the FTO gene has been recently reported to be a major candidate for human obesity,"[22] even though the exact method by which it causes obesity is unknown. This gene has been shown to be associated with BMI, hip circumference, body weight,[23] and type 2 diabetes.[24] Others disagree by claiming the LEP, NMB and ADRB3 genes are the most consistent predictors of changes in body fat, in adults.[25] Finally, research has "found evidence of a maternal effect on chromosome 12 and a paternal effect on chromosome 13."[26] It should be obvious there are genes that cause some people to have a tendency towards obesity, but in the next section it will become equally obvious there are other contributing environmental factors, and those contributing factors may have the ability to overpower much of the genetic influence.

As further research is conducted there will be more genes discovered that affect energy expenditure, appetite and fat metabolism. As these genes are found it is reasonable to believe more personalized recommendations regarding diet, exercise and drug therapy will be forthcoming. As of today, genetic research is not capable of predicting with certainty who will or will not gain weight, but it is "useful for the identification of individuals at high risk for gaining body fat over time."[27]

Obesity related genetic disorders all pretty much affect the motivation to eat. "Estimates from the most rigorous studies suggest more than 50% of the variance in eating disorders and disordered eating behaviors can be accounted for by genetic effects."[28] For example, "binge eating disorder appears to aggregate in families and have a significant genetic component."[29] "Thus, human food intake should not be considered as an entirely voluntarily controllable phenomenon, but rather one driven by powerful biological signals."[30] The question left unanswered by these studies is just how powerful is the genetic motivation to eat? If it is only a mildly influencing factor the motivation for good health or to maintain a socially desirable appearance may be capable of overriding it. If on the other hand it is quite strong these motivations may not be sufficient to help us maintain a reasonable body weight. It could be an unknown interaction between the various genes that is the culprit. "Gene/gene interactions are likely to become common in complex genetic diseases including obesity."[31]

A really important question is whether or not obesity should be considered a genetic disorder. "It clearly is in some relatively rare cases."[32] Whenever obesity is caused by a defect in one or more genes it obviously has a genetic origin, but it should be noted, only a minority of obesity cases can be explained by genetics.[33] Genetically caused obesity only results in about five percent of the obesity cases.[34] What about the other 95 percent?

Many non-genetic factors have been shown to contribute to individual weight gain, which are referred to as environmental factors. In most cases these environmental factors work in conjunction with a genetic predisposition for weight gain. Many research findings suggest environmental factors are very powerful in influencing weight gain. "In the presence of a genetic predisposition to obesity, the severity of the disease is largely determined by lifestyle and environmental conditions."[35] "Common obesity arises when individual's genetic makeup is susceptible to an environment that promotes energy consumption over energy expenditure."[36] The fact is developed societies have an environment favoring weight gain rather than weight stabilization because of an abundance of food, often high calorie food, and a lack of exercise. "In most humans genes do not directly cause obesity, but they predispose to becoming obese in the changed environment of the modern world."[37]

"Although genetic variation is responsible for a large portion of the variation in BMI, it is equally clear expression of the genotype will depend on the environment."[38] In other words, when considering the differences in body type and weight gain, the environmental role is paramount, while the genetic role is subordinate. There are also a variety of psychosocial and socioeconomic problems that frequently lead to weight gain; among them are "divorce, solitude, poor economy and low education, unemployment, and problems at work."[39]

Here are some interesting facts about the genetic impact on obesity:

- "Genes can powerfully influence human eating behavior."[40] Since this is true a concentration on behavior modification could help achieve a weight-loss objective.

- "Genes seem to be important in the development of most severe early-onset forms of obesity."[41] There is a greater tendency for genes to affect early-onset forms of obesity than for them to affect obesity acquired later in life.[42]

- There appears to be an inverse relationship between total body fat and central abdominal fat and alcohol consumption. It has been shown women who drank between one to one and a half drinks per day had a lower total body fat and central abdominal fat then did nondrinkers.[43] "The gene-environment interaction suggests women with the greatest genetic risk of abdominal obesity may benefit more from this level of alcohol consumption than those at lower risk."[44]

- Genes may have a stronger influence on the distribution of fat in the lower body in women than in men of African origin.[45] There is also evidence to indicate the "importance of considering men and women separately in genetic analysis."[46]

- Obese individuals are characterized by common personality profiles. These profiles "could be genetically transmitted, as would be expected according to modern views on the fundamental inherited nature of personality."[47]

Summary

I realize the relative importance placed on genetics vis-à-vis environmental factors is a matter of debate. Most research results cannot tear the genetic component away from the environmental one. People with a family history of obesity can still respond well to increased exercise, even though they may have a strong genetic tendency towards weight gain.[48] Several genes (together with environmental factors) may be in control of body fat stores,[49] "no gene has yet been confirmed as a susceptibility or modifying locus for central obesity."[50] A genetic tendency towards obesity supports the idea that the entire physical, psychological, physiological and biochemical makeup of an individual is significantly influenced by genetic factors. These factors must work in concert with one another to cause obesity.

The solution to losing weight is far simpler than having to figure out the complexities of your genetic makeup and trying to make some sort of genetic correction. By determining which environmental conditions have the greatest impact on the problem (e.g. excess caloric intake, inadequate exercise, a hormonal imbalance, a psychological disturbance) and taking appropriate steps to alter them, you can make major improvement in your situation. "The most likely environmental factor contributing to the current obesity epidemic is a continuing decline in daily energy expenditure that is not matched by an equivalent reduction in energy intake."[51]

Genetic research has not progressed to the point where a useful profiling of individual genetic backgrounds can be of much value. Up to this point "the scientific evidence for most associations between genetic variants and disease risk is insufficient to support useful applications."[52] At the present time there is no targeted obesity therapy available.[53] It could be many years before scientific knowledge and experience have progressed to the point where researchers can effectively use medical intervention coupled with lifestyle to effectively develop useful genetic profiles.[54] In short, genetic knowledge is not advanced enough to allow its reasonable application to the problem of obesity.

Here's a silly thought, what if over-eating and lack of exercise could alter proper genetic function? Bougneres concluded that it could when he stated, a "sedentary life and caloric abundance has created new physiological conditions capable of changing the level of expression of a number of genes involved in fuel metabolism and body weight regulation."[55] Gene expression is mainly dependent on environmental and behavioral factors.[56] It seems clear the way genes perform is directly affected by the environmental conditions they are subjected to. Perhaps the biggest potential genetic solution to obesity can be found between our ears, that is, the genetics that control how we approach solving the problem.

Finally, it has been suggested that rather than searching for genes that cause us to be overweight researchers might be better off searching for genes that cause muscularity and leanness.[57] The identification of DNA associated with obesity should be considered as only "the beginning of the long series of steps needed to elucidate disease pathways and to establish the specific role individual genes may play in the process."[58]

Endnotes

1. L.A. Barness, J.M. Opitz, E. Gilbert-Barness, "Obesity: Genetic, molecular, and environmental aspects," *Am J Med Genet* Part A 143A (2007) 3016-3034.
2. J.V. Neel, "The thrifty genotype," Nutri Rev 57 (1999) S2-S9.
3. K.K. Davison, L.L. Birch, "Obesigenic families: parents' physical activity and dietary intake patterns predict girls' risk of overweight," *Int'l J Obes* 26 (2002) 1186-1193.
4. A.G. Comuzzie, B.D. Mitchell, S. Cole, L.J. Martin, W-C Hsueh, D.L. Rainwater, L. Almasy, M.P. Stern, J. Hixson, J.W. Maccluer, J. Blangero, "The genetics of obesity in Mexican Americans: the evidence from genome scanning efforts in the San Antonio Family Heart Study," *Hum Bio* 75 (2003) 635-646.
5. J.A. Jacobsson, P. Danielsson, V. Svensson, J. Klovins, U. Gyllensten, C. Marcus, H.B. Schioth, R. Fredriksson, "Major gender difference in association of FTO gene variant among severely obese children with obesity and obesity related phenotypes," *Biochem Biophy Res Comm* 368 (2008) 476-482.
6. Ibid.
7. A. Peeters, S. Beckers, A. Verrijken, P. Roevens, P. Peeters, L. Van Gaal, W. Van Hul, "Variants in the FTO gene are associated with common obesity in the Belgian population," *Mole Gen Metab* 93 (2008) 481-484.
8. A. Lev-Ran, "Human obesity: an evolutionary approach to understanding our bulging waistline," *Dia/Met Res & Rev* 17 (2001) 347-362.
9. E.J. Applegate, *"The Anatomy & Physiology Learning System,"* 2nd ed, (Philadelphia, PA: Saunders, 2000) 33-34.
10. "Gene," *Dorland's Illustrated Medical Dictionary*, 30th ed: 762.
11. Ibid.
12. "Chromosome," *Dorland's Illustrated Medical Dictionary*, 30th ed: 362.
13. E.J. Applegate, *"The Anatomy & Physiology Learning System,"* 2nd ed, (Philadelphia, PA: Saunders, 2000) 43.
14. B.K. Cornes, G. Zu, N.G. Martin, "Sex differences in genetic variation in weight: a longitudinal study of body mass index in adolescent twins," *Behav Genet* 37 (2007) 648-660.
15. K. Schouboe, P.M. Visscher, B. Erbas, K.O. Kyvik, J.L. Hopper, J.E. Henriksen, B.L. Heitmann, T.I.A. Sorensen, "Twin study of genetic and environmental influences on adult body size, shape, and composition," *Int'l J Obes* 28 (2004) 39-48.
16. H.N. Lyon, J.N. Hirschhorn, "Genetics of common forms of obesity: a brief overview," *Am J Clin Nutri* 80 (2005) 215S-217S.
17. S. Stone, V. Abkevich, D.L. Russell, R. Riley, K. Timms, T. Tran, D. Trem, D. Frank, S. Jammulapati, C.D. Neff, D. Iliev, R. Gress, G. He, G.C. Frech, T.D. Adams, M.H. Skolnick, J.S. Lanchbury, A. Gutin, S.C. Hunt, D. Shattuck, "TBC1D1 is a candidate for a severe obesity gene and evidence for a gene/gene interaction in obesity predisposition," *Hum Mole Gen* 15 (2006) 2709-2720.

18. K. Silventoinen, K.H. Pietilainen, P. Tynelius, T.I.A. Sorensen, J. Kaprio, R. Rasmussen, "Genetic and environmental factors and relative weight from birth to age to 18: the Swedish young male twins study," *Int'L J Obes* 31 (2007) 615-621.

19. N.F. Butte, G. Cai, S.A. Cole, A.G. Comuzzie, "Viva la familia study: genetic and environmental contributions to childhood obesity and its comorbidities in the Hispanic population," *Am J Clin Nutr* 54 (2006) 646-654.

20. K. Schouboe, P.M. Visscher, B. Erbas, K.O. Kyvik, J.L. Hopper, J.E. Henriksen, B.L. Heitmann, T.I.A. Sorensen, "Twin study of genetic and environmental influences on adult body size, shape, and composition," *Int'l J Obes* 28 (2004) 39-48.

21. J.A. Martinez, M.D. Parra, J.L. Santos, M.J. Moreno-Aliaga, A. Marti, M.A. Martinez-Gonzalez, "Genotype-dependent response to energy-restricted diets in obese subjects: towards personalized nutrition," *Asia Pac J Clin Nutr* 17 (2008) 119-122.

22. A. Lopez-Bermejo, C.J. Petry, M. Diaz, G. Sebastiani, F. de Zegher, D.B. Dunger, L. Ibanez, "The association between the FTO gene and fat mass in humans develops by the postnatal age of two weeks," *J Clin Endocrinol Metab* 93 (2008) 1501-1505.

23. A. Scuteri, S. Sanna, W.M. Chen, M. Uda, G. Albai, J. Strait, S. Najjar, R. Nagaraja, M. Orru, G. Usala, M. Dei, S. Lai, A. Maschio, F. Busonero, A. Mulas, G.B. Ehret, A.A. Fink, A.B. Weder, R.S. Cooper, P. Galan, A. Chakravarti, D. Schlessinger, A. Cao, E. Lakatta, G.R. Abecasis, "Genome-wide association scan shows genetic variants in the FTO Gene are associated with obesity related traits," *PloS Genetics* 3 (2007) 1200-1210.

24. R. Do, S.D. Bailey, K. Desbiens, A. Belisle, A. Montpetit, C. Bouchard, L. Perusse, M.C. Vohl, J.C. Engert, "Genetic variants of FTO influence adiposity, insulin sensitivity, leptin levels, and resting metabolic rate in the Québec family study," *Diabetes* 57 (2008) 1147-1150.

25. L. Bouchard, A. Tremblay, C. Bouchard, L. Perusse, "Contribution of several candidate gene polymorphisms in the determination of adiposity changes: results from the Québec family study," *Int'l J Obes* 31 (2007) 891-899.

26. C. Dong, W.D. Li, F. Geller, L. Lei, D. Li, O.Y. Gorlova, J. Hebebrand, C.I. Amos, R.D. Nichols, R.A. Price, "Possible genomic imprinting of three human obesity-related genetic loci," *Am J Hum Gen* 76 (2005) 427-437.

27. L. Bouchard, A. Tremblay, C. Bouchard, L. Perusse, "Contribution of several candidate gene polymorphisms in the determination of adiposity changes: results from the Québec family study," *Int'l J Obes* 31 (2007) 891-899.

28. K.L. Klump, W.H. Kaye, M. Strober, "The evolving genetic foundations of eating disorders," *Psych Clin N Am* 24 (2001) 215-225.

29. K.N. Javaras, N.M. Laird, T. Reichborn-Kjennerud, C.M. Bulik, H.G. Pope, Jr., J.I. Hudson, " Familiality and heritability of binge eating disorder: results of a case-control family study and a twin study," *Int'l J Eat Disord* 41 (2008) 174-179.

30. I.S. Farooqi, S. O'Rahilly, "Genetics of obesity in humans," *Endocrinol Rev* 27 (2006) 710-718.

31. S. Stone, V. Abkevich, D.L. Russell, R. Riley, K. Timms, T. Tran, D. Trem, D. Frank, S. Jammulapati, C.D. Neff, D. Iliev, R. Gress, G. He, G.C. Frech, T.D. Adams, M.H. Skolnick, J.S. Lanchbury, A. Gutin, S.C. Hunt, D. Shattuck, "TBC1D1 is a candidate for a severe obesity gene and evidence for a gene/gene interaction in obesity predisposition," *Hum Mole Gen* 15 (2006) 2709-2720.

32. R.J.F. Loos, C. Bouchard, "Obesity - is it a genetic disorder," *J Int Med* 254 (2003) 401-425.

33. P. Boutin, "Genetics of human obesity," *Clin Endocrinol Metab* 15 (2001) 391-404.

34. R.J.F. Loos, C. Bouchard, "Obesity - is it a genetic disorder," *J Int Med* 254 (2003) 401-425.

35. Ibid.

36. D.M. Mutch, K. Clement, "Unraveling the genetics of human obesity," *PloS Genetics* 2 (2006) 1956-1963.

37. H.R. Berthoud, C. Morrison, "The brain, appetite, and obesity," *Ann Rev Psych* 59 (2008) 55-92.

38. N.F. Butte, G. Cai, S.A. Cole, A.G. Comuzzie, "Viva la familia study: genetic and environmental contributions to childhood obesity and its comorbidities in the Hispanic population," *Am J Clin Nutr* 54 (2006) 646-654.

39. R. Rosmond, C. Bouchard, P. Bjorntorp, "5-HT$_{2A}$ Receptor gene promoter polymorphism in relation to abdominal obesity and cortisol," *Obes Res* 10 (2002) 585-589.

40. I.S. Farooqi, S. O'Rahilly," Genetic factors in human obesity," *Obes Revs* 8 (2007) 37-40.

41. C.G. Bell, A.J. Walley, P. Froguel, "The genetics of human obesity," *Nat Revs Genetics* 6 (2005) 221-234.

42. Ibid.

43. J.R. Greenfield, K. Samaras, A.B. Jenkins, P.J. Kelly, T.D. Spector, L.V. Campbell, "Moderate alcohol consumption, dietary fat composition, and abdominal obesity in women: evidence for gene-environment interaction," *J Clin Endocrinol & Metab* 88 (2003) 5381-5386.

44. Ibid.

45. I. Miljkovic-Gacic, X. Wang, C.M. Kammerer, C.H. Bunker, A.L. Patrick, V.W. Wheeler, L.H. Kuller, R.W. Evans, J.M. Zmuda, "Sex and genetic effects on upper and lower body fat and associations with diabetes in multigenerational families of African heritage," *Metab Clin & Exper* 57 (2008) 819-823.

46. J.J. McCarthy, J. Meyer, D.J. Moliterno, L.K. Newby, W.J. Rogers, E.J. Topol, "Evidence for substantial effect modification by gender in a large-scale genetic association study of the metabolic syndrome among coronary heart disease patients," *Hum Gen* 114 (2003) 87-98.

47. J.M. Martins, A. Trinca, A. Afonso, F. Carreiras, J. Falcao, J.S. Nunes, S. doVale, J.C. daCosta, "Psychoneuroendocrine characteristics of common obesity clinical subtypes," *Int'l J Obes* 25 (2001) 24-32.

48. K. Samaras, P.J. Kelly, M.N. Chiano, T.D. Spector, L.V. Campbell, "Genetic and environmental influences on total-body and central abdominal fat: the effect of physical activity in female twins," *Ann Int Med* 130 (1999) 873-882.

49. P. Arner, "Hunting for human obesity genes? Look in the adipose tissue!" *Int'l J Obes* 245 (2000) S57-S62.

50. R. Rosmond, " Association studies of genetic polymorphisms in central obesity: a critical review," *Int'l J Obes* 27 (2003) 1141-1151.

51. A. Marti, M.J. Moreno-Aliaga, J. Hebebrand, J.A. Martinez, "Genes, lifestyles and obesity," *Int'l J Obes* 28 (2004) S29-S36.

52. A. Cecile, J.W. Janssens, M. Gwinn, L.A. Bradley, B.A. Oostra, C.M. vanDuijn, M.J. Khoury, "A critical appraisal of the scientific basis of commercial genomic profiles used to assess health risks and personalize health interventions," *Am J Hum Gen* 82 (2008) 593-599.

53. M.J. Moreno-Aliaga, J.L. Santos, A. Marti, J.A. Martinez, "Does weight loss prognosis depend on genetic make-up?" *Obes Revs* 6 (2005) 155-168.

54. A. Cecile, J.W. Janssens, M. Gwinn, L.A. Bradley, B.A. Oostra, C.M. vanDuijn, M.J. Khoury, "A critical appraisal of the scientific basis of commercial genomic profiles used to assess health risks and personalize health interventions," *Am J Hum Gen* 82 (2008) 593-599.

55. P. Bougneres, "Genetics of obesity and type 2 diabetes: tracking pathogenic traits during the predisease period," *Diabetes* 51 (2002) S295-S303.

56. E. Jequier, "Pathways to obesity," *Int'l J Obes* 26 (2002) S12-S17.

57. M.W. Peeters, M.A. Thomis, R.J.F. Loos, C.A. Derom, R. Fagard, A.L. Claessens, R.F. Vlietinck, G.P. Beunen, "Heritability of somatotype components: a multivariate analysis," *Int'l J Obes* 31 (2007) 1295-1301.

58. S.K. Sieberts, E.E. Schadt, "Moving toward a system genetics view of disease," *Mamm Genome* 18 (2007) 389-401.

Part Two

Consider Your Options

3   The Importance of Food Choices

What we eat and drink and the reasons behind this food acquisition behavior are not only interesting but are extremely important to our health and weight management. It is also a topic that doesn't get adequate attention. As a result it is one we frequently understand only superficially. The problem is a limited understanding can lead us to inadequacies in our personal health practices that have possible long-term consequences. This chapter is not intended to turn you into a dietitian or nutritionist; however, if you gain the basic knowledge offered and apply the simple principles outlined your weight loss effort will go much smoother and you will be far more successful.

A drug is "any substance that affects the structure or functioning of a living organism."[1] Food fits the definition of a drug and in many cases it is useful to think of food as a drug, since we use food to promote health, sustain life and heal the sick. Nutrients are, "substances that provide energy or building material for the survival and growth of a living organism,"[2] and nutrients are what we need from the food we eat. Macronutrients are nutrients providing calories and energy. The three generally recognized macronutrients are fat, protein and carbohydrates.[3] Although alcohol is not usually considered part of a normal food plan, researchers sometimes include it as a fourth macronutrient, because Americans obtain three to five percent of their total daily calories from its consumption.[4] I will give alcohol, limited discussion from this point.

The 21st century diet is dramatically different from that of our ancestors. In addition to the abundance of food and snacks available today the macronutrient composition of our food has changed. Not all of these changes are good, for example:

- Our carbohydrate intake has increased at the expense of protein.[5]

- The carbohydrate composition, which used to be primarily from wild plants, fruits and vegetables,[6] is now comprised of many processed and refined products (e.g. corn flakes, pancakes and fried potatoes, all of which have a high glycemic index). "The glycemic index (GI) is a physiologically based measure of carbohydrate quality - a comparison of carbohydrates...based on their immediate effect on blood-glucose levels... carbohydrates that break down quickly during digestion have high GI values... carbohydrates that break down slowly, releasing glucose gradually into the bloodstream, have a low glycemic index."[7]

- The composition of our fat intake has changed substantially:
  o Omega-6 fatty acid intake has increased dramatically at the expense of omega-3 fatty acid, and this is because:
    ▪ Modern diets contain little fish, which is high in omega-3,
    ▪ Modern diets contain more oils from corn, sunflower, safflower, cottonseed and soy, all of which are high in omega-6,
    ▪ The fat composition of meat often reflects an abnormal animal diet.[8]
  o Our intake of trans fats and altered fats is increasing at an astonishing rate, which may be because "high-fat, more calorie-dense diets promote over eating and overweight...one reason may be that palatability and the energy density of food are closely correlated with human food preferences."[9]

One important question becomes what is the optimum dietary ratio of macronutrients? Although there is disagreement, many experts recommend a diet consisting of approximately 50 percent carbohydrates, 30 percent fat, and 20 percent protein.[10] The correct balance for any individual depends on a variety of factors, such as age, lifestyle, exercise habits, existing health conditions, personal goals, etc.[11] The fact is a professional athlete has completely different requirements than grandma. Because this is true, it stands to reason that the macronutrient recommendations mentioned clearly need to be customized to your fit individual needs.

We have all heard the axiom, losing weight is nothing more than burning more calories than what you take in. With that in mind, effective food planning should consider the difference between the energy in the food we eat, compared to the amount of energy our bodies burn during our daily activities. So, by planning for a negative energy balance we can accomplish weight loss.[12] Losing weight is not automatically a direct function of reducing how much you eat. Scientists have demonstrated the type of food you eat determines what will be burned and what will be stored as fat,[13] (e.g. hot peppers will fire up your metabolism and help you lose weight).

Diets and Dieting

The whole concept of diets and dieting is one that raises the hair on the back of my neck. Some of the reasons I feel that way are:

- The word *diet* is fraught with images of starvation or deprivation, and need not be,

- Going on a diet implies going off a current diet, whereas a modest adjustment may be all that's necessary,

- "During weight loss, dietary quality may be compromised,"[14] since diets are all too often nutritionally unbalanced and inadequate,

- Those promoting dieting are often concerned with weight loss at the expense of nutritional health and reading what they say about their diets frequently convinces me they don't know the difference,

- "The diet industry does not offer accurate information about the efficacy... of diets, thereby preying upon people's fantasies about weight loss,"[15]

- A low calorie diet (LCD), (800 to 1,200 calories/day) or worse yet a very low calorie diet (VLCD) (less than 800 calories/day),[16] remind me of trying to save gas by putting less in the tank, how foolish,

- Fasting or severe dieting causes a starvation syndrome where the body attempts to store all the energy it can for future use, most of which is stored as fat.

I favor the idea of sensible *food planning* instead of dieting.

Reasons for Dieting

A close look at the realities of dieting leads to the conclusion there are basically three fundamental reasons for dieting: (1) dieting to improve health, (2) dieting to improve appearance, and (3) dieting to appease a third party. It is not unusual to find different strategies are required to successfully address each. As you look closer at these reasons for dieting keep in mind they have been organized in the order of probability of success:

- Dieting to Improve Health - People who diet to improve their health find it easier to adopt healthy eating habits, stay on target towards their objective and avoid dysfunctional eating, than do dieters who are trying to improve their appearance or meet someone else's expectations. Dieting for this reason is the easiest to do and results in the best success.

- Dieting to Improve Appearance - Growing up in a home in which the parents engaged in dieting behavior, is generally associated with chronic dieting aimed at changing one's appearance.[17] People who diet for appearance purposes tend to exhibit greater body dissatisfaction and lower self-esteem than those dieting for health, and often use such strategies as skipping meals, eating only one type of food, forced vomiting and abuse of laxatives and diuretics.[18] One danger is if the eating pattern of forced vomiting and abuse of laxatives and diuretics is adopted it can lead to an eating disorder.

- Dieting to Appease a Third Party - Certainly the most difficult weight-loss objective is to lose weight to pacify a third-party. Frequently this happens as a result of a physician suggesting weight loss or at the suggestion of a family member and usually results in the least success of the three options.

Types of Diets

Diets fall into a variety of types, for example we frequently hear of people who are on a low-fat diet, a low carb diet, a low glycemic load diet, a vegetarian diet or perhaps a vegan diet, and finally the best, although the least popular diet, the one the creator made for us, know as the balanced diet. As you can see by the names, some of these diets tell you right away they are trying to minimize certain macronutrients, many of which are essential to proper bodily function. Here's a brash opinion, generally speaking, I feel low fat, low carb, vegetarian, and vegan diets are pure and simple foolishness. Let me explain.

Fat and carbohydrates are the body's preferred energy sources. Protein, which is the building block of the cells, provides a far less efficient and effective source of energy. Fat has nine calories/gm) while carbohydrates and protein each have 4 calories/gm).[19] Obviously reduced fat in your food plan could be beneficial for reducing calories; however, it is vital to understand: (1) how much fat is in the diet, and (2) what type of fat it is. I would agree with those who believe there is an over consumption of fat in Western culture, but here's where rushing into a low-fat diet becomes unreasonable. To just arbitrarily eliminate fat from the diet reduces essential fats, often called essential fatty acids, along with the non-essential fats. Essential fats are those the body cannot make for itself but must have for proper function. For example, the brain and nervous system are among the biggest users of essential fats and must have them supplied through the diet. Without them in the diet brain and nervous system function deteriorate. Women who systematically avoid fat in their diets have been shown to have lower self-esteem, higher scores on body dissatisfaction, more cases of bulimia and a tendency toward interpersonal distrust.[20] "These associations suggest that fat avoidance may be a predictor of eating pathology and psychosocial problems in college-aged women."[21] If anyone suggests you need a low-fat diet, without knowing how much fat you are currently eating and what type of fat it is, that should be a hint they're lost and I suggest you get away from them quickly and find someone who has at least a minimal understanding of nutrition!

The flip side of this situation is just as absurd. The high fat approach may be useful for weight loss in the short-term, but the potential harmful effects of such a diet over the long term remained a big concern.[22] Probably the most popular of the high-fat diets is the Atkins diet. For those brave souls using this diet, with its huge meat consumption and little or no fiber intake, they should expect constipation to be one of the unpleasant side effects and it would be a good idea for them to keep a close eye on their cholesterol and triglyceride levels. Weight loss could be accomplished with a moderate energy restricted diet containing normal fat content.[23]

Only a limited amount of research has been conducted on low carbohydrate diets. An extremely low carbohydrate, high fat diet consisting of only eight percent carbohydrates with over 60 percent fat and 30 percent protein was found to cause body fat loss, but the mechanism appeared to be through abnormal manipulation of the endocrine system. The problem is the study only ran for six weeks and the study participants were men of normal weight rather than obese subjects.[24] This leaves the study results suspect in terms whether or not they even apply to the obese.

Instead of a low-fat diet, a high fat diet or low carbohydrate diet, monitoring the glycemic index of the foods eaten offers a more sensible approach to weight loss. One reason may be diets based on low glycemic index foods appear to delay the onset of hunger.[25] When compared with a high glycemic index, low-calorie diet a low glycemic energy restricted diet attained by proper food selection can assist in achieving a negative energy balance during obesity treatment, which favors weight loss and weight maintenance.[26] In addition, it has been shown a low glycemic diet reduces both hunger and metabolic risk factors.[27] There may be several reasons why a low glycemic index diet suppresses hunger:

- Low glycemic index foods remain in the digestive track longer, signaling satiety,

- High glycemic index foods may stimulate hunger because of the rapid rise and fall in blood sugar levels, which appear to stimulate responses intended to counteract the drop in sugar,

- After a high glycemic index food is eaten both adrenaline and cortisol are released, which stimulates appetite,

- Low glycemic index foods contain abundant fiber, thereby increasing the bulk in the intestinal track, which leads to satiety,[28] and this is important for obese people because it has been shown "obese men and women have significantly lower dietary fiber intakes than do lean men and women."[29]

There is even better news about the low glycemic index diet. When compared with a low-fat diet, high-fat diet or low-carbohydrate diet, it offers a lot of nutrition, and good nutritional balance, because of the high fruit and vegetable intake.

Then there are those who recommend a very low-calorie diet (VLCD) (i.e. less than 800 calories/day) for the obese. Although short-term weight loss can be achieved using a VLCD, long-term maintenance of weight loss is generally poor. A VLCD coupled with the drug sibutramine was found to help the patient maintain weight loss better than patients that didn't use the drug.[30] Then on the other hand you could try a VLCD coupled with another dietary aid called Nutrilett, which is intended to offset the nutritional deficiency, but since that will constipate you, you'll need to take a fiber supplement called Fiberform.[31] I think you're probably seeing an ugly trend here. The VLCD, by its nature, is so deficient in nutrition, while you're on it you'll have to: (1) take a whole bunch of additional nutritional supplements to keep it from killing you, and (2) at the same time deal with the inherent side effects of the recommended pharmaceuticals.

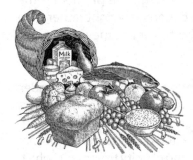

I can't be sure just how much nonsense you are willing to put up with in order to eat an extremely unhealthy VLCD but I can guarantee you I wouldn't buy into any of these nutritionally compromised diets. "Because reduced calorie diets could exacerbate nutritional problems in older persons, dietary intervention should be oriented toward improving diet quality by increasing intake of nutrients-dense foods such as fruits, vegetables, and calcium rich foods while reducing consumption of energy-dense foods."[32] I think it takes no stretch of the imagination to believe their findings could easily apply to other overweight populations (e.g. younger women, men, adolescents).

It always comes back to the basic idea of a balanced food plan, with fewer calories consumed each day than what your body actually uses, plus adequate exercise. "A multidisciplinary weight reduction program that combines a VLCD, followed by a balanced hypocaloric diet, with a moderate-intensity progressive exercise program and behavior modification is an effective means for weight reduction in obese children and adolescents."[33] It has even been claimed an initial VLCD period doesn't affect long-term weight loss,[34] so rather than beginning with the VLCD and shortly thereafter moving to a low-calorie diet seems foolish. Why not just adopt the low-calorie diet in the first place, balance your nutrition and begin an exercise program?

There are two closely related diets that are fairly popular with dieters these days. They are the vegetarian diet and the even stricter vegan diet. The typical vegetarian diet is composed primarily of plant-based foods with some animal-based foods, such as milk and eggs added. The strict vegetarian eats no meat. The vegan diet is a stricter variation of the vegetarian diet, which includes no animal-based foods. These diets are frequently used because they are low in calories and have been shown to result in significant weight loss.[35] The big problem with both diets is they can be quite nutritionally deficient if you are not knowledgeable about how to use them. Because of their diet both vegetarians and vegans are generally in need of more protein, vitamin D, vitamin B12, vitamin K, folic acid, calcium, phosphorus, selenium and zinc,[36] as well as iron, essential amino acids and essential fats, all of which are found in meat. I don't favor either of these diets because of the complexity involved in maintaining the necessary nutritional balance. Later in the nutrition section of this chapter, I will discuss a much easier yet effective technique for weight control.

I guess if you're going to fool around with a diet that will lead to all types of nutritional deficiencies, I probably should mention malnutrition. There are two types of malnutrition: (1) kwashiorkor, and (2) marasmus.

- Kwashiorkor - develops quickly and as a result of acute illness. Surprisingly, this type of malnutrition can be hard to detect because the person's body weight may remain normal. Physical signs may include edema, skin problems, and poor wound healing. Appropriate nutritional treatment should help support the individual but the metabolic disruption will not normalize until the underlying illness or injury is resolved.[37] I would argue: (1) living your life in a continuous nutritionally deficient state is a chronic illness, and (2) many obese people, even though they may appear robust, are suffering from malnutrition.

- Marasmus - is commonly known as starvation. This type of malnutrition is the result of decreased energy intake relative to energy expenditure. Marasmus usually develops over months or even years. An inadequate energy intake can be the result of eating habits or the result of disease (e.g. cancer). Physical signs may include fat loss coupled with muscle wasting.[38] Loss of body fat may be a desirable situation but the greater concern comes from a loss of lean muscle mass. The obvious goal is to walk a fine line between losing weight healthfully and being malnourished. The joy of losing weight while not realizing you are suffering from malnutrition comes with a high cost. Just think of this scenario! We all know hospitals are loaded with doctors, nurses, technicians, nutritionists and dietitians, and all of them are supposed to know something about nutrition. Holmes reported in the UK 40 percent of the adult patients and 15 percent of children suffered from malnutrition while in the hospital. It affects medical and surgical patients, the young and the old, and to make matters worse the longer they stay in the hospital the worse it gets, all delaying recovery and increasing hospital costs.[39] The point I hope to make with that information is, if malnutrition is as rampant as Holmes reports it to be, inside a hospital, with all those supposed nutritional experts available, you get some idea of how touchy it could be for you to get your own nutritional balance correct. Don't give up it isn't impossible. There will be more discussion on how to solve this situation in the following section on nutrition.

In addition, dieting strategies that are inflexible oftentimes lead to symptoms of eating disorders including mood disturbances and higher anxiety.[40] It all comes back to the benefits of a balanced diet. Ironically, "substantial weight loss can be obtained even with a moderately energy-restricted diet."[41] It has also been demonstrated people attempting to lose weight through self-directed dieting struggle significantly compared to those that seek help.[42]

Caloric Balance

Several times earlier in this chapter I mentioned energy balance. So what does that mean, how does it relate to your diet and how can you make it work to your advantage? Your body requires energy to:

- Move about, much like your automobile requires gasoline,
- Think,
- Repair itself from damage (e.g. work, injury, exercise),
- Create the white blood cells necessary to kill foreign invaders like bacteria, fungus, and virus.

The way we get energy into our bodies is through the food we eat and the things we drink. The measurement of the energy we consume is what we know as the calorie. Everything we eat and drink has calories, except for pure water. Some things have few calories, like lettuce, and some have many calories, like chocolate cake. If during any given day you take in more calories than what your body uses, you have a positive calorie/energy balance, which the body doesn't just eliminate but rather stores as fat for future use. If you keep this process up long enough you can gain a tremendous amount of weight. Here's a cool idea! If you are trying to lose weight, it makes sense to take in fewer calories than your body consumes. This causes your body to go into the fat warehouse and take out some of the fat it needs for energy. "To lose one pound of body fat, you must burn an extra 3,500 calories beyond what you are consuming."[43] Just think about it, for someone who wants to lose ten pounds they need a deficit of 35,000 calories and to lose 100 pounds they need a staggering deficit of 350,000 calories. That is a lot when you consider that the average person eats between 2,500 to 3,500 calories per day. Once you've reached the weight you desire the obvious way to maintain your weight is to consume approximately the same number of calories each day that your body needs to function.

When researchers talk about burning calories they really mean oxidizing them or using them for the body's energy needs. "Thermogenesis is the production of heat in response to food intake."[44] There are basically three components that constitute our daily energy expenditure. They are:

- Resting Metabolic Rate (RMR) - is the energy required to sustain bodily functions and maintain body temperature at rest. The good news is muscle is metabolically active tissue, which means the more lean muscle mass you have the more calories you use while at rest. Amazingly, RMR accounts for between 60 and 75 percent of daily energy consumption.

- Thermic Effect of Food (TEF) - is the energy required to ingest, digest and store food. TEF accounts for approximately ten percent of daily energy consumption.

- Thermic Effect of Activity (TEA) - is the energy required to perform physical activity beyond that required for RMR and TEF. TEA accounts for between 15 and 35 percent of daily energy consumption.[45] Since we have the most control over the TEA, it will be discussed at greater length in the chapter on exercise.

Capsaicin, green tea and CH-19 sweet pepper (containing capsicum annuum L) have a thermogenic effect when consumed. Although these foods have a thermogenic effect they also help dieters by suppressing hunger.[46]

Successful Dieters

Successful dieters have greater impulse regulation, a greater tendency towards perfectionism and more fluctuation in weight than do unsuccessful dieters, and the more weight the person is trying to lose the more prone they are to lapses in restraint.[47] But there is good news. Dieters who are fearful of yo-yo dieting find by changing their diets to eat more healthy foods without the underlying intent of dramatically altering their bodies, they are less likely to experience bouts of over eating or other eating disorders.[48] Although diets can lead to short-term weight loss those losses are generally not maintained. Frequently, with the passage of time the lost weight is regained, unfortunately it rarely stops at the pre-diet weight but actually increases beyond.[49] Successful dieters tend to hold more rigid beliefs about food and therefore seem better able to control their eating behavior.[50] It is also clear more than diet alone is needed. The real answer lies in proper food planning combined with exercise and other interventions such as psychological counseling and hormone balancing.

The Downside of Dieting

Dieting has more than one downside. Let's take a look at some of the more important failures of dieting.

- The biggest difficulty with dieting is its close relationship with nutritional deficiency. Dieting often leads to classic malnutrition, while at the same time the dieter generally remains oblivious to what is happening. The nutritional aspects of healthy weight loss and weight maintenance are given in-depth consideration later in this chapter.

- Dieting tends to coexist with a number of other health risk behaviors. Teen dieting may be an indicator of low self-esteem, body dissatisfaction and depressive symptoms and has been reported to parallel higher rates of smoking.[51] Encouraging healthy eating among individuals who suffer from any of these psychosocial conditions should help them improve their situation.[52]

- Restrained eaters are those individuals who eat less than desired and normally try to reduce their caloric intake in order to control their body weight.[53] Since most dieters rely on dietary restriction as their primary strategy, this can backfire if the dieter becomes preoccupied with food or begins eating in the absence of hunger, all of which increases the probability of further weight gain rather than weight-loss and makes weight maintenance doubtful.[54] Most successful dieters view food with a heightened awareness of the nutritional and psychological aspects of the food.[55] The so called trust model has been claimed to be effective for weight loss because it is comprised of: (1) unconditional permission to eat when hungry and whatever food is desired, (2) eating for physical rather than emotional reasons, and (3) reliance on internal hunger and satiety cues to determine when and how much to eat.[56] A word of caution is needed here. Item (1) above says individuals may eat whatever they want when they are hungry. I don't believe that for a minute. As you will see later in the section on nutrition what you eat and when you eat it both have a tremendous impact on the body's ability to shed excess pounds.

- "In the civilian population, meal skipping is a common method of attempted weight management, although it has no proven efficacy, is usually associated with obesity, and has many adverse effects on performance."[57] In fact, nearly 50 percent of female adolescent dieters report skipping meals although additional study data suggests meal skipping is less prevalent among adults.[58] Breakfast is especially important. People who eat breakfast regularly are much more likely to have nutritionally sound diets and that may be especially true for older adults, because breakfast provides a higher proportion of their total daily nutritional intake.[59] Meal skipping is not only part of the malnutrition model but is one of the quickest ways to throw the body into starvation mode.

- A starvation issue begins to arise when the food deprivation is large or of long duration. Severe food deprivation, (e.g. fasting, extreme dieting, meal skipping), signals the body to begin a starvation mode, causing several detrimental weight loss events to occur. In technical terms, the body's attempt to conserve energy, as a result of food deprivation, brings in to play two distinct regulatory thermogenic control systems:

  o Nonspecific Thermogenesis - the body reacts "rapidly to starvation stress by functioning as a buffer against energy imbalance and hence spares both lean and fat tissue."[60]

  o Fat-Specific Thermogenesis - when fat storage levels drop significantly the body's primary "function is specifically to spare body fat when fat stores become severely depleted and to ensure its rapid replenishment with increased food availability."[61]

In plain words here is what happens:

o   Once the body thinks starvation is in progress it begins to conserve energy by storing it as fat. Initially this process preserves both fat stores and lean muscle mass.

o   At the same time fat storage begins the body dials down the resting metabolic rate, which serves to consume fewer calories while the body is at rest.

o   If the starvation lasts long enough, muscle tissue begins to break down to be used as a fuel source and as lean muscle mass deteriorates the body dials back the resting metabolic rate even more.

o   Once the body has been trained to be very efficient with energy conservation when you returned to normal eating the energy consumed is efficiently stored as fat, and worse yet, normal eating will not only return you to your previous bodyweight but will pack on even more pounds than before.

After conducting extensive research on dozens of popular diets researchers concluded, all of the diets could result in weight loss but, "the majority of individuals who lose weight are losing the struggle to keep the weight off."[62] The most obvious reason is the diet is only one component to weight loss. Without the inclusion of the additional considerations discussed in this book, diet alone weight loss efforts are generally doomed to failure.

Nutrition - It's a Bigger Deal Than You Might Think

Today there are many fad diets masquerading as good, sound, balanced weight-loss plans, when in fact many of them are nothing more than very nutritionally poor examples of how desperate some so called experts have become in their quest to create and sell weight loss products. "One of the greatest hazards of fad diets is that they may be nutritionally inadequate,"[63] and I suggest these authors were very kind when they used the words may be nutritionally inadequate.

Caveat - In 1943 the Food & Drug Administration (FDA) developed what it called Recommended Dietary Allowances (RDA), which it updates regularly. The RDA was intended to indicate the daily dietary intake level of nutrients considered adequate to meet the requirements of most healthy individuals. More recently it has begun calling these minimum daily recommendations, the Reference Daily Intake or Recommended Daily Intake (RDI). The name change is not terribly important but there is one critical point that needs to be made. Since the FDA promotes these minimum daily requirements as the minimum requirements needed to sustain the health of an already healthy individual, that means they are intended to just keep the already healthy person alive. Most knowledgeable health care professionals recognize they are woefully inadequate for most of the population. In fact if a person is trying to build lean muscle mass, overcome a disease, or prevent future illness, their nutritional needs will greatly exceed the FDA requirements. Keep in mind these recommendations are exactly what they claim to be minimums, so use them only as a guide for your nutrition planning but consider increasing them substantially, perhaps as much as 50 to 100 percent or more, according to your needs.

Many diets are suggested by well meaning professionals, without any real thought being given to the current nutritional status of the dieter. I believe it is pure and utter nonsense for any healthcare professional or diet guru to suggest a diet incorporating reduced calories, very low calories, reduced fat or reduced carbohydrates, without first establishing a baseline understanding of the current nutritional status of the patient. The classic example is a recommendation for fat consumption. All too often healthcare professionals direct the obese person to reduce their fat intake without ever gathering a shred of evidence about the person's current level of fat consumption. This is a classic case of prescribing a remedy before making a diagnosis (i.e. the cart before the horse). The correct conversation needs to shift the emphasis away "from dieting and drastic weight-control measures toward the long-term implementation of healthful eating and physical activity behaviors."[64] Let's consider what that might look like.

Fuel the Engine - Healthy Eating

When I think about providing my body with the necessary nutrition to make it operate properly I am reminded of the saying, *the Ferrari won't run well on low octane fuel*. You can polish the Ferrari, change the oil regularly, change the filters, check the fluids, inflate the tires, etc., but the overall *performance* and *longevity* of that expensive engine is determined by the quality of the fuel used. Your body is no different. Both may run for a short time on less than optimal fuel, but if you insist on using low-grade fuel in either one, the day of reckoning will come sooner rather than later.

The foundation for losing weight, maintaining a consistent weight and maintaining good health, is good nutrition and exercise. I will discuss exercise in the next chapter; let's look at healthy eating. Earlier in this chapter we discussed the fact that macronutrients are nutrients providing fuel for the engine, and the three basic macronutrients are carbohydrates, fat and protein. We also established a starting point for recommended macronutrient balance in a normal diet (i.e. 50 percent carbohydrates, 30 percent fat, and 20 percent protein). If metabolic syndrome exists it is not just the caloric balance in our diet that is important but it is the macronutrient composition that helps in its management.[65]

I mentioned earlier food fits the definition of a drug. In line with that thought some researchers talk about medical nutrition therapy. "Medical nutrition therapy consists of two steps, - conducting a nutrition assessment and developing and implementing a nutrition care plan."[66] While it is true this conversation is usually held with seriously ill medical patients, it still can be effectively applied in a weight loss plan. How might that be done?

The easy way of beginning a simple nutrition assessment is to record your food intake (i.e. keep a food journal). In the food journal you write down all of the food and drinks you consume, usually over the period of the week or more. Keeping a food journal is valuable for a number of reasons: (1) it increases food consumption awareness, (2) it emphasizes what changes need to be made, (3) it guides those changes, and (4) it becomes a monitoring tool.[67] At the end of the recording period you review the journal. You'll find it doesn't take a nutritionist to tell you where some of the glaring problems are. For example, if you eat fries and a burger for lunch every day by looking at the journal you can quickly determine you might be eating too much fat, (primarily altered fat). If you eat cookies and ice cream every night before you go to bed, the thought that you're eating too much sugar should jump off the pages of the journal. With this knowledge it becomes obvious a slight alteration will make a substantial improvement in your food plan. This process will help you become aware of some of the excesses in your food plan so you can make the adjustments. People who carefully and accurately maintain a food journal: (1) lose significantly more weight than those who do not, and (2) they actually lose double the weight of those who only recorded sporadically.[68] In a later section of this chapter you will see my Rule of Thirds, which will help you improve your food planning.

What to Include in Your Food Plan

Before considering what foods to include in your food plan you must come to grips with the reality that the same two fundamentals guiding your overall weight loss plan, also apply when developing your food plan. They are:

- Balance - "The most sensible eating plans are those that involve a wide selection of foods..."[69] which simply means you cannot just eat what you like. You must bring variety into your food plan (e.g. fat, carbohydrates, protein, green foods, red foods, yellow foods, vegetables, fruit, meat, raw foods). You must avoid eating the same breakfast, lunch or dinner, day after day, because: (1) you like it, (2) it is convenient, or (3) it is cheap. Variety is of great importance since no two foods have exactly the same nutritional complex.

- Lifestyle - I've tried to avoid the words *lifestyle change* primarily because there is a natural tendency to resist when we hear the word *change* or think about having to change. I like to think of the quest for a healthier lifestyle as a process of slowly moving toward a more useful, self-serving lifestyle, offering the possibility of better health, more functionality, increased longevity and improved happiness. People seeking help to resolve a weight problem must understand a successful outcome requires a lifelong effort.[70] Also be aware, a lifestyle adjustment will generally not work, if it is someone else's idea that is thrust upon you. If you are attempting to lose weight and have any hope of being successful, you will find some lifestyle modification is going to be necessary! One of those centers around food planning.

Specifically, what should be included in a good food plan? It is not as difficult as it often seems. Here is what I recommend:

- Natural Foods - The creator provided mankind with a whole variety of wonderful natural foods to eat. Among those are fruits, vegetables, herbs and meat, (if you're a meat eater, and I hope you are). Nowhere among those natural foods do we find such things as French fries, cookies, candy, donuts or potato chips. A lot of these processed concoctions are so devoid of nutrition they shouldn't even be called food. "Switching from a diet of imitation foods, such as those found in the typical low-fat and high carbohydrate diets or those imitation foods high in partially hydrogenated vegetable oils, to a diet of real foods with normal levels of natural fats, will result in a gradual and sustained weight loss in most overweight people."[71]

  Here's a simple food test. Unwrap a candy bar and set it on the kitchen counter alongside a couple of strawberries, a slice of apple or a piece of an orange. Within a few weeks insects and/or mold will have eaten the fruit. They recognize these items as nutritious food. On the other hand you could leave the candy bar there for six months and nothing would touch it. If it didn't melt from being in the sun it would still be in the same condition it was the day you put it there. If insects, bacteria or mold refuse to eat the candy bar, consider whether or not it is good for you. Please, take your food plan in the direction of real, natural foods. Oh, and obtain them as fresh as possible.

- A Variety of Foods - A variety of foods are essential for a variety of nutrition. Different foods contain different percentages of the various nutrients needed by the body. It is interesting to note, the reason foods vary so much in color is the result of the differences in their nutrient content. By eating a one-dimensional diet, large quantities of certain nutrients may be consumed, which can easily become more than what is needed, while others may drop to a deficiency level or be ignored altogether. **Caveat** - a balanced diet is not a cookie in each hand!

- Green Foods - Today when many people talk about green foods they are generally referring to health supplements that include chlorella, spirulina, sea algae, kelp, barley grass and wheat grass, which are usually taken in capsule, powder or liquid form. While these are wonderful sources of nutrition, at this point I am more interested in edible green plants, to be consumed as a food source. Green foods have a lot to offer all food plans, and here are some of the reasons. Green foods:

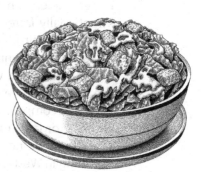

- o Help the body eliminate toxins,
- o Encourage the growth of good bacteria in the digestive system,
- o Boost immunity,
- o Support cellular metabolism,
- o Purify the blood,
- o Are rich in protein, vitamins, minerals and some fatty acids,
- o Are very alkalizing to the body.

Nutritionally "green vegetables are the most highly prized, yielding larger percentages of vitamins and minerals and more protein than most other vegetables."[72] Green foods contain chlorophyll, which neutralizes acids and toxins in the blood, thereby giving them a reputation as a powerful blood purifier. If you are looking for a very large dose of nutrition each day, buy a juicer, juice vegetables and drink between 12 and 24 ounces of this juice per day.

- • Organic Foods - Before I discuss organic foods let me acknowledge they are considerably more expensive than conventionally grown foods. I know this because I eat an organic diet myself. Aside from the expense, organic foods are better for you than conventionally grown foods, for several reasons:

  - o Organic plants aren't contaminated with large amounts of chemical fertilizers and pesticides like their conventional counterparts.

  - o More importantly organic plants provide superior nutrition. In 2008, Hubert and van de Vijver determined there were over 100 previous nutrition studies that compared organically grown foods with conventionally grown and on average organically grown foods have higher levels of anti-oxidants, vitamin C and minerals and the same or better protein quality.[73] Here's why! Plants are intended to nurse from the breast of mother earth for a predetermined period of time, which we know as the plants' normal growing season. Conventionally grown plants whose growth is hyper stimulated by chemical fertilizers grow in a much shorter period of time. By rushing the plants' growth and harvesting it sooner, the plant is nutritionally deficient because it has not had the time it needed to fully absorb the proper amount of nutrition, from the earth. The nutritional deficiency of the plant is the same nutritional deficiency you get when you eat it.

o   Similar results hold true for naturally raised animals. Animals fed a conventional diet are often fed foods not even remotely related to the animals' normal diet. For example, corn is not part the normal diet for cows or pigs, yet farmers intentionally fatten them by feeding them corn. The animal not only gets fatter but their fat content is altered. They pack on many pounds of what researchers call white fat, which leads to a condition in the animal, called fatty degeneration and which in turn negatively affects our health when we eat the animal.[74] Research done in the UK suggests there are sizable differences in fatty acid composition between conventionally and organically raised lambs, with the organic meat having a higher omega-3 content,[75] and omega-3 is something we need more of in our diets, since omega-3 levels have been declining in Western diet for years.

- Specific Considerations -

o   **Fat** - In Western society today we are crazed with the idea of too much fat in our diets. The reality is fat has gotten an unjustifiably bad rap. We have all heard the commentary about the negative side of fat, for example: (1) high fat diets cause heart disease, (2) high cholesterol diets cause heart disease, (3) high fat diets elevate cholesterol, and (4) eating fat causes us to be fat. The first three have been shown to be complete myths,[76] while the fourth is misleading.

The fat we eat does not float around in our system and look for a place to attach itself to our body. The problem is this; although fat is needed to sustain life and is the desired source of energy it provides the body with more than twice the calories per gram than carbohydrates and protein. What is true is in order to lose weight we need to: (1) assess our total dietary fat intake, and (2) adjust it downward if it is contributing excess calories. But during the process of lowering dietary fat, beware.

Our obsession with dietary fat has another bad side. Many people are encouraged to reduce their dietary fat intake without considering the distinction between *essential fats* and *nonessential fats*. The body does not produce essential fats; therefore they must be obtained from the diet. The body is able to manufacture nonessential fats from other nutrients. This distinction turns out to be very important for those professionals arbitrarily suggesting that you reduce fat from your diet. If you are not careful it becomes synonymous with throwing the baby out with the bathwater, since by arbitrarily minimizing total dietary fat you may be eliminating the essential fats your body can't make.

The question becomes, what are the essential fats and what foods should you include in your diet in order to get them? There are two primary groups of essential fats:

- Linoleic Acid (Omega-3) - Common sources are flax seeds, pumpkin seeds, canola oil, soybeans, dark leafy greens and cold-water fish such as salmon, trout, mackerel and sardines.
- Alpha-Linolenic Acid (Omega-6) - Common sources are flax seeds, pumpkin seeds, sunflower seeds, sesame seeds, soybeans and meat.[77]

In addition, a balance problem exists with the essential fatty acid intake in our Western diet. Erasmus suggests a healthy diet should consist of two grams of Omega-6 for each gram of Omega-3,[78] or in plain words they should be consumed in a 2:1 ratio. The reality is our diet actually consists of 10 to 20 grams of Omega-6 for each gram of omega-3.[79] One simple way to start to bring these essential fatty acids back into balance is to decrease the consumption of red meat while increasing the consumption of cold-water fish and dark leafy greens.

Finally, the fat conversation would not be complete without some consideration of saturated fat. Saturated fat is frequently maligned as the real evildoer among fats. But a closer look reveals the problem may not be so much the consumption of saturated fat as it is the environment or lifestyle of the person eating it. If saturated fat were the villain it is made out to be, the Masai tribesmen of Kenya and the Samburus of Uganda, who consume more than twice as much saturated fat as Western experts recommend, would suffer from the chronic ailments we do. For example, their cholesterol should be sky high, but it isn't, it's among the lowest ever measured on earth.[80]

Similar examples exist closer to home, (e.g. the Alaskan Eskimo and the Inuit of Greenland). So what is going on here? The answer lies in multiple environmental and lifestyle factors. If like the Masai's and Samburus, we: (1) got massive amounts of exercise, (2) lived a more stress-free lifestyle, (3) didn't smoke, and (4) ate all organic foods; we like them, might experience a whole lot less obesity, heart disease, stroke, cancer, etc.

Several other things are in play here. Domestic animals are generally fatter than wild animals because of their inbreeding, artificial feeding and limited exercise. Although the East Africans have domesticated their animals, but because they are not inbred,[81] eat a natural diet, get more exercise and aren't forced to grow at a drug induced hyper fast rate, they are as lean as their wild counterparts. The lesson is we could improve our overall health and weight status if we paid more attention, to these factors.

o **Carbohydrates** - For years carbohydrates have been broken down into two sub-classes know as *simple carbohydrates* and *complex carbohydrates*. Sugars because of their small molecules were considered simple carbohydrates while starches with their bigger molecules were considered complex carbohydrates. For 50 years, based on their small molecular size, simple carbohydrates were believed to digest quickly and be absorbed quickly into the bloodstream, causing a rapid rise in blood sugar. The contrary belief was held for complex carbohydrates. In recent years these beliefs about the speed of digestion have been seriously questioned.[82] Today a numerical scoring system, called the glycemic index, is used to describe the speed that carbohydrates in individual foods affect blood glucose levels. Here's what the numbers mean:

- Low Glycemic Index (Desirable) = 0-55
- Intermediate Glycemic Index = 56-69
- High Glycemic Index (Undesirable) = above 70[83]

Eating low glycemic foods has a couple of advantages for people trying to lose weight: "(1) they fill you up and keep you satisfied longer, (2) they help you burn more body fat and less muscle."[84] The foolishness of either a low carb diet or a very low carb diet is that while you are reducing carbs from your diet either fat or protein or both are increasing. If you continue to eat the normal volume of food you will now have a low carb diet with a high fat or a high-protein diet. All of these situations are detrimental to weight loss and good health. If you are attempting to follow a low carb diet you need to understand the nutritional risks of such an unbalanced diet.[85]

Based on two million years of human evolution, it is possible the human body is not intended to metabolize large amounts of carbohydrates, especially high glycemic index carbs that are rapidly digested and drive high levels of insulin secretion.[86] Most fruits and vegetables are fairly high in carbohydrates, low in fat, moderate to low in protein and extremely low on the glycemic index. Considering that the Western diet is high in fat and protein this makes fruits and vegetables ideal foods for good health and weight loss.

Men between 20-59 eat less than one third of the recommended amount of fruit while only half of them get the recommended amount of vegetables.[87] This highlights the need for men in this age range to improve their dietary habits, helping them lose weight and improve other related health factors. Men respond well to specific dietary targets, which promote greater consumption of fruits, vegetables and dairy products.[88]

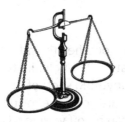

Finally, excess consumption of carbohydrates may contribute to depression.[89] As I have said before, **it's all about balance**!

o **Protein** - Protein molecules are made up of subunits or building blocks called amino acids. There are both nonessential and essential amino acids. *Nonessential amino acids* are those the body can make from other nutrients. *Essential amino acids* are those that must be obtained from the diet, since the body cannot manufacture them. There are between 8 and 11 essential amino acids, depending on our age. A *complete protein* is a protein containing all the essential amino acids, and an *incomplete protein* is a protein that does not contain all of them.

In some circles there is a belief we in the West eat too much protein. It has been claimed "the health benefits previously observed with high protein diets can be derived from a much more modest and manageable level of protein intake."[90] Later research questioned the adequacy of the current recommended daily allowance for dietary protein intake in older adults and went on to say, while animal protein sources are not only complete protein sources they are also a source of high biological-value protein, neither of which is true for vegetable proteins.[91] Following closely on the heels of those two studies, in 2009 Layman emphasized the importance of protein for maintaining body composition, bone health and glucose homeostasis in adults,[92] and went on to outline the following dietary protein guidelines:

- "Protein is a critical part of the adult diet,
- Protein needs are proportional to bodyweight; NOT energy intake,
- Adult protein utilization is a function of intake at individual meals,
- Most adults benefit from protein intakes above the minimum RDA."[93]

Many vegetarian or vegan food plans include soy-protein as a substitute for meat. The good news is soy-protein is a fairly good source of protein with an intermediate glycemic index. High soy-protein consumption with limited fat and carbohydrates has been shown to improve the body composition in overweight and obese people, while preserving muscle mass.[94]

Caveat. Because of the phytoestrogens in soy-protein it may work well for women, but men should approach its use with caution, because it may upset the very delicate male estrogen balance.

What to Limit in Your Food Plan

Although there is a wide variety of food to eat on planet earth, good health and weight control suggests there are some foods that should be eaten in moderation if not eliminated altogether. Understand, I am not some radical food purist that never puts anything short of the perfect food in my mouth. First, that's foolish because of the constant pressure you have to subject yourself too, and second it's not necessary. There are times when you can go off your food plan and not do damage to your weight loss program (e.g. vacations, special occasions), providing you don't deviate too far for too long. Remember, **it's all about balance**, with a little moderation thrown in! So, what should you really be careful of?

- Processed Foods - Grocery stores are full of foods that are processed. Processed foods come in all shapes and sizes are packaged in cans, bags, boxes and bottles, and often come in unnatural colors, smells and textures. Generally these manufactured misfits have one thing in common, they are made from one or more of the following: (1) white flour, (2) white sugar, (3) white rice, or (4) altered oils. The first three were made white by processes like polishing, buffing, mashing, grinding, bleaching, deodorizing, etc., and during these processes they were stripped of their nutritional value. So how much loss of nutrition might there be?

  In his book *Fats that Heal, Fats that Kill*, Erasmus cited two researchers who have studied how nutritionally deficient processed flour really is, and here is what they found. Processing reduced the following nutrients in wheat: calcium (60 percent), chromium (40 percent), cobalt (89 percent), copper (68 percent), iron (76 percent), magnesium (85 percent), manganese (86 percent), molybdenum (48 percent), phosphorus (71 percent), potassium (77 percent), selenium (16 percent), strontium (95 percent), zinc (78 percent), vitamins B_1, B_2 and B_3 (72-81 percent), vitamin B_6 (72 percent), pantothenic acid (50 percent), folacin (67 percent), vitamin E (86 percent), Omega-6 (95 percent), Omega-3 (95 percent), protein (33 percent), and fiber (95 percent).[95] To me that is an unthinkable degradation of what started out as healthy, nutritious wheat.

  Ballantine suggests three steps when moving toward a natural diet: (1) replace refined sugar with raw sugar, honey, maple sugar or molasses, (2) replace refined white flour with whole-grain flour, and (3) replace refined vegetable oils and shortening with real butter.[96]

  In addition, the inclusion of a mixture of brown and black rice in the food plan may result in more effective weight control than white rice alone.[97]

  I realize many products made from these degraded imitations frequently advertise they are enriched or fortified. What that really means is once the manufacturer has removed all the nutrition, they sprinkled back a little bit, in an effort to be able to tell you their product is enriched, all of which is intended to fool you into thinking it's better than the original. Their claims are nothing more than low-grade, false advertising perpetrated on the unknowing. Later in this chapter I will discuss how to read food labels. A little knowledge of how to use food labels will greatly aid you in determining what is in processed foods and help you to find those items you want and those you want to avoid.

In addition to these white foods there are other processed food items that are literally dangerous to your health and will hold you back in your weight loss effort. Examples of some highly altered food items that are advertised as better for you than the natural ones are: (1) margarine (claimed by some chemists to be only one molecule away from being plastic), (2) hydrogenated vegetable oils (where hydrogen was bubbled through the oil to make it solid at room temperature and to give it a much longer shelf life), and (3) irradiated meat (meat that has been radiated to kill bacteria, not to mention killing all of the enzymes and a lot of the nutrients).

• Low Anything - As you embark on your weight loss program you will come across many things that begin with the word *low*. You will hear people talk about low calorie diets, low carb diets, low fat diets, low protein diets and on and on. To me the word *low* usually means below the minimum requirements needed to maintain your health. If you eat a food plan low in one macronutrient then, one or both of the others have to be high, putting you out of dietary balance. I suggest you avoid *low anything*. Remember, **it's all about balance**.

• Altered Fats - There are several ways to change the composition of the fats we eat, making them questionable for human consumption. Following are two of the most prominent, which I have chosen to discuss here, because you will find them everywhere and they are easy to recognize and minimize during your food planning. Four things do great damage to otherwise healthy fats. They are exposure to: (1) heat, (2) light, (3) oxygen, and (4) chemicals. Isn't it ironic nature packages many of its best oils in seeds that protect against these four problems?

    o Trans Fats - Trans fats exist in a number of different forms, primarily determined by their molecular bonding structure. The trans fats you should be most concerned with are the altered fats resulting from bubbling the gas hydrogen through them. These are typically cheap, low quality vegetable oils referred to as *hydrogenated* or *partially hydrogenated* oils. The process not only adds hydrogen to the oil but also involves high temperature heating of the oil. The two main reasons for hydrogenating oil is to dramatically extend its shelf life and to make it solid at room temperature, so it may be used in such products as margarine, chocolate, baked goods, etc.

The resulting oil has raised many health questions since the human body is unable to handle it in the same way it does natural oil. You may be thinking, surely the food industry wouldn't provide an unsafe or unhealthy food product, so it can't possibly be bad to consume hydrogenated trans fat, can it? Guess again! Here are just some of the reported adverse effects:

- Lowered good (HDL) cholesterol,
- Elevated bad (LDL) cholesterol,
- Elevated total cholesterol,
- Reduced birth weight in human infants,
- Increased blood insulin level in humans,
- Decreased levels of testosterone in male animals,
- Decreased response of red blood cells to insulin, (a potential difficulty for diabetics),
- Adverse alterations in the activities of important enzyme systems that metabolize chemical carcinogens,
- Alterations in fat cell size and number,
- Increased adverse effects of essential fatty acid deficiency,
- Promotes childhood asthma.[98]

If part of your weight loss program is to cut down on fats, trans fats would be a good place to start.

○ Modified Fats - A lot of the food we eat involves frying, which requires cooking oils to be heated to high temperatures. When cooking temperatures exceed 320°F the molecular structure of the oil is actually modified, resulting in toxic substances being created. As a matter of fact "deep-fried oils create a great health hazard for human beings."[99] In addition, they even degrade further when they are not replaced frequently, (e.g. in the French frying vat at your local fast food restaurant).

About the only oil that isn't damaged by frying temperatures is motor oil, but it may not be a good choice for your French fries. The next logical question then becomes, if I still insist on occasionally frying foods, which oils might be the least resistant to damage from heat. Here are some:

- Butter,
- Tropical Fats,
- Peanut oil,
- Sesame oil,
- Olive oil.[100]

Similar to trans fats, if you want to cut down on fats, modified fats might be another good place to take action. If in addition to weight loss your health is of any concern, you will certainly want to take a close look at your consumption of both trans fats and modified fats and minimize them.

- Chemical Contaminated Foods - Today's Western conventionally grown plant-based food supply is contaminated with pesticides and chemical fertilizers in excess of anything you might imagine. Following is a bit of my experience supporting that statement. Back in the early 1980's I moved to Traverse City, Michigan, the cherry capital of the world. This part of Michigan is literally covered with fruit trees. I bought a house that had 14 peach trees on the property. Not being a farmer, I set out to find out how to care for those trees. I went to the local Farm Bureau and consulted with a couple of farmers who willingly guided me. Being the good student that I am, I did as they directed. I purchased the liquid pesticide-fertilizer, took it 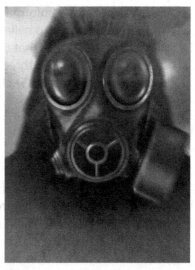 home and read the directions. As a result I clothed myself from head to toe in a long-sleeved shirt, long pants, gloves, hat, goggles and respirator and waited until a day without wind. I then proceeded to spray these trees to the point of saturation. I did this several times throughout the summer and wound up with the most beautiful peaches imaginable. They were the size of softballs and totally flawless. They had grown quickly and no pest could get within a quarter-mile of my property.

The majority of those deadly chemicals soaked directly into the fruit. Any residue that was washed off onto the ground by rain, soaked into the ground where it was picked up by the roots of the tree and transported to the fruit. Any way you look at it my fruit was extremely contaminated. Naïvely I did what the farmers told me to do, and without thinking further I simply rinsed the peaches off in the kitchen sink before eating them. I must have been nuts to think those peaches were even close to being safe to eat!

This, by the way is similar to how commercial cherry orchards are sprayed. The farmers have enormous tanks of chemicals that they tow behind their tractors. Each tank has a large fan on the back end of it with fan blades at least five feet long, which are used to blow thousands of gallons of this stuff into the trees. For days before the orchards are sprayed the farmers notify local residents to keep their windows closed and their children and pets inside. Now, if you are thinking to yourself I don't believe this guy, because I am confident the US Department of Agriculture is looking out for me, and conventional growing practices couldn't possibly result in such a dangerous food; then you might want to stop here and skip to the next section.

So what produce might be the worst? Not all reference sources have identically the same top ten or twelve items on their list of the most pesticide-contaminated products. Here is the test I use when trying to evaluate such information. I look at a variety of sources of information and when I begin to see a common thread running through them, I tend to believe there might be a kernel of truth in that commonality. Here are three sources that rank the twelve worst pesticide contaminated fruits and vegetables.[101] [102] [103] All three agree on ten. Here they are: (1) apples, (2) pears, (3) bell peppers, (4) celery, (5) cherries, (6) grapes (especially imported), (7) nectarines, (8) peaches, (9) strawberries, and (10) potatoes. Interestingly, cherries and peaches are included on all three! In addition, red raspberries and spinach made two of the three lists.

Just for fun let's look at what these sources consider to be the least contaminated produce. The same three sources rank the twelve least pesticide contaminated fruits and vegetables. All agree on nine. Here they are: (1) asparagus, (2) avocados, (3) bananas, (4) broccoli, (5) onions, (6) kiwi fruit, (7) mangoes, (8) papaya, and (9) pineapple. In addition, sweet peas, corn and cauliflower made two of the three lists.

The take-away messages are. First, I realize this is a weight-loss book, so if weight loss is your only concern and health is not a big item, you can ignore this section on pesticide contaminated food, Second, if health and weight loss are both important to you, and your food budget allows it, eat organic. If you can't do that at least buy organic when purchasing items from the list of most contaminated products. Third, if you are not going to eat organic, for good health it makes sense to try and eat more items from the least contaminated list and fewer items from the most contaminated list, but keep in mind some valuable nutrition will be sacrificed.

- Others - The list of foods that should be limited in our diets is endless; however, there are three that have become so dominant in our diets and are so worthless as a source of nutrition I will mention them here. Natural healers are almost unanimous in their agreement that: (1) white sugar, (2) white flour, and (3) white rice are three foodstuffs best eliminated from the diet. The reason the word *white* is attached to each of the three, when white is not their natural color, indicates they have been made white, by some intervention.

The question is what is the purpose in making them white? In our puritanical past white things were believed to be good, so enterprising food processors jumped on the bandwagon and in an attempt to give the consumer a more desirable looking product they began to bleach sugar, flour and rice. As you might expect a process as severe as bleaching makes them pure all right, in fact it virtually sterilizes them, leaving them nutritionally worthless. In their unrefined states all three have a valuable place in human nutrition, but once they are refined they actually become hazardous. Let's look at them individually in their refined state.

- **White Sugar** - So what's the big deal with refined sugar? Refined sugar has a number of health concerns not typically found in the use of whole sugars such as honey, molasses, unrefined cane sugar, etc.).

  - Because refined sugar is comprised of empty calories (i.e. calories with no nutritional value) it provides the body with worthless calories adding to the body's caloric load and displacing nutritionally valuable calories. These calories still need to be burned by the body and when they aren't burned they are stored as fat.[104]

  - Refined sugar complicates the sugar regulation mechanism of the body. Refined sugar enters the bloodstream quicker than natural sugar, resulting in a spike in the amount of insulin being dumped into the bloodstream. Over time this continued insulin-spiking process can result in the body's cells becoming insulin insensitive, which in turn leads to varying symptoms of metabolic syndrome, especially diabetes.[105]

  - Spikes in blood sugar cause a number of chemical reactions in the body creating inflammation,[106] and inflammation is a precursor to aging.

  - Another problem sugar causes is toxicity in the body. It is argued by some that sugar combines with proteins and forms complexes detrimental to the body, especially the blood vessel system.[107]

  Sugar consumption in the US has grown dramatically in recent years. Here is how it has progressed:

  - 1815 =   15   pounds / year / person,[108]
  - 1900 =   26   pounds / year / person,[109]
  - 1996 =   153   pounds / year / person.[110]

- **White Flour** - To increase product shelf life flour processing strips away the inner and outer layers of the grain, where most of the nutrients are concentrated, leaving only the starchy center.[111] Also by removing 80 percent of the valuable phosphorus and nearly all of the vitamins from the raw product, insects will have little interest in bothering it during shipment or storage.[112] That is a really bad sign because if insects won't eat it most likely we shouldn't either. Refined white flour generally contains only a modest 13 percent of the chromium, 9 percent of the manganese, and 19 percent of the iron found in whole wheat, and to make matters worse after all the fiber is removed some unscrupulous processors will add in ground wood fiber, so they can claim their product is fiber enriched.[113] Wood fiber may be good for woodpeckers but is not good for us!

o **White Rice** - One of the prime processing techniques for rice is called polishing. Somehow, I have never wished to have my food polished. Well come to find out it isn't really polishing any way. Polishing is simply a term given to a process where the rice is pounded until the outer husk is removed. Unfortunately the outer husk contains most of the protein, vitamins and minerals. Of course, this is important to all of us who eat rice expecting to get nutrition from it, but it becomes extremely important for vegetarians and vegans who rely on rice as a source of protein.

What this all boils down to is, if you are trying to lose weight you need proper nutrition from your diet. In order to get proper nutrition you need to eat natural sugars, which come from such foods as fruit, honey, molasses, whole-grain flour and rice. If you don't do this you'll need to get your nutrition somewhere else, and in the process your daily caloric intake is likely to remain higher than optimal for you.

It is Easier Than You Think (The Rule of Thirds)

In 21st century many people frequently lack the ability to take something complicated and boil it down into simple, understandable terms. We all too often come to realize the truth may be somewhat elusive when we:

- Hear our politicians trying to explain what they think is best for us,
- Hear our teenagers trying to explain a misbehavior,
- Listen to our bosses trying to explain how they want some particular task handled,
- Have someone try to explain to us how to improve our eating or exercise habits in order to lose weight. When this happens I bet they believe in such nonsense as:
  o In order to lose weight you need to eat less than X calories a day, in fact "calorie counting is often a waste of time...one can most accurately judge his caloric needs from the signals his body provides,"[114]
  o You need to count the calories you eat,
  o You shouldn't have more than X percent of your calories from fat,
  o If you want to keep track of your caloric intake, buy a calorie calculator and calculate the calories you eat at each meal,
  o You need to write down your daily caloric intake,
  o A piece of meat the size of your fist is approximately equal to X calories.

My response is *Ya Right*. The questions I imagine you have already asked yourself are: (1) How would I do that, (2) where would I start, and (3) do I have enough time in my life to tackle a complicated task like this one? If you find the whole thing nauseating, you have just joined the millions of people before you who have failed to lose weight and keep it off because the experts have developed tools for accomplishing the task that are so complicated they are unworkable for most of us mortals. Part of the difficulty in helping people lose weight is that the necessary changes in knowledge and in nutrition related behavior is insufficient to get the desired results,[115] and part of the reason is a complexity of the systems employed.

If you are a degreed nutritionist you can skip the rest of this section, otherwise understand there is an easier way. Although, what I am about to show you is conceptually easy to understand and implement, because you don't have to have any knowledge of nutrition, you will still need a bit of self determination. I have developed what I call the <u>Rule of Thirds</u>.

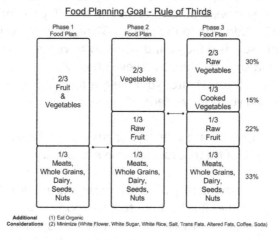

As you can see the <u>Rule of Thirds</u> contains three vertical columns. Reading from left to right you will see phase 1, phase 2 and phase 3. It is all very simple yet effective.

- **Phase 1** - When you sit down to eat look at what you're about to eat. You should see two-thirds fruit and vegetables, and one-third meat, whole grains, dairy, seeds and nuts. Stay on phase 1 until you are consistently eating this way.

- **Phase 2** - Once you have determined you are consistent with the phase 1 food plan it's now time to try to improve on it. The important thing about phase 2 is improvement involves breaking the phase 1 fruit and vegetable group in two-thirds vegetables and one-third raw fruit. What this means is you may need to make two slight adjustments from the phase 1 plan First, concentrate on eating two-thirds vegetables and one-third fruit from the fruit and vegetable group of phase 1. Second, the fruit you eat will be raw fruit not canned, cooked or in some other way processed.

Phase 2 should not be terribly difficult to accomplish, however moving to Phase 3 will become more challenging.

- **Phase 3** - Continue to eat the same volume of raw fruit, meat, whole grains, dairy, seeds and nuts you were eating in phase 2. The adjustment is in the vegetables you eat. Move toward more raw vegetables than cooked or processed. The goal is to achieve two-thirds raw vegetables to one-third cooked. I know this may be a tough adjustment, but by cooking your vegetables you kill the enzymes your body needs to properly digest them and you damage many of the other nutrients. Although you may never fully get phase 3 down perfect, it is still a good goal.

  By looking to the right of the third column you can see the percentage each food group consists of. If you are eating perfectly according to the Rule of Thirds you are eating 30 percent raw vegetables, 15 percent cooked vegetables, 22 percent raw fruit and 33 percent meats, whole grains, dairy, seeds and nuts. This situation may still be improved if you were able to eliminate the 15 percent cooked vegetables and eat those raw, in addition to the already 30 percent raw vegetables in the food plan. Achieving phase 3 is difficult and you may never get there, but don't let that stop you. Even if you are only able to achieve phase 2, coupled with proper exercise, that should enable you to: (1) alter your weight as you desire, and (2) at the same time get the nutrition your body needs.

  Caveat - Be sure when you are selecting foods for the lower third of the rule you don't overdue any one of them, especially meat and dairy.

One additional consideration is the theory of food combining. It holds that since different foods require different digestive enzymes it is best not to have foods requiring an acidic environment and foods requiring a more alkaline environment in the stomach at the same time. Most food combining devotees feel it is best: (1) not to eat protein and carbohydrates at the same meal, and (2) to eat sugary foods by themselves. While I am neither promoting nor denouncing this theory, if you want to understand it further you will need to explore it on your own.

This food plan is also in alignment with research data showing effective dietary changes work best when food groups or clusters of foods are changed at one time rather than trying to change several individual food items.[116] Notice too, the Rule of Thirds doesn't put any restrictions on how much you eat. Weight control is certainly not about starvation, if you are hungry eat, just maintain the proper ratios.

This still leaves one unanswered question. If I follow the Rule of Thirds are some fruits, vegetables, grains and meats better than others? The answer may be debatable, but the more than 6,000 year-old[117] East Indian tradition of Ayurvedic healing answers with an emphatic, yes! In Ayurveda there are three primary life forces in the body called doshas. They are known as Vata, Pitta and Kapha. Ayurveda claims that one of these three forces is predominant in each one of us. In his outstanding book, Ayurvedic Healing, Frawley offers a simple test to determine which Dosha is predominant in you.[118] He then presents a set of tables showing which foods in each food group should be emphasized and which should be deemphasized for the predominant dosha.[119] Once you are comfortable working the Rule of Thirds, this added Ayurvedic experience might help you further refine your food planning for a higher level of health and weight loss.

Nutritional Supplements / Meal Replacements / Diet Aids

We are all bombarded with advertising promising weight loss by taking the advertised product, usually a liquid or powder concoction. Many are nutritional supplements. In addition to being marketed as a foundation of good health they are also touted as weight control aids. Many supplements can have a positive affect on weight loss, but they all should raise the same questions for each of us: (1) what is it, (2) how does it work, (3) what does it do to my body, and (4) are there negative long term effects I should know about? One of the reasons for these questions is, "most of the weight-loss supplements taken contain stimulants."[120]

It is not my intent to analyze the different products on the market today, but I will: (1) mention a few of the most popular ones, and (2) give you a more general overview of what to look for and expect from their use. Before I do that please understand:

- Anything good for your body, also has the potential to do harm. Vitamins, minerals, amino acids and enzymes that the body normally needs in specific amounts, can become detrimental if taken excessively,

- All of the sales fluff surrounding the use of these products is intended to appeal to us for one of two, or possibly both, of the following reasons:
    o Laziness - we want an easy solution to the problem, and/or
    o Cost - we want a cheap solution.

After all the hype we are still faced with the reality that, **it's all about a balanced approach.** For example, many of these products are intended to make you feel full so you eat less, but eating less can easily result in diminished nutrition. If your nutritional intake is not up to par before you begin reducing your food intake, your nutritional intake will really take a hit if you consume less of the already diminished nutrients, (refer back to the Rule of Thirds).

In addition to the potential health risks associated with an excessive or imbalanced use of nutritional supplements, meal replacements or diet aids, there is evidence they present an increased risk of developing an eating disorder. One study of a group of college women reported that their "data demonstrate that college women with a high risk of developing eating disorders report high rates of diet aid use."[121]

Many of these products work by causing the body to work in a way it wasn't intended too. One well-known example is the stimulating effect of the ephedra and ephedrine containing supplements. These put the body in a hyper active state by constricting blood vessels and increasing blood pressure and heart rate.[122] Most health care practitioners deem that to be problematic.[123]

Nutritional Supplements

On the positive side, "long-term use of multivitamins, vitamins B_6 and B_{12}, and chromium were significantly associated with lower levels of weight gain."[124] Fat oxidation, also referred to as beta-oxidation, is the body's way of breaking down large fat molecules into smaller ones so they can more readily be used as sources of energy. It has been shown an inverse relationship exists between vitamin C intake and fat oxidation.[125] Similarly, men who engage in moderate-intensity exercise may improve the amount of weight they lose by increasing their calcium intake. Unfortunately increased calcium consumption doesn't have a similar effect in women.[126] In addition, it has been suggested stimulant-free dietary supplements containing Glucomannan, Chitosan, Fenugreek, Gymnema Sylvestre, or Vitamin C may be capable of delaying glucose absorption, eliciting lipid malabsorption, reducing caloric intake, and improving insulin sensitivity,[127] all of which are advantageous for weight control.

When you looked at the Rule of Thirds you saw a food plan dominated by unprocessed green foods. There are two reasons for this:

- Green foods contain no altered fats, no trans fats, minimal if any sugar, and the carbohydrates they contain are unrefined,
- Green foods also contain phyto-nutrients full of vital antioxidants, vitamins, minerals,[128] and omega fatty acids,[129] all good things. These things are important for weight loss because of their high nutrition and low caloric content, but in addition, their health benefits include elimination of toxins, increasing levels of good bacteria and improving immunity.[130]

Meal Replacements

In recent years meal replacements have gained a lot of popularity among people trying to lose weight or maintain weight loss. Meal replacements work in several ways. First, meal replacements are used to assist the dieter in controlling caloric intake. Second, they have been thought to promote a thermogenic response, even though the result is generally regarded as minimal.[131] A thermogenic response is one producing heat in the body,[132] which burns excess calories and promotes a negative energy balance.[133] Third, they are used to supply increased nutrition in what oftentimes is a nutritionally depleted food plan.

Some of the reasons why meal replacements have become so popular, are they: (1) provide a fixed amount of food with a known calorie content, (2) simplify food choices, (3) require little or no preparation, (4) help dieters avoid problem foods,[134] and (5) are cheaper than the food typically purchased by many obese dieters.[135] One of the benefits of meal replacements is they tend to help the dieter improve their food planning. Those who use meal replacements often take their overall nutritional needs more seriously. Dieters using meal replacements not only lose weight by lowering their caloric intake but they also reduce their cholesterol.[136]

A study of an unidentified, commercially available, high-protein, low-carbohydrate, low-fat food supplement combined with both aerobic and resistance exercise, found after ten weeks several things happened: (1) as might be expected, the macronutrient profiles of the subjects changed in the direction of the meal replacement, (2) total energy intake decreased, (3) physiological adaptations to exercise were improved, (4) fat mass decreased, (5) muscle mass increased, and (6) time to exhaustion during exercise increased.[137] I would suggest the same results could most likely be obtained using similar meal replacements.

Are there differences between liquid and solid meal replacements? It seems: (1) people who used a liquid meal replacement have a higher than normal food intake at their next meal, (2) because of that under weight elderly people might benefit from consuming liquid meal replacements, and (3) overweight people might benefit more from consuming solid meal replacements.[138] These differences exist because the liquid meal replacements require less energy to digest, leaving more of their energy available for the needs of the body, Conversely the solid meal replacements require more energy to digest, thereby consuming more of the available energy.

Just how good are meal replacements as a tool for weight maintenance? Two studies have shown: (1) meal replacements used as weight maintenance tools frequently lead to healthier eating but did not necessarily translate into improved weight maintenance,[139] and (2) the popular meal replacement SlimFast did help people lose weight initially, but as a weight maintenance tool its effect diminished over time.[140]

Diet Aids

Diet aids normally consist of natural products that are believed to have some basic nutritional value but are generally not thought of as nutritional supplements (e.g. herbs, spices, teas).

For years green tea has been known to be high in antioxidants. It has recently been shown to have a positive impact on weight loss. Studies have concluded green tea could reduce body fat in obese subjects by increasing energy expenditure, fat oxidation,[141] and thermogenesis.[142] It is interesting to note the green tea, frequently used in trials is not green tea, as we know it, but is an herbal extract of green tea. Chantre at al studied a green tea extract (brand name AR25 Exolise), and found it aided weight reduction by inhibiting fats and stimulating thermogenesis.[143] Tests of a green tea extract (brand name Herbal One), found a single 250 mg capsule taken after each of the three major meals resulted in measureable weight loss.[144]

This leaves open three questions. First, would drinking green tea be as effective as the extract? No, because the extract can be concentrated to the point where it would take dozens of cups of green tea daily, to get the same effect as a daily supply of green tea extract capsules. Second, are all green tea extracts the same? No, because manufacturing practices vary significantly and the quality of the green tea being harvested is dependent upon climatic and soil conditions in the locale in which it was grown. Third, how can you figure out which if any green tea extract is right for you? Experiment! Network with other people to find out what experience they have had with various products. One good place to start is your local health food store. Try different products, be sure to buy them from reputable manufacturers and see which, if any of them benefits you.

Spices may provide a similar result to that of green tea. "Consumption of spiced foods or herbal drinks leads to greater thermogenesis and in some cases to greater satiety."[145] However, the benefits of using spices for weight loss seem to: (1) be more heavily steeped in theory than they are in reality, and (2) offer limited benefit.

One of the most popular diet aids today is Hoodia. Hoodia has been shown to be an effective appetite-suppressant. However, there are some problems with Hoodia. First, there are numerous species of Hoodia, the most popular of which is Hoodia Gordonii.[146] Because of the many species of Hoodia, it may be difficult for you to determine which species gives you the best result. Second, when the manufacturer mixes more than one species it becomes difficult to determine which species is primary in the product being purchased. Third, because Hoodia is scarce adulteration has become a major problem.[147]

While nutritional supplements, meal replacements and diet aids all hold the possibility of being helpful with weight reduction, a few words of caution are needed.

- Even though these products may not normally exhibit the side effects associated with drugs, they may nevertheless cause undesirable reactions in the body. For example, several of these items produce a thermogenic reaction, caused by the caffeine in the product (e.g. green tea). The positive thermogenic benefits can be quickly off set by: (1) unwanted cardio stimulation, (2) increased blood pressure,[148] and (3) caffeine addiction. In addition, meal replacements often get their good taste from excessive amounts of refined sugar.

- In order to get the desired affect, frequently an abnormally high dose of the product is needed (e.g. green tea). Excessive use of these aids may drive the body into an unbalanced condition.

In the long run I think it is much safer to make sensible dietary adjustments, than it is to try and get fast, easy weight loss by using nutritional supplements, meal replacements or diet aids as a mainstay in your program. If you decide to use one of these products to jumpstart weight-loss, as you become more knowledgeable and experienced with your own body's needs, wean yourself off it.

Don't forget, **it's all about balance**!

Read the Labels

There are food labels on packaged foods entitled *Nutrition Facts*. There are a few things on the label that are quite important to understand. All of the values listed on the label are for a single serving and at the top of the label you will find the number of servings in the container. If you want to more fully understand the nutrition facts, on the label, you might want to do some additional study on this subject. The Internet is a good place to begin, and you will find www.cfsan.fda.gov/label.html helpful.

I suggest you concern yourself with the following:

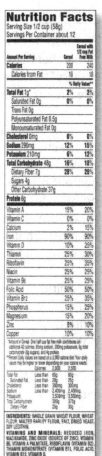

- Look at total fat, total carbohydrate and protein - As mentioned earlier in this chapter many, experts suggest a diet consisting of approximately 50 percent carbohydrates, 30 percent fat and 20 percent protein. Looking at these three items on the nutrition facts label will give you an accurate perspective of how much you will consume by eating this food. Factor that into your overall daily food plan.

- Look at trans fats - Keep them low. Remember, trans fats and altered fats are bad.

- Look at sodium - Here is a key point. Understand what the label refers to as sodium, is really sodium chloride, which is simply table salt. Sodium and sodium chloride are not the same thing! Sodium is generally a very good thing for the body but refined table salt is not. Since the nutrition facts label is really referring to refined table salt, keep it low. The American Heart Association suggests no more than 3,000 mg of refined table salt per day, for healthy adults,[149] and that is arguably quite high.

- Look at fiber - Currently most labels refer to dietary fiber. Keep it high. A few years ago dietary fiber was broken down into two subcategories designated as soluble fiber and insoluble fiber, but today they are frequently lumped together and referred to as dietary fiber.[150] If the label does distinguish between soluble and insoluble fiber lean towards the product with the most soluble fiber. Insoluble fiber is strictly what mom called roughage. The only thing it does is to help prevent constipation. Soluble fiber does the same thing plus it absorbs and removes toxicity and cholesterol that have entered the intestinal system for disposal.

By now you may have made a couple of additional observations.

- I have not suggested you should be overly concerned with the calories listed on the product label. The reason is if you are following the Rule of Thirds and eating normal food portions, your caloric intake will take care of itself.

- Food labels only appear on some foods. Foods that have been created or altered in a manufacturing plant require government mandated food labels. Foods in their natural state (e.g. fruits, vegetables) don't need food labels.

Summary

The importance of a proper diet in a weight loss program is difficult to overstate. Some researchers argue, "dietary changes contribute more to weight-loss than increased physical activity,"[151] while others believe a combined approach utilizing both diet and exercise, is more effective at reducing weight than an approach focusing on either one alone.[152]

One big consideration is the macronutrient composition of the diet. Realizing experts disagree on exactly what the ideal macronutrient composition should be in a nutritionally sound diet, a good starting point is a diet consisting of 50 percent carbohydrates, 30 percent fat, and 20 percent protein. The important point to remember here is to use this guideline as a beginning point only, and to adjust your macronutrient intake according to your changing needs. For maximum success, weight-loss programs must be customized to the individual.[153] [154] For example, an increasingly demanding exercise regime might require a protein increase at the expense of some fat and/or carbohydrates.

In addition to macronutrient composition, the quality of the macronutrients being consumed must be considered. As mentioned earlier today's western diet has swung in favor of many refined, high glycemic carbohydrates and an abundance of altered fats. Both situations are not only detrimental to a weight loss effort but are damaging to good health. Over the last decade, while the calorie intake of successful weight losers has remained stable, the composition of their food intake has shifted to an increased fat intake and a corresponding decreased carbohydrate intake.[155] What this implies is there is more than one macronutrient intake program that supports weight loss.

Here's what some of the popular diets try to control:

- Weight Watchers Diet - Restrict portion size and count calories,
- Atkins Diet - Minimize carbohydrate intake without fat restriction,
- Zone Diet - Balance macronutrient intake and glycemic load,
- Ornish Diet - Restrict fat intake.[156]

Closely related to diet quality is the quantity of calories consumed in the diet. There is no question in order to lose weight you must consume less calories each day than your daily activities burn up. This is referred to as a negative caloric balance. Similarly, if you want to maintain your current body weight, you're calorie intake must be equal to the number of calories burned.

Attempting to accomplish the proper balance raises two important questions:

- Isn't the only way to achieve a proper caloric balance to suffer an unpleasant deprivation of food? No! To avoid this problem follow the Rule of Thirds. A changed pattern of food intake itself might help a weight loss effort, independent of energy intake.[157]
- How will you know when you have achieved a proper caloric balance? Keep a close eye on your body weight and follow the Belt Hole Rule.

There are additional benefits to eating a balanced diet. "When dietary treatment encourages a balanced diet without drastic restrictions, improvements in self-esteem, alimentary diseases, and lifestyle may occur, leading to weight loss and reduction in health-risking factors."[158]

The most commonly overlooked aspect of *dieting* is the importance of adequate nutrition. Weight loss, weight maintenance, a high energy level, desired bodily function and cell repair and maintenance all depend on providing the body with adequate nutrition. There are a number of ways to ensure nutritional balance in your diet. Here are a few:

- The best way to ensure nutritional balance is to hire the services of a trained and experienced nutritionist,
- Another option is to study nutrition yourself and then integrate what you've learned into your daily practice, and while it is true educating yourself in good nutrition doesn't automatically translate into optimal eating practices, Nowak demonstrated students with better food knowledge ate recommended foods more often than those with less knowledge,[159]
- A simpler way is to utilize the Rule of Thirds,
- Finally one of the most powerful ways to get a lot of high quality nutrition is to get a juicer and juice a variety of fruits and vegetables (heavy on the vegetables). Consuming 12 to 24 ounces of fresh juice per day will boost your nutritional intake significantly, but be careful not to over do it.

As discussed earlier in this chapter good food planning includes a variety of choices. Carefully consider:

- Natural unprocessed foods,
- A wide variety of foods,
- Green foods,
- Organic foods,
- Which fats you include,
- Which carbohydrates you include,
- Sources of protein.

The unfortunate reality is "food choices are more likely to be made on the basis of taste, cost, and convenience than for health-related reasons."[160] If your intention is to optimize your nutritional intake you must give these choices reasonable consideration. They should become the foundation of your daily food planning process.

Concentrate more on the right foods to eat rather than foods to avoid,[161] since psychologically the process of focusing on the outcome you want helps you achieve it. Because solid foods suppress appetite longer than liquids do, it may be beneficial to incorporate more solid food in your food planning strategy.[162]

Once the composition of the food plan has been determined another important factor is portion size. The trend toward increased portion sizes, both at home and in restaurants, began in the 1970's and has continued to spiral out of control since then.[163] The concept of *Super Size Me* has caught on very well and is one of the factors contributing to a national weight control crisis. *Portion distortion,*[164] as it has been dubbed, becomes a double whammy when unrealistically large portions are consumed and those portions are comprised of the wrong foods and beverages. Since "accurate portion control is an important factor in weight loss success... use of packaged entrees is in effective method of achieving this."[165] This is the place to put the Rule of Thirds to work, since it concentrates so heavily on the right foods to eat that portion control becomes less of a problem.

Just as there are things that need to be included in food and nutritional planning, there are a number of things that need to be minimized. The one thing that will help you the most is to read the nutrition facts labels. When preparing your food plan consider minimizing the use of:

- Processed foods,
- Low anything (e.g. low calorie, low fat, low carbohydrate),
- Altered fats, trans fats, and modified fats,
- Pesticide and chemical fertilizer contaminated foods,
- White sugar,
- White rice,

- White flour,
- Table Salt.

So which approach is best? "There is no compelling evidence for any specific dietary mixture other than energy restriction with respect to long-term weight maintenance."[166] To think a single diet will work for everyone is unrealistic,[167] and perhaps downright dangerous. Essentially most dietary plans will have some degree of success if they are coupled with appropriate exercise. As mentioned numerous times before, I find it much easier and more effective to simply follow the Rule of Thirds.

Endnotes

1. W.J. Willey, "*Better than steroids*," (Pocatello, ID: *The Fitness Medicine Clinic, PC*, 2007) 40.
2. "Nutrient," *Dorland's Illustrated Medical Dictionary*, 30th ed: 1295.
3. McKinley Health Center-University of Illinois at Urbana-Champaign, http://www.mckinley. illinois.edu/Handouts/macronutrients.htm
4. R.L. Atkinson, "Role of nutrition planning in the treatment for obesity," *Endocrin Metab Clinics N Am* 25 (1996) 955-964.
5. L. Madsen, B. Liaset, K. Kristiansen, "Macronutrients and obesity: views, news and reviews," *Future Lipidol* 3 (2008) 43-74.
6. Ibid.
7. J. Brand-Miller, T.M.S. Wolever, K. Foster-Powell, S. Colagiuri, "*The New Glucose Revolution: the authoritative guide to the glycemic index*," (NY, NY: Marlowe & Company, 2003) x.
8. L. Madsen, B. Liaset, K. Kristiansen, "Macronutrients and obesity: views, news and reviews," *Future Lipidol* 3 (2008) 43-74.
9. C. Davis, R.D. Levitan, P. Muglia, C. Bewell, J.L. Kennedy, "Decision-making deficits and overeating: a risk model for obesity," *Obes Res* 12 (2004) 929-935.
10. R.J. deSouza, J.F. Swain, L.J. Appel, F.M. Sacks, "Alternatives for macronutrient intake and chronic disease: a comparison of the OmniHeart diets with popular diets and with dietary recommendations," *Am J Clin Nutr* 88 (2008) 1-11.
11. F. Muzio, L. Mondazzi, W.S. Harris, D. Sommariva, A. Branchi, "Effects of moderate variations in the macronutrient content of the diet on cardiovascular disease risk factors in obese patients with the metabolic syndrome," *Am J Clin Nutr* 86 (2007) 946-951.
12. T.C. Crowe, H.A. LaFontaine, C.J. Gibbons, D. Cameron-Smith, B.A. Swinburn, "Energy density of foods and beverages in the Australian food supply: influence of macronutrients in comparison to dietary intake," *Euro J Clin Nutr* 58 (2004) 1485-1491.
13. J. Brand-Miller, T.M.S. Wolever, K. Foster-Powell, S. Colagiuri, "*The New Glucose Revolution: the authoritative guide to the glycemic index*," (NY, NY: Marlowe & Company, 2003) 175.
14. K.J. Melanson, T.J. Angelopoulos, V.T. Nguyen, M. Martini, L. Zukley, J. Lowndes, T.J. Dube, J.J. Fiutem, B.W. Yount, J.M. Rippe, "Consumption of whole-grains during weight loss: effects on dietary quality, dietary fiber, Magnesium, Vitamin B$_6$, and obesity," *J Am Diet Assn* 106 (2006) 1380-1388.
15. T. McFarlane, J. Polivy, R.E. McCabe, "Help, not harm: psychological foundation for a nondieting approach toward health," *J Soc Issues* 55 (1999) 261-276.

16.   *"Lifestyle and weight management consultant manual-American Council on Exercise,"* (San Diego, CA: *American Council on Exercise,* 2005) 254.

17.   E. Putterman, W. Linden, "Appearance versus health: does the reason for dieting affect dieting behavior," *J Behav Med* 27 (2004) 185-204.

18.   Ibid.

19.   *"Personal trainer manual-American Council on Exercise,"* 3rd ed, (San Diego, CA: *American Council on Exercise,* 2003) 117.

20.   M. Liebman, B.A. Cameron, D.K. Carson, D.M. Brown, S.S. Meyer, "Dietary fat reduction behaviors in college students: relationships to dieting status, gender and keys psychosocial variables," *Appetite* 36 (2001) 51-56.

21.   Ibid.

22.   K.A. McAuley, C.M. Hopkins, K.J. Smith, R.T. McLay, S.M. Williams, R.W. Taylor, J.I. Mann, "Comparison of high fat and high-protein diets with a high-carbohydrate diet in insulin-resistant obese women." *Diabetologia* 48 (2005) 8-16.

23.   M.F. Rolland-Cachera, H. Thibault, J.C. Souberbielle, D. Soulie, P. Carbonel, M. Deheeger, D. Roinsol, E. Longueville, F. Andisle, P. Serog, "Massive obesity in adolescents: dietary interventions and behaviours associated with weight regain at 2-y follow-up," *Intl J Obes* 28 (2004) 514-519.

24.   J.S. Volek, M.J. Sharman, D.M. Love, N.G. Avery, A.L. Gomez, T.P. Scheett, W.J. Kraemer, "Body composition and hormonal responses to a carbohydrate-restricted diet," *Metabolism* 51 (2002) 864-870.

25.   S.G. Aldana, *"The culprit & the cure,"* (Mapleton, UT: *Maple Mountain Press,* 2005) 130.

26.   I. Abete, D. Parra, J.A. Martinez, "Energy restricted diets based on a distinct food selection affecting the glycemic index induced different weight loss and oxidative response," *Clin Nutr* 27 (2008) 545-551.

27.   Z. Fajczak, A. Gabor, V. Kovacs, E. Martos, "The effects of a 6-week low glycemic load diet based on low glycemic index foods in overweight/obese children-pilot study," *J Am College Nutr* 27 (2008) 12-21.

28.   J. Brand-Miller, T.M.S. Wolever, K. Foster-Powell, S. Colagiuri, *"The New Glucose Revolution: the authoritative guide to the glycemic index,"* (NY, NY: Marlowe & Company, 2003) 183.

29.   J.L. Slavin, "Dietary fiber and body weight," *Nutrition* 21 (2005) 411-418.

30.   E.M.H. Mathus-Vliegen for the Balance Study Group, "Long-term maintenance of weight loss with sibutramine in a GP setting following a specialist guided very-low-calorie diet: a double-blind, placebo-controlled, parallel group study," *Euro J Clin Nutr* 59 (2005) S31-S39.

31.   K.R. Ryttig, H. Flaten, S. Rossner, Long-term effects of a very low calorie diet (Nutrilett) in obesity treatment: a prospective randomized, comparison between the VLCD and a hypocaloric diet + behavior modification and their combination," *Intl J Obes* 21 (1997) 574-579.

32.   G.L. Jensen, M-A Roy, A.E. Buchanan, M.B. Berg, "Weight loss intervention for obese older women: improvements in performance and function," *Obes Res* 12 (2004) 1814-1820.

33.   M.S. Sothern, J.N. Udall, Jr., R.M. Suskind, A. Vargas, U. Blecker, "Weight loss and growth velocity in obese children after very low-calorie diet, exercise, and behavior modification," *Acta Paediatr* 89 (2000) 1036-1043.

34.   H. Lantz, M. Peltonen, L. Agren, J.S. Torgerson, "A dietary and behavioural programme for the treatment of obesity: a 4-year clinical trial and a long-term posttreatment follow-up," *J Int Med* 254 (2003) 272-279.

35.   G.M. Turner-McGrievy, N.D. Barnard, A.R. Scialli, "A two-year randomized weight loss trial comparing a vegan diet to a more moderate low-fat diet," *Obesity* 15 (2007) 2276-2281.

36. Ibid.

37. D.D. Hensrud, "Nutrition screening and assessment," *Med Clins N Am* 83 (1999) 1525-1546.

38. Ibid.

39. S. Holmes, "Nutrition: a necessary adjunct to hospital care," *J Royal Soc Prom Health* 119 (1999) 175-179.

40. T.M. Stewart, D.A. Williamson, M.A. White, "Rigid versus flexible dieting: association with eating disorder symptoms in nonobese women," *Appetite* 38 (2002) 39-44.

41. M.F. Rolland-Cachera, H. Thibault, J.C. Souberbielle, D. Soulie, P. Carbonel, M. Deheeger, D. Roinsol, E. Longueville, F. Andisle, P. Serog, "Massive obesity in adolescents: dietary interventions and behaviours associated with weight regain at 2-y follow-up," *Intl J Obes* 28 (2004) 514-519.

42. K. Presnelll, E. Stice, J. Tristan, "Experimental investigation of the effects of naturalistic dieting on bulimic symptoms: moderating effects of depressive symptoms," *Appetite* 50 (2008) 91-101.

43. *"Lifestyle and weight management consultant manual-American Council on Exercise,"* (San Diego, CA: *American Council on Exercise*, 2005) 196.

44. E.J. Applegate, *"The Anatomy & Physiology Learning System,"* 2nd ed, (Philadelphia, PA: Saunders, 2000) 361.

45. *"Personal trainer manual-American Council on Exercise,"* 3rd ed, (San Diego, CA: *American Council on Exercise*, 2003) 105.

46. H.C. Reinbach, A. Smeets, T. Martinussen, P. Moller, M.S. Westerterp-Plantenga, "Effects of capsaicin, green tea and CH-19 sweet pepper on appetite and energy intake in humans in negative and positive energy balance," *Clin Nutr* 28 (2009) 260-265.

47. E. Putterman, W. Linden, "Appearance versus health: does the reason for dieting affect dieting behavior," *J Behav Med* 27 (2004) 185-204.

48. Ibid.

49. T. Mann, A.J. Tomiyama, E. Westling, A.M. Lew, B. Samuels, J. Chatman, "Medicare's search for effective obesity treatments: diets are not the answer," *Am Psych* 68 (2007) 220-233.

50. S.F.L. Kirk, A.J. Hill, "Exploring the food beliefs and eating behavior of successful and unsuccessful dieters," *J Hum Nutr & Diet* 10 (1997) 331-341.

51. S. Crow, M.E. Eisenberg, M. Stone, D. Neumark-Sztainer, "Psychosocial and behavioral correlates of dieting among overweight and non-overweight adolescents," *J Adol Health* 38 (2006) 569-574.

52. M. LeBarzic, "Le syndrome de restriction congnitive: de la norme au desordre du comportement alimentaire," *Dia Metab* 27 (2001) 512-516.

53. A. Jansen, E. Louwerse, N. Leemans, E. Schouten, "Self-esteem as a better predictor of restrained eaters' food intake than attributional style and disinhibition tendency," *Euro J Person* 12 (1998) 43-56.

54. I.U. Eneli, P.A. Crum, T.L. Tylka, "The trust model: a different feeding paradigm for managing childhood obesity," *Obes* 16 (2008) 2197-2204.

55. S.F.L. Kirk, A.J. Hill, "Exploring the food beliefs and eating behavior of successful and unsuccessful dieters," *J Hum Nutr & Diet* 10 (1997) 331-341.

56. I.U. Eneli, P.A. Crum, T.L. Tylka, "The trust model: a different feeding paradigm for managing childhood obesity," *Obes* 16 (2008) 2197-2204.

57. J.J. Harrow, R.I. Cordoves, R.B. Hulette, "Attitudes toward intentional weight loss and dietary behavior among US Armyreserve soldiers during annual training," *Mil Med* 171 (2006) 678-683.

58. K. Presnell, E. Stice, J. Tristan, "Experimental investigation of the effects of naturalistic dieting on bulimics symptoms: moderating effects of depressive symptoms," *Appetite* 50 (2008) 91-101.

59. P. Williams, "Breakfast and the diets of Australian adults: an analysis of data from the 1995 national nutrition survey," *Intl J Food Sci Nutr* 56 (2005) 65-79.

60. A.G. Dulloo, J. Jacquet, "Adaptive reduction in basal metabolic rate in response to food deprivation in humans: a role for feedback signals from fat stores," *Am J Clin Nutr* 68 (1998) 599-606.

61. Ibid.

62. J. Rankins, M.S. Williams, D.J. Montgomery, D.B. Wilton, "Demystifying weight loss diets," *Ecol Food Nutr* 45 (2006) 379-430.

63. *"Lifestyle and weight management consultant manual-American Council on Exercise,"* (San Diego, CA: *American Council on Exercise*, 2005) 101.

64. D. Neumark-Sztainer, M. Wall, J. Guo, M. Story, J. Haines, M. Eisenberg, "Obesity, disordered eating, and eating disorders in a longitudinal study of adolescents: how do dieters fare 5 years later?" *J Am Diet Assn* 106 (2006) 559-568.

65. F. Muzio, D. Sommariva, L. Mondazzi, A. Branch, "Long-term effects of low-calorie diet on the metabolic syndrome in obese nondiabetic patients," *Diabetes Care* 28 (2005) 1485-1586.

66. J.L. Gilbreath, C. Biesemeier, "Medical nutrition therapy: a powerful tool in disease management," *Am J Managed Care* 5 (1999) 81-86.

67. M.D. Corbalan, E.M. Morales, M. Canteras, A. Espallardo, T. Hernandez, M. Garaulet, "Effectiveness of cognitive-behavioral therapy based on the Mediterranean diet for the treatment of obesity," *Nutrition* 25 (2009) 861-869.

68. Ibid.

69. R.L. Atkinson, "Role of nutrition planning in the treatment for obesity," *Endocrin Metab Clinics N Am* 25 (1996) 955-964.

70. M.R. Naghii, "The importance of body weight and weight management for military personnel," *Mil Med* 171 (2006) 550-555.

71. M.G. Enig, *"Know Your Fats,"* (Silver Spring, MD: Bethesda Press 2000) 188.

72. R. Ballentine, *"Diet & Nutrition,"* (Honesdale, PA: *The Himalayan Institute Press* 1978) 283.

73. M. Huber, L.P.L. van de Vijver, "State-of-the-art research on organic nutrition and health promotion," *Euro J Integrative Med* 8 (2008) S63.

74. U. Erasmus, *"Fats that Heal Fats that Kill,"* (Burnaby, BC, Canada: *Alive Books*, 1986) 223, 226.

75. K.M. Angood, J.D. Wood, G.R. Nute, F.M. Whittington, S.I. Hughes, P.R. Sheard, "A comparison of organic and conventionally-produced lamb purchased from three major UK supermarkets: price, eating quality and fatty acid composition," *Meat Sci* 78 (2008) 176-184.

76. U. Ravnskov, *"The Cholesterol Myths,"* (Washington, DC: *New Trends Publishing, Inc.* 2000) 15-115.

77. U. Erasmus, *"Fats that Heal Fats that Kill,"* (Burnaby, BC, Canada: *Alive Books*, 1986) 21, 43.

78. Ibid., 316.

79. Ibid., 433.

80. U. Ravnskov, *"The Cholesterol Myths,"* (Washington, DC: *New Trends Publishing, Inc.*, 2000) 32.

81. U. Erasmus, *"Fats that Heal Fats that Kill,"* (Burnaby, BC, Canada: *Alive Books*, 1986) 224.

82. J. Brand-Miller, T.M.S. Wolever, K. Foster-Powell, S. Colagiuri, *"The New Glucose Revolution: the authoritative guide to the glycemic index,"* (NY, NY: Marlowe & Company, 2003) 22.

83. Ibid., 33.

84. Ibid., 174.

85. D.M. Winham, C.B. Collins, A.M. Hutchins, "Dietary intakes, attitudes toward carbohydrates of postmenopausal women following low carbohydrate diets," *Can J Diet Prac Res* 70 (2009) 44-47.

86. J.B. Miller, "The glycemic index: where are we now and where are we going?" *Food Aus* 57 (2005) 200-204.

87. A.S. Hagler, G.J. Norman, M.F. Zabinski, J.F. Sallis, K.J. Calfas, K. Patrick, "Psychosocial correlates of dietary intake among overweight and obese men," *Am J Health Behav* 31 (2007) 3-12.

88. A. Booth, C. Nowson, A. Worsley, C. Margerison, M. Jorna, "Dietary approaches for weight loss with increased intakes of fruit, vegetables and dairy products," *Nutr & Diet* 65 (2008) 115-120.

89. R.E. Roberts, W.J. Strawbridge, S. Deleger, G.A. Kaplan, "Are the fat more jolly?" *Ann Behav Med* 24 (2002) 169-180.

90. P.J. Arciero, C.L. Gentile, R. Pressman, M. Everett, M.J. Ormsbee, J. Martin, J. Santamore, L. Gorman, P.C. Fehling, M.D. Vukovich, B.C. Nindl, "Moderate protein intake improves total and regional body composition and insulin sensitivity in overweight adults," *Metab Clin Exp* 57 (2008) 757-765.

91. D.K. Houston, B.J. Nicklas, J. Ding, T.B. Harris, F.A. Tylavsky, A.B. Neuman, J.S. Lee, N.R. Sahyoun, M. Visser, S.B. Kritchevsky, "Dietary protein intake is associated with lean mass change in older, community-dwelling adults: the health, aging, and body composition (Health ABC) study," *Am J Clin Nutr* 87 (2008) 150-155.

92. D.K. Layman, "Dietary guidelines should reflect new understandings about adult protein needs," *Nutr Metab* 6 (2009) 1-6.

93. Ibid.

94. P. Deibert, D. Konig, A. Schmidt-Trucksaess, K.S. Zaenker, I. Frey, U. Landmann, A. Berg, "Weight loss without losing muscle mass in pre-obese and obese subjects induced by a high-soy-protein diet," *Intl J Obes* 28 (2004) 1349-1352.

95. U. Erasmus, *"Fats that Heal Fats that Kill,"* (Burnaby, BC, Canada: *Alive Books*, 1986) 76.

96. R. Ballentine, *"Diet & Nutrition,"* (Honesdale, PA: *The Himalayan Institute Press*, 1978) 293.

97. J.Y. Kim, J.H. Kim, D.H. Lee, S.H. Kim, S.S. Lee, "Meal replacement with mixed rice is more effective than white rice in weight control, while improving antioxidant enzyme activity in obese women," *Nutr Res* 28 (2008) 66-71.

98. M.G. Enig, *"Know Your Fats,"* (Silver Spring, MD: Bethesda Press, 2000) 85.

99. U. Erasmus, *"Fats that Heal Fats that Kill,"* (Burnaby, BC, Canada: *Alive Books,* 1986) 113.

100. Ibid., 129.

101. *"The most contaminated foods / the least contaminated foods,"* (Economic Research Service / USDA – Agricultural Outlook 1997) http://www.avianweb.com/organicfoods.html

102. *"The 12 most contaminated and the 12 least contaminated foods, "* (The Environmental Working Group) http://www.enviroalternatives.com/foodcontaminated.html

103. *"Twelve riskiest foods,"* (Living and raw foods) http://www.living-foods.com/articles/twelvelist.html

104. *"3 reasons to care about excess sugar consumption,"* (Kitchen Table Medicine) http://www.kitchentablemedicine.com/3-reasons-to-care-about-excess-sugar-consumption/

105. *"3 reasons to care about excess sugar consumption,"* (Kitchen Table Medicine) http://www.kitchentablemedicine.com/3-reasons-to-care-about-excess-sugar-consumption/

106. N. Perricone, *"The Perricone Prescription,"* (New York, NY: *HarperCollins Publishers, Inc.,* 2002) 34.

107. *"3 reasons to care about excess sugar consumption,"* (Kitchen Table Medicine) http://www. kitchentablemedicine.com/3-reasons-to-care-about-excess-sugar-consumption/

108. R. Ballentine, *"Diet & Nutrition,"* (Honesdale, PA: *The Himalayan Institute Press,* 1978) 59.

109. B. Jensen, "Dr. Jensen's Guide to Body Chemistry & Nutrition," (Lincolnwood, IL: *Keats Publishing,* 2000) 33.

110. *"US sugar consumption continues to grow,"* (Economic Research Service / USDA - Agricultural Outlook 1997) http://www.ers.usda.gov/publications/agoutlook/mar1997/ao238g.pdf

111. R. Ballentine, *"Diet & Nutrition,"* (Honesdale, PA: *The Himalayan Institute Press,* 1978) 70.

112. W. Price, *"Nutrition and Physical Degeneration,"* (La Mesa, CA: *Price-Pottenger Nutrition Foundation, Inc.,* 1989) 493.

113. R. Ballentine, *"Diet & Nutrition,"* (Honesdale, PA: *The Himalayan Institute Press,* 1978) 72.

114. Ibid., 89.

115. A.C. Bell, B.A. Swinburn, H. Amosa, R.K. Scragg, "A nutrition and exercise intervention program for controlling weight in Samoan communities in New Zealand, "Intl *J Obes* 25 (2001) 920-927.

116. D.P. Keenan, R. AbuSabha, M. Sigman-Grant, C. Achterberg, J. Ruffing, "Factors perceived to influence dietary fat reduction behaviors," *J Nutr Ed* 31 (1999) 134-144.

117. D. Frawley, "Ayurvedic Healing," 2nd ed (Twin Lakes, WI: Lotus Press, 2000) 6.

118. Ibid., 31-34.

119. Ibid., 83-98.

120. H.M. Blanck, M.K. Serdula, C. Gillespie, D.A. Galuska, P.A. Sharpe, J.M. Conway, L.K. Khan, B.E. Ainsworth, "Use of nonprescription dietary supplements for weight loss is common among Americans," *J Am Diet Assoc* 107 (2007) 441-447.

121. C.I. Celio, K.H. Luce, S.W. Bryson, A.J. Winzelberg, D. Cunning, R. Rockwell, A.A. Celio-Doyle, D.E. Wilfley, C.B. Taylor, "Use of diet pills and other dieting aids in a college population with high weight and shape concerns," *Intl J Eat Disord* 39 (2006) 492-497.

122. *"Lifestyle and weight management consultant manual-American Council on Exercise,"* (San Diego, CA: *American Council on Exercise,* 2005) 207.

123. J.T. Dwyer, D.B. Allison, P.M. Coates, "Dietary supplements in weight reduction," *J Am Diet Assoc* 105 (2005) S80-S86.

124. M.C. Nachtigal, R.E. Patterson, K.L. Stratton, L.A. Adams, A.L. Shattuck, E. White, "Dietary supplements and weight control in the middle-age population," *J Alter Comp Med* 11 (2005) 909-915.

125. C.S. Johnston, C. Corte, P.D. Swan, "Marginal vitamin C status is associated with reduced fat oxidation during submaximal exercise in young adults," *Nutr Metab* 3 (2006) 1-5.

126. B.W. Bailey, D.K. Sullivan, E.P. Kirk, S. Hall, J.E. Donnelly, "The influence of calcium consumption on weight and fat following 9 months of exercise in men and women," *J Am Coll Nutr* 26 (2007) 350-355.

127. D.E. Woodgate, J.A. Conquer, "Effects of a stimulant-free dietary supplement on body weight and fat loss in obese adults: a six-week exploratory study," *Current Ther Res* 64 (2003) 248-262.

128. *"Health benefits of green foods,"* (Share Guide The Holistic Health Magazine and Resource Directory) http://www.shareguide.com/greenfoods.html

129. *"Benefits of green foods,"* (Health Searches) http://www.healthsearches.org/Categories_of_Q&A/ Integrative_&_Alternative_Medicine/1333_2.php

130. J.J. Gormley, *"Green foods green gold: unearthing the nutritional benefits of green foods,"* - (Frontiers of Science) - brief article," http://www.findarticles.com/p/articles/mi_m0FKA/is_2_64/ai_83033015/

131. C.B. Scott, R. Devore, "Diet induced thermogenesis: variations among three isocaloric meal-replacement shakes," *Nutrition* 21 (2005) 874-877.

132. "Thermogenesis," *Dorland's Illustrated Medical Dictionary*, 30th edition: 1900.

133. M. Westererp-Plantenga, K. Diepvens, A.M.C.P. Joosen, S. Berube-Parent, A. Tremblay, "Metabolic effects of spices, teas, and caffeine," *Physio & Behav* 89 (2006) 85-91.

134. T. Wadden, "Lifestyle modification for the management of obesity," *Gastroenterology* 132 (2007) 2226-2238.

135. S. Huerta, Z. Li, H.C. Li, M.S. Hu, C.A. Yu, D. Heber, "Feasibility of a partial meal replacement plan for weight loss in low income patients," *Intl J Obes* 28 (2004) 1575-1579.

136. J.W. Anderson, J. Fuller, K. Patterson, R. Blair, A. Tabor, "Soy compared to casein meal replacement shakes with energy-restricted diets for obese women: randomized controlled trial," *Metab Clin Exp* 56 (2007) 280-288.

137. C.M. Lockwood, J.R. Moon, S.E. Tobkin, A.A. Walter, A.E. Smith, V.J. Dalbo, J.T. Cramer, J.R. Stout, "Minimal nutrition intervention with high-protein/low-carbohydrate and low-fat, nutrient-dense foods supplement improves body composition and exercise benefits in overweight adults: a randomized controlled trial," *Nutr Metab* 5 (2008) 1-15.

138. A.J. Stull, J.W. Apolzan, A.E. Thalacker-Mercer, H.B. Iglay, W.W. Campbell, "Liquid and solid meal replacement products differentially affect postprandial appetite and food intake in older adults," *J Am Diet Assoc* 108 (2008) 1226-1230.

139. R.A. Annunziato, C.A. Timko, C.E. Crerand, E.R. Didie, D.L. Bellace, S. Phelan, I. Kerzhnerman, M.R. Lowe, "A randomized trial examining differential meal replacement adherence in a weight loss maintenance program after one-year follow-up," *Eat Behav* 10 (2009) 176-183.

140. T. Wadden, "Lifestyle modification for the management of obesity," *Gastroenterology* 132 (2007) 2226-2238.

141. P. Auvichayapat, M. Propochanung, O. Tunkamnerdthai, B. Sripanidkulchai, N. Auvichayapat, B. Thinkhamrop, S. Kunhasura, S. Wongpratoom, S. Sinawat, P. Hongprapas, "Effectiveness of green tea on weight reduction in obese Thais: a randomized controlled trial," *Physio & Behav* 93 (2008) 486-491.

142. A.G. Dulloo, C. Duret, D. Rohrer, L. Girardier, N. Mensi, M. Fathi, P. Chantre, J. Vandermander, "Efficacy of a green tea extract rich in catechin polyphenols and caffeine in increasing 24-h energy expenditure and fat oxidation in humans," *Am J Clin Nutri* 70 (1999) 1040-1045.

143. P. Chantre, D. Lairon, "Recent findings of green tea extract AR25 (Exolise) and its activity for the treatment of obesity," *Phytomed* 9 (2002) 3-8.

144. P. Auvichayapat, M. Propochanung, O. Tunkamnerdthai, B. Sripanidkulchai, N. Auvichayapat, B. Thinkhamrop, S. Kunhasura, S. Wongpratoom, S. Sinawat, P. Hongprapas, "Effectiveness of green tea on weight reduction in obese Thais: a randomized controlled trial," *Physio & Behav* 93 (2008) 486-491.

145. M. Westerterp-Plantenga, K. Diepvens, A.M.C.P. Joosen, S. Berube-Parent, A. Tremblay, "Metabolic effects of spices, teas, and caffeine," *Physio & Behav* 89 (2006) 85-91.

146. F.R. van Heerden, "Hoodia Gordonii: a natural appetite suppressant," *J Ethnopharmacology* 119 (2008) 434-437.

147. Ibid.

148. M. Westerterp-Plantenga, K. Diepvens, A.M.C.P. Joosen, S. Berube-Parent, A. Tremblay, "Metabolic effects of spices, teas, and caffeine," *Physio & Behav* 89 (2006) 85-91.

149. *"Lifestyle and weight management consultant manual-American Council on Exercise,"* (San Diego, CA: *American Council on Exercise*, 2005) 199.

150. J.L. Slavin, "Dietary fiber and body weight," *Nutrition* 21 (2005) 411-418.

151. C.L. Dunn, P.J. Hannan, R.W. Jeffery, N.E. Sherwood, N.P. Pronk, R. Boyle, "The comparative and cumulative effects of a dietary restriction and exercise on weight loss," *Intl J Obes* 30 (2006) 112-121.

152. Ibid.

153. L. Kaul, J.J. Nidiry, "Management of obesity in low-income African Americans," *J Nat Med Assoc* 91 (1999) 139-143.

154. A.M. Herriot, D.E. Thomas, K.H. Hart, J. Warren, J. Truby, "A qualitative investigation of individuals' experiences and expectations before and after completing a trial of commercial weight loss programs." *J Hum Nutr Diet* 21 (2008) 72-80.

155. S. Phelan, H.R. Wyatt, J.O. Hill, R.R. Wing, "Are the eating and exercise habits of successful weight losers changing?" *Obesity* 14 (2006) 710-716.

156. M.L. Dansinger, J.A. Gleason, J.L. Griffith, H.S. Selker, E.J. Schaefer, "Comparison of the Atkins, Ornish, Weight Watchers, and Zone Diets for weight loss and heart disease risk reduction," *JAMA* 293 (2005) 43-53.

157. M. Nakade, J.S. Lee, K. Kawakubo, Y. Amano, K. Mori, A. Akabayashi, "Correlation between food intake change patterns and body weight loss in middle-aged women in Japan," *Obes Res Clin Prac* 1 (2007) 79-89.

158. C.B. Nonino-Borges, R.M. Borges, M. Bavaresco, V.M.M. Suen, A.C. Moreira, J.S. Marchini, "Influence of meal time on salivary circadian cortisol rhythms and weight loss in obese women," *Nurtition* 23 (2007) 385-391.

159. M. Nowak, "The weight-conscious adolescent: body image, food intake, and weight related behavior," *J Adol Health* 23 (1998) 389-398.

160. C. Davis, R.D. Levitan, P. Muglia, C. Bewell, J.L. Kennedy, "Decision-making deficits and over eating: a risk model for obesity," *Obes Res* 12 (2004) 929-935.

161. Ibid.

162. H.J. Leidy, J.W. Apolzan, R.D. Mattes, W.W. Campbell, "Food form and portion size affect postprandial appetite sensations and hormonal responses in healthy, nonobese, older adults," *Obesity* 10 (2009) 1-7.

163. C.C. Tangney, K.A. Gustashaw, T.M. Stefan, C. Sullivan, J. Ventrelle, C.A. Filipowski, A.D. Heffernan, J. Hankins, "A review: which dietary plan is best for your patience seeking weight loss and sustained weight management?" *Dis Mon* 51 (2005) 284-316.

164. H.M. Seagle, G.W. Strain, A. Makris, R.S. Reeves, "Position of the American Dietetic Association: weight management," *J Am Diet Assoc* 109 (2009) 330-346.

165. S.M. Hannum, L. Carson, E.M. Evans, K.A. Canene, E.L. Petr, L. Bui, J.W. Erdman, Jr., "Use of portion-controlled entrées enhances weight loss in women," *Obes Res* 12 (2004) 538-546.

166. C.C. Tangney, K.A. Gustashaw, T.M. Stefan, C. Sullivan, J. Ventrelle, C.A. Filipowski, A.D. Heffernan, J. Hankins, "A review: which dietary plan is best for your patience seeking weight loss and sustained weight management?" *Dis Mon* 51 (2005) 284-316.

167. J.S. Volek, J.L. VanHeest, C.E. Forsythe, "Diet and exercise for weight loss," *Sport Med* 35 (2005) 1-9.

4   The Power of Exercise

Politics and religion are perhaps the only subjects engendering more mixed feelings and possibly more controversy than exercise. Exercise, with all its inherent benefits is often misunderstood and frequently maligned, for three common reasons:

- Existing research and exercise literature is often conflicting and/or unclear,
- People lack the knowledge needed to:
    - Understand the benefits they can derive from exercise,
    - Determine what their specific exercise needs are,
    - Figure out how to develop an exercise program that will benefit them,
- There are many exercise gurus who oversell the benefits of exercise, either for their own personal financial gain or because they simply don't know any better.

Before we go any further I think it is important to make, what I consider to be, a vital distinction. This distinction is not only important for you to understand my thinking but will prove critical to the success of your weight loss program. Much of the research cited in this chapter uses the terminology "physical activity," and frequently researchers use the words physical activity and exercise interchangeably. I believe that is an unfortunate mistake and here's why. *Physical activity* and *exercise* are two different things.

Physical Activity - The US Department of Agriculture (USDA) defines physical activity as "movement of the body that uses energy."[1] The World Health Organization goes a little further by defining it as "any bodily movement produced by skeletal muscles that requires energy expenditure."[2] By applying these definitions of physical activity to our daily lives you can see they include everything from running a marathon to stumbling to the refrigerator to get another beer, and if both of these activities meet the definition and we are given a choice you know which one it will be. As you will see later most researchers believe 30 minutes of moderate physical activity a day, and they define moderate physical activity to include such things as gardening, housecleaning, taking care of the kids, walking, etc., done most days of the week, will work wonders for your weight loss effort and overall health. As you can probably guess that won't cut it in the exercise definition. I believe these are life events we do as part of daily living, and for reasons to be explained below, have little if anything to do with exercise. Here is one of the reasons I make that claim. When researchers attempted to reduce the blood fat content, in healthy men eating a high-saturated fat diet, using high-volume, low-intensity physical activity they found no improvement, because the intensity was too low.[3]

I have heard it claimed one way to know if you're getting adequate, healthy physical activity is if you are performing a *fun, sweaty activity*. That particular idea would not include swimming, (no sweat there) but would include one of my favorite activities, which is a nap in the sun after feasting at the cruise ship lunch buffet (lots of fun and sweat there). It goes without saying this yardstick is not terribly useful.

Exercise - To rise to the level of an exercise a physical activity needs to clear a number of hurdles. It:

- Must work your body harder than your normal level of daily activity,
- Must contribute significantly to overall physical fitness,
- Must be controllable by monitoring such parameters as VO_{2max}. Researchers frequently use the words maximum heart rate and VO_{2max} interchangeably.
- Results in a health related benefit (e.g. reduced body weight, lower blood pressure, lower risk of metabolic syndrome).

Let's be clear about one thing! I am not saying the energy expended during normal physical activity doesn't count toward the energy deficit required to lose weight and live a healthy life, rather what I am saying is it may only have a minimal impact on weight loss and improved health when compared to a planned and structured exercise routine. Arguably any exercise is better than none and more is probably better.[4] One of the reasons more is better is it leads to a better quality of weight loss, because intense exercise results in a greater loss of body fat while conserving more lean muscle mass.[5] If Aldana, is correct, fitness is important because "sedentary individuals are eight times more likely to die from cardiovascular disease and five times more likely to die from cancer than people who have high levels of fitness."[6] It should be obvious a combination of the two is better than either one alone. In other words, "energy expenditure, not only through voluntary exercise but also through spontaneous, daily, physical activities can have a positive effect on reducing body weight."[7]

Given these distinctions the first question becomes, what does the research say about how exercise will help you lose weight?

Why Exercise is Important

There is a lot of research supporting the idea, "physical activity is one of the most important contributors to long-term weight loss,"[8] and "is one of the most important components of the overall approach to treating obesity."[9] However, one problem is men and women understand a lack of exercise is a very important reason for their weight gain, but still show little or no interest in increasing their level of exercise.[10] We already know from the previous chapter "physical activity in daily life in conjunction with a controlled diet can have a positive effect on reducing body weight,"[11] therefore, imagine the additional benefit of adding a true exercise regime.

Fat Oxidation

Fat oxidation, or beta-oxidation when it occurs inside the cell's mitochondria, (i.e. the cell's energy production engines) is the process of breaking down fatty acids to produce energy.[12] Furthermore, "weight loss and physical activity in previously sedentary obese adults is associated with enlargement of mitochondria and an increase in the mitochondrial content in skeletal muscle."[13] During the fat oxidation process, large fat molecules are taken from storage and broken down into smaller molecules that can be used for energy production. "Exercise increases the demand for energy and...this means an increase in fat... oxidation both during and post-exercise."[14] This same increased oxidation also helps decrease fat balance (fat intake - fat burned = fat stored).[15]

Obese individuals typically exhibit an impaired capacity for fat oxidation, which improves significantly with relatively acute exercise training.[16] Obese women who participate in endurance exercise training, experience improvements in fatty acid oxidative capacity.[17] In fact, exercise increases fatty acid oxidation,[18] with the key exercise determinant being intensity and duration.[19] "Maximal rates of fat oxidation occur at an exercise intensity of 65% of VO_{2max}."[20] So, calculate VO_{2max} using this formula (220 - your age x 65 percent = 65 percent of VO_{2max}) and monitor your heart rate to ensure that you are in the recommended range. A leisurely stroll in the park will not get the desired rate.

It should also be noted considerable individual variation exists in both the maximum rate of fat oxidation and the intensity at which it occurs.[21] Understanding the individual nature of a recommended target, like the suggested 65 percent of VO_{2max}, is important because through experimentation you may find you get better success with a slightly different VO_{2max} rate. Never hesitate to use the VO_{2max} rate that gives you the best results, as long as you don't go too high. For the average person too high a VO_{2max} would probably be above 80 percent.

Reduced Health Risk Factors

The US Centers for Disease Control and Prevention ranks Heart Disease as the number one cause of death in the US at 26 percent, with Cancer close behind at 21 percent, and Diabetes and

Alzheimer's considerably farther down the list at 3 percent.[22] Is it reasonable to believe while we are exercising to lose weight the same exercises might help reduce the health risk factors leading to these dreaded diseases? The answer is an emphatic yes.

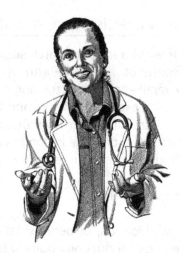

Exercise "not only contributes to an increased energy expenditure and fat loss but also protects against a loss of lean muscle mass, improves cardiorespiratory fitness, reduces obesity-related cardiometabolic health risks, and evokes sensations of well-being."[23] In fact, epidemiological data has shown exercise reduces the incidence of at least 20 unhealthy conditions, (including cardiovascular disease, hypertension, type 2 diabetes, obesity, osteoporosis, sarcopenia, cognitive disorders and some forms of cancer), most of which are considered risk factors for chronic disease.[24] A study of 508 postmenopausal women showed "the extent of weight loss was directly related to the reduction of risk factors."[25] It seems like the more excess weight you lose the lower your risk factors go. Another study confirmed that this inverse dose response relationship definitely existed between cardiorespiratory fitness and metabolic syndrome.[26] When all is said and done exercise research makes a very compelling case for the fact that irrespective of weight loss, the resulting reduction in metabolic syndrome risk factors is a major benefit.[27]

There is an important point to be made here. In the details of some research studies it becomes apparent exercise participants gained a health benefit while not losing weight. How is it possible health benefits could be achieved without weight loss? The answer lies in a shifting of body composition. If you are exercising hard enough, using weight resistant exercises and you are only moderately overweight (e.g. 10 to 20 pounds), your exercise program could be replacing fat loss with corresponding gains in lean muscle mass. As a result your health markers would be improving and you're calorie-burning capability improving, even though total body weight remains constant. This works fine as long as you are only moderately overweight. If on the other hand you were 100 pounds overweight you cannot replace 100 pounds of fat loss with 100 pounds of lean muscle mass gain. In this case you should be gaining some lean muscle mass, losing lots of body fat and experiencing an overall weight loss and health improvement.

Exercise Can be a Predictor

Exercise can be a predictor of certain weight related outcomes. For example:

- Exercise levels can be a predictor of total body and central abdominal fat mass.[28]

- Exercise levels can be a predictor of general level of health and potential longevity.[29]

- A satisfactory exercise outcome, in children and adolescents, can be predicted if they have previously participated in an exercise group.[30]

- Independent of body mass index (BMI), a higher level of fitness predicts a lower risk of cardiovascular disease and mortality. In addition here's an impressive list of affected health markers: (1) lower blood pressure, (2) better blood fat profiles, (3) reduced belly fat, (4) less systemic inflammation, (5) better cardiac function, (6) healthier blood vessels, and (7) higher heart rate variability).[31]

- Motivation to improve body shape is a good predictor of weight loss behavior among women exercising in health and fitness clubs.[32]

Finally, here's an additional side benefit of exercise, not related to weight loss. It has been shown men who maintain physical fitness are less likely to require doctor visits and hospital stays when compared to unfit men.[33]

Psychological Benefits

The purpose of this section is not to compete with the next chapter, which deals with the broad topic of the psychological aspects of weight loss, but rather to deal with the narrower topic of the psychological benefits of exercise. In general exercising can:

- Decrease hypertension,[34]
- Have an indirect psychological effect on weight loss as a result of improvement in self appraisal and mood factors,[35]
- Improve emotional well-being,[36]

Specifically in men research has shown making exercise an integral part of one's weight loss program may psychologically impact the exerciser in three of ways. Exercise:

- Tends to decrease hunger,
- Can promote a psychological boost encouraging increased calorie output during exercise,
- May strengthen the normal restraint coping mechanism.[37]

Much of the improved mood and increased self-esteem emanates from the so-called *Runner's High*, which was first seen in distance runners and later recognized to a lesser extent in a variety of other exercise participants.[38] The runner's high is a mild state of euphoria often experienced by strenuous exercisers, which is attributed to an increased pituitary gland and hypothalamus production of endorphins. While endorphins are brain chemicals that have a number of functions, "one function appears to be mediation of pain perception."[39] The good news for those who have never experienced the relaxation, piece of mind and elevated mood associated with a strenuous exercise session, it is there for your taking. There is no secret if you put in the proper effort you too can experience the benefit and enjoyment of an endorphin rush.

Disease Prevention and Treatment

As discussed earlier, being overweight is accompanied by a number of health risk factors. As we progress you will discover the majority of those health risk factors can be mitigated through weight loss. So the real question is, while we are exercising are there additional benefits to be gained, and if so, what are they? During our investigation of the topics that follow, the weight loss portion of the discussion cannot be easily separated from the health improvement component. For example, heart disease prevention and treatment benefits equally from both weight loss and exercise, while the prevention and treatment of cancer appears to benefit significantly more from weight loss than it does directly from exercise. During the following discussions in this chapter no further attempt will be made to separate the two. While you are exercising to lose weight you will also be minimizing, reversing and hopefully eliminating a number of health risk factors.

Heart Disease

With heart disease the number one cause of death in the US, let's take a closer look at what exercise can do to reduce that possibility. Generally, "excess body fat is associated with increased cardiovascular disease (CVD) risk."[40] Unfortunately even the kids are involved. The endothelial cells are the layer of cells that line the cavities of the heart and blood vessels,[41] which promote unrestricted blood flow because they are smoother than most other cells of the body. Study data concluded six months of exercise restored endothelial function in obese children, which was associated with an improved cardiovascular risk profile.[42] Another study of sedentary patients demonstrated, "exercise not only has favorable effects on blood pressure but also prevents the development of left ventricular hypertrophy."[43] "Left ventricular hypertrophy is enlargement (hypertrophy) of the muscle tissue that makes up the wall of your heart's main pumping chamber (left ventricle),"[44] which often develops as a result of high blood pressure.[45]

If you have already had a heart attack or have been diagnosed with some form of coronary heart disease you may have entered a cardiac rehabilitation program. "Cardiac rehabilitation improves exercise capacity and induces significant weight loss in obese patients."[46] "High-calorie expenditure exercise is substantially more effective than standard cardiac rehabilitation exercise at inducing weight loss and risk factor change in overweight patients with coronary heart disease."[47] Wow, just think about that! If you are participating in a cardiac rehab program you get both heart health and weight loss benefits.

While inflammation is discussed later in greater detail it is related to heart health. "Studies suggest that inflammation is important in arteriosclerosis... the process in which fatty deposits build up in the inner lining of arteries."[48] C-reactive protein (CRP) is one of the proteins that increase during the body's inflammation process.[49] Obesity has been closely linked to a variety of measures of inflammation including CRP. Weight reduction directly influences CRP levels in both overweight and obese individuals,[50] and "lifestyle modification emphasizing regular exercise training significantly decreases hs-CRP."[51] It seems clear anything that helps you lose weight will improve your CRP profile, and of course exercise is one of the primary tools.

In addition to improving a wide array of generally accepted cardiovascular risk factors, exercise can also favorably alter other heart related functions. For example, heart rate recovery is the measurable rate of decrease in heart rate after exercise, which has been shown to: (1) be a powerful predictor of mortality in healthy adult men with risk factors for cardiovascular disease and diabetes, and (2) be improved by weight loss.[52] Additionally, in obese subjects, nutrition and exercise induced weight loss also results in improved arterial elasticity, which could reduce cardiovascular events and mortality.[53] Finally, in overweight and obese adults aerobic exercise has been shown to decrease triglycerides.[54]

When it comes to exercise, it is possible the overall benefit the heart receives may exceed the weight-loss benefit!

Cancer

Since cancer is the second leading cause of death in the US, let's explore the possible benefits of exercise. There is no confusion about the fact that certain kinds of cancer can either be prevented or have their treatment assisted by exercise and/or weight loss. What is troublesome is the magnitude of the existing problem, claimed by the researchers. Study data suggests one in five cancer deaths in the US, may be attributed to obesity.[55] "The International Agency for Research on Cancer estimates 25% of cancer cases worldwide are caused by overweight or obesity and a sedentary lifestyle."[56] Although the first study discussed US cancer deaths and the second study discussed worldwide cancer cases, both seem alarming in their magnitude.

The next important question is what specific cancers are we talking about? Here are the cancers researchers claim might be linked to obesity:

- Colorectal, breast (in postmenopausal women), prostate, endometrial, lung,[57]
- Esophagus, stomach, gallbladder,[58]
- Kidney, gastric cardia.[59]

Here are some interesting statistics related to some of these cancers.

- <u>Prostate Cancer</u> - A study of over 10,000 men undergoing prostate biopsies suggested obese men with prostate cancer tended to have a much more aggressive form of the cancer than did leaner men.[60]

o Breast Cancer - It appears the post-menopausal period is problematic. A "consistent, independent and positive association has been found between obesity and breast cancer in postmenopausal women,"[61] and between 6-19 percent of obese women are estimated to have a potential for this cancer.[62] If you fit this profile and are diabetic as well, you have a 16 percent higher risk of breast cancer than your non-diabetic counterparts.[63] It gets even worse if you are an obese Hispanic woman because these higher statistics apply to you even if you aren't post-menopausal.[64]

o Ovarian Cancer - I realize you don't have any control over what might have happened to you in infancy, but it is interesting to note that study data has shown women who died of ovarian cancer frequently had high rates of weight gain in infancy.[65] I only bring this up to emphasize the importance of controlling your current lifestyle in order to mitigate your risk factors and to suggest you help overweight female children lose weight.

Why might exercise exert such a cancer protective influence, on the body? It has been suggested exercise may work by:

- Decreasing gastrointestinal transit time,
- Consuming calories that might otherwise be used for tumor growth,
- Improving the functioning of the immune system,
- Postponing the onset of puberty.[66]

The link between exercise and cancer is certainly more difficult to make than the ones between exercise and heart disease or exercise and diabetes, but similar to what you will see later in the discussion of exercise vis-à-vis brain function, the strong, overriding reason for exercise is to lose weight. Ultimately the critical link is not the one between exercise and cancer but rather the one between excess body weight and cancer.

Diabetes

To begin with, here are some important definitions:

- Diabetes (proper name Diabetes Mellitus) - is a common condition in which the body either does not produce enough insulin or cannot properly use insulin,[67] which in turn results in the blood stream carrying too much glucose,
- Insulin - is a hormone produced in the pancreas and used as a vehicle to transport glucose from the bloodstream into the cells,[68]
- Glucose - is a blood sugar used by the cells to produce energy,
- Insulin Resistance - is the resistance of the cell receptor sites to the action of insulin.

There are two types of diabetes, type 1 diabetes and type 2 diabetes.

- <u>Type 1 Diabetes</u> - is also referred to as: (1) juvenile-onset diabetes, because it usually begins before age 20, or (2) insulin-dependent diabetes, because it results from an insulin deficiency. Type 1 diabetes only comprises about ten percent of the diabetes cases.[69] It is commonly thought to be an autoimmune disease where the body's own immune system attacks and destroys the beta cells in the pancreas, which are responsible for the production of insulin. Type 1 diabetes is believed to be the result of a flaw in the DNA, therefore, it is generally accepted that it can only be controlled through medical intervention (e.g. drug therapy). While that is not to say lifestyle changes cannot or will not make improvement in this condition the main focus of our consideration will be type 2 diabetes, where lifestyle can make all the difference.

- <u>Type 2 Diabetes</u> - is also referred to as: (1) adult-onset diabetes, because it usually begins after age 20, or (2) non-insulin-dependent diabetes, because it is not the result of an insulin deficiency. Type 2 diabetes comprises about 90 percent of the diabetes cases.[70] Type 2 diabetics typically have adequate blood insulin levels, but the insulin has difficulty transporting the glucose into the cells either because of a loss of insulin receptor sites or their defective functioning. In somewhat more technical terms, "reduced insulin sensitivity is a central mediator of the pathophysiology leading to type 2 diabetes."[71]

Scientists realize the inextricable link between excess body weight and type 2 diabetes and as you will see in the cited research, it becomes clear that lifestyle is the problem, when they say such things as:

  o "Excess consumption of palatable food and reduced exercise have been incontrovertibly associated with insulin resistance,"[72]
  o "Modifications to diet and implementing an exercise program, are first-line treatments for type 2 diabetes,"[73]
  o Six months of weight loss plus aerobic exercise, *but not weight loss alone,* "results in significant increases in glucose utilization and insulin sensitivity in obese postmenopausal women,"[74]
  o "3 months of dynamic strength training improves insulin sensitivity in obese middle-aged males."[75]

Two possible scenarios exist. First, you don't have type 2 diabetes and you would like to prevent it. Second, you have diabetes and you would like to get rid of it. What should you do? Interestingly, the data is absolutely clear that both situations require the same approach.

If you'd like to lower your risk of developing type 2 diabetes, the reduction of belly fat, improved physical fitness, improved glucose tolerance and improved body composition all have been shown to reduce the risk of developing type 2 diabetes in elderly, obese subjects.[76] As you will see in the paragraphs below exercise is the key ingredient, since it results in better physical fitness and body composition both of which positively influence glucose tolerance and belly fat, in fact it has been claimed exercise is essential for belly fat loss.[77] Here is how strongly one scientist feels about the subject. "Physical activity is of direct benefit, perhaps even essential to preventive and curative medicine in relation to insulin resistance and type 2 diabetes."[78] It gets even better! A study of non-obese (but ever so slightly overweight BMI 23.5-29.9), non-diabetic, healthy, middle aged men and women concluded, "exercise training and calorie restriction induced weight loss are effective means for improving glucose tolerance and insulin action,"[79] in this already healthy group.

But what if you are already overweight or obese and have type 2 diabetes? The research makes clear exercise can have several benefits, including:

- Improve insulin sensitivity,[80]
- Improve glucose utilization,[81]
- Reduce obesity and related co-morbid conditions,[82] (co-morbid means "a disease or other pathological process that occurs simultaneously with another);"[83] here the co-morbid conditions are obesity and type 2 diabetes,
- It tends to particularly zero in on abdominal fat, which: (1) correlates the most with insulin resistance, and (2) carries with it a higher health risk than fat in other parts of the body,[84]
- Improve oxidative capacity in older adults.[85]

The *take away message* here is if you are overweight, have type 2 diabetes and are really determined to get rid of it, you must:

- Never let anyone convince you there's nothing you can do about it, because it is likely the result of your lifestyle and habits not the result of some misguided fate of the universe,
- Get on an exercise program,
- Lose weight.

As soon as you begin losing weight your diabetes markers will begin to improve and given time and persistence you should be able to overcome type 2 diabetes completely.

Brain Function

The overall benefits of exercise on brain function are only now beginning to be realized. Of course our principal reason for engaging in an exercise program is to lose or maintain body weight, but isn't it neat to find out there are a myriad of other related health benefits? As you saw in the preceding pages, one of the psychological benefits you can get from exercise is the runner's high, but the benefits go further. Exercise can even have a positive impact on certain aspects of your mental health.

Annesi reported that exercise participants benefit psychologically, they experience an improved mood, and the mood changes they experience appear to have a direct relation to their commitment to their exercise program and to their reductions in BMI.[86] It is interesting to realize that by participating in an exercise program you can not only lose weight and gain a wide array of additional health benefits but you can also improve your mood. The bigger issue is, can exercise affect a deeper element of brain function? The answer is yes.

Research data links exercise with improvement in brain function and cognition. "Physical activity, and aerobic fitness training in particular, can have a positive effect on multiple aspects of brain function and cognition."[87] For example, it has been shown a weight loss of as little as five percent was associated with reduced levels of depression and hostility.[88] In addition, there is convincing evidence regular exercise can not only reduce depression and the decline in cognition associated with aging, but as far-fetched as it might seem it can also provide the brain with protection against traumatic and toxic insults.[89] I find it remarkable that a sensible exercise regime could have such a positive impact on the brain.

Dementia is defined broadly as, "a general loss of cognitive abilities including impairment of memory"[90] and it includes a whole host of well publicized conditions like Alzheimer's disease, Parkinson's disease, etc.[91] Jagust suggests regions of the brain vulnerable to Alzheimer's disease undergo a generalized atrophy in obese people, [92] and this atrophy has been associated with cognitive decline.[93] He is not the first or only researcher to reach this conclusion; in fact he cited four other studies claiming a definite connection between obesity and the risk of cognitive decline and dementia, especially Alzheimer's disease.[94] With our society becoming more sedentary and more overweight, is it any wonder the dementia related diseases are increasing rapidly? The study data cited gives us a glimpse of what our future might hold, in terms of dementia, with all its specific, insidious diseases.

Bone Density

With osteoporosis being a hot topic today, you probably are hearing a lot about declining bone density. Bone density is the amount of bone tissue in a given volume of bone. The concern is a lower than normal bone density can lead to bone fractures that might not otherwise occur. While some purists would argue with the choice of terminology, frequently researchers and medical practitioners refer to *bone density* as *bone mineral density* and sometimes as *bone mass*. Hereafter, I will use the terminology *bone density* unless I am quoting researchers using other terminology.

Although, there are inconsistencies in the research studies that have looked at how exercise might affect bone density, which may be the result of the type, frequency and duration of the exercise studied,[95] it has been known for years physical activity enhances the mechanical competence of bone.[96] But be careful here, as I have argued elsewhere there are a lot of physical activities that may not pass the beneficial exercise test. Study results "suggest that more intense exercise of longer duration may be required to enhance bone mineral density in older persons."[97] The National Osteoporosis Foundation arranges bone healthy exercise into the following three categories:

- Weight-bearing (high impact) exercises (e.g. dancing, high impact aerobics, hiking, jogging/running, jumping rope, stair climbing, tennis),

- Weight-bearing (low-impact) exercises (e.g. elliptical training machines, low impact aerobics, stair-step machines, walking),

- Resistance and strength training exercises (e.g. functional movements such as standing and rising up on your toes, lifting weights, using elastic exercise bands, using weight machines, lifting your own body weight).[98]

Postmenopausal women involved in weight-loss programs that utilize aerobic exercise, have shown improvement in their bone mineral density.[99] Other studies have gone further in saying, "the best exercises for building bone density are weight-or-load-bearing exercises."[100] In simple terms weight-or-load-bearing exercises fall into two categories: (1) weight resistance training, or (2) anything else that makes you struggle against gravity. When it comes to bone density it has been suggested your extra body weight might be your friend, due to the increased skeletal loading; however, obesity coupled with the weight-loss process are associated with low-grade systemic inflammation, which increases bone density loss.[101] So it would appear the one possible benefit to obesity is negated by an offsetting detriment. In the end that still leaves us with no overall benefit to obesity.

Bone structure and geometry adapt to mechanical loading, and the redistribution of bone mineral within the bone as well as the resulting changes in bone geometry are in direct relation to the number and intensity of daily impacts.[102] Even small gains in bone geometry can result in large improvements in bone strength.[103] Weight-bearing exercise, when coupled with other weight-loss interventions, increases markers of bone formation.[104] Different types of exercises appear to exert different influences on men and women. Women increase their bone density the most by increasing their aerobic capacity, while men who increase their strength and lean muscle mass achieved greater gains in bone density.[105]

Weight bearing exercises provide a loading on the bones causing them to retain normal bone density and it is for that reason astronauts in a weightless environment rapidly lose bone density. NASA says space biomedical researchers have found, "the microgravity environment of space causes men and women of all ages to lose up to 1% of their bone mass per month due to disuse atrophy, a condition similar to osteoporosis."[106] The University of California studied 13 astronauts who lived on the International Space Station between four-six months and found on average their bone strength decreased 14 percent, while three of the astronauts had alarmingly greater decreases of between 20 and 30 percent.[107] This alone doesn't totally make the case for the benefits of weight bearing exercise but there is further research.

It may be insightful to stratify some of the data by age group. When dealing with adolescents the idea is to get them started early building bone density, which will carry over into their later years. For example, Hind & Burrows reported boys and girls are at an opportune stage in their development to augment bone mineral accrual through exercise,[108] although they left unanswered the question of the most desirable type, intensity and duration of exercise to employ. By combining resistance and impact training in growing children they experience a more favorable bone response than with either type of exercise by itself.[109] It has been estimated in the US, three million women participate in high school, college and professional sports, with an additional 14 million age 25-44 participating in regular vigorous exercise.[110] Unfortunately in recent years many female high school varsity sports have been deemphasized. Bush argues in favor continued emphasis on these varsity sports when she says, "adolescent female athletic participation should be encouraged to increase bone mineral density and consequently reduce future fracture risk."[111]

The foundation for peak bone mass in adulthood has been laid in childhood by both genetic factors and exercise habits. In order to develop peak bone mass during childhood and adolescence, children must be monitored to ensure they have a proper calcium, protein, and vitamin D intake and they regularly engage in weight-bearing exercises.[112] This should not imply your adult stage bone density is completely controlled by what happened during childhood. If some of these requirements were not completely met during childhood there's still plenty you can do. Here's what I suggest:

- Evaluate your current calcium, protein, and vitamin D intake and assess your exercise program to ensure they are adequately meeting your needs,

- If you are over 55 or 60 years old, consult a doctor specializing in anti aging in order to ensure your hormone levels are appropriate for your age,

- Ensure you are eating in accordance with the Rule of Thirds.

Finally, here is some interesting research. Generally heart transplantation patients receive glucocorticoid therapy to help alleviate heart rejection. As a result of this therapy, within two months of heart transplant surgery, three percent of whole-body bone mineral density is lost, the majority of which is lost in the lumbar region of the spine. Obviously, the reversibility of glucocorticoid therapy induced bone loss becomes very important to the heart transplant patient. A combination of resistance exercises targeted at both: (1) the lumbar region of the back, and (2) all major muscle groups, restores bone mineral density toward pre-transplantation levels.[113]

Inflammation

Inflammation is "a localized protective response elicited by injury or destruction of tissues, which serves to destroy, dilute, or wall off (sequester) both the imperious agent and the injured tissue."[114] According to the Cleveland Clinic "inflammation is a process by which the body's white blood cells and chemicals protect us from infection and foreign substances such as bacteria and viruses."[115] Simply put inflammation is the basic way the body reacts to an injury or foreign invader. A problem exists when the body's immune system inappropriately triggers an inflammatory response when there is no foreign substance present. In this situation, commonly known as autoimmune disease, (e.g. rheumatoid arthritis, multiple sclerosis) the immune system turns against the body and damages its own normally healthy tissues.

Recent research demonstrates there is a direct connection between inflammation and most chronic degenerative diseases. Perricone offers the following rather exhaustive list of these diseases, "arthritis, multiple sclerosis, atherosclerosis, diabetes, Alzheimer's disease, osteoporosis, asthma, cirrhosis of the liver, bowel disorders, meningitis, cystic fibrosis, cancer, stroke, psoriasis, and, of course aging."[116]

Until recently there has been disagreement among researchers as to whether or not exercise can help reduce unwanted, systemic inflammation. Some claim weight loss resulting from dietary intervention reduces overall inflammation, however additional study is needed to assess the effects of exercise on inflammation.[117] Others have found "a high-fiber, low-fat diet combined with daily aerobic exercise, results in significant reductions in...inflammatory proteins in postmenopausal women."[118] They were more emphatic when they claimed impressive improvement in inflammatory response from individuals who engaged in intensive lifestyle modification.[119] Still others found, "diet plus exercise, but not diet alone, is effective in reducing markers of inflammation in older obese women."[120] One group claimed they found only modest changes in inflammation markers in older women with type 2 diabetes, as the result of a weight-loss diet and exercise program, but went on to suggest perhaps more dramatic weight loss or other clinical interventions would be helpful.[121] Since their exercise program consisted solely of walking three to four times per week for 60 minutes I would suggest a more rigorous exercise regime might get a better result.

Later three studies further confused the issue when the first concluded, "exercise training improved cardiorespiratory fitness but had no consistent effect on inflammatory marker levels,"[122] the second concluded a "hypocaloric diet and moderate physical activity resulted in a significant general decrease in the level of inflammation,"[123] and the third reported aerobic exercise was not only critical to improve VO_{2max} in postmenopausal women participating in a weight-loss program, but aerobic exercise was necessary to decrease inflammation and increase bone mineral density.[124]

It doesn't appear the cited research settles the issue but what does seem clear is this:

- Inflammation at the right time and in the right place is a good thing; however, prolonged inflammation raises havoc with the body,

- While there is some belief that during exercise we induce a minimum amount of low-grade inflammation into the body, it is also believed to dissipate rapidly,

- There is research that is emphatic about the positive benefits of exercise in reducing systemic inflammation,

- I have found no research suggesting exercise might have a negative effect on long-term, systemic inflammation.

The real advantage for you is while you are losing weight you also have the potential to improve your markers of systemic inflammation.

Other

As you have seen there is a lot of research dealing with the relationship between exercise and the six high profile disease risk factors discussed above; however, there isn't a lot beyond that point. I will cite a few research studies on less popular health related conditions. This short list is not intended to be all-inclusive, but hopefully will spur you on to do additional research, should you have a medical condition not discussed in this chapter.

- Good cholesterol (HDL) - Study data shows vigorous exercise, moderate alcohol consumption, and reasonable weight loss can all have the beneficial impact of boosting HDL, the odd thing is those individuals with already high HDL seem to benefit the most from these factors, while those most at risk due to low HDL benefit the least.[125]

- Growth Hormone (GH) - Pituitary gland production of GH diminishes with age; however, intense physical exercise has been shown to stimulate more output, but exercise intensity and duration, as well as gender and the level of both fitness and obesity affect the GH response to exercise.[126]

- Polycystic Ovary Syndrome - Obese women with polycystic ovary syndrome, (which is claimed to be the most frequent cause of infertility in adult women), show improved biochemical profiles from both endurance and resistance exercise.[127]

Exercise Specifics

There is a difference in our individual exercise needs, which is based on such things as age, sex, race, current weight status, total calories consumed per day and personal objectives. It is not the intention of this section to lay out a specific exercise program, with the hope it will fit everyone. The ideas presented below are intended to: (1) give you a basic understanding of what your exercise counselor should be trying to accomplish, in the design and implementation of your personal training program, and (2) make you knowledgeable enough to ask them intelligent questions.

In the research studies that follow you will see a lot of reference to VO_{2max}, aerobic exercise and anaerobic exercise. Right now is a great time to distinguish the three:

- VO_{2max} - is "the total capacity to consume oxygen at the cellular level,"[128] also frequently referred to as the body's: (1) maximum oxygen consumption, (2) maximum oxygen uptake, (3) aerobic capacity, or (4) VO_{2peak}. Your personal VO_{2max} is the maximum amount of oxygen your body is capable of processing from the time oxygen is inhaled into your lungs from the external environment, transferred onto your bloodstream's red blood cells, transported to your body's cells where it is extracted by the cells and used for energy production. As you might expect the speed of this process controls the intensity and duration of an exercise session. The good news is VO_{2max} can be increased by exercise.

- Aerobic - means operating "with, or in the presence of oxygen."[129] Normally when you are performing any aerobic exercise your body will be operating well below your normal VO_{2max} and it will produce cellular energy utilizing fatty acids and/or glucose combined with oxygen. If you are exercising aerobically (e.g. walking briskly might require 50-60 percent of VO_{2max}) you should be able to continue for a fairly long period of time before tiring. Once you begin to approach your VO_{2max} (e.g. perhaps above 60 percent of VO_{2max}) you enter a zone called your anaerobic threshold, which represents a transition point where you begin to move from aerobic to anaerobic cellular energy production. In this mode of exercise you will only be able to continue for a limited period of time because of oxygen starvation. As the words imply, once you reach your anaerobic threshold, you are becoming partially anaerobic energy dependent.

- Anaerobic - means operating "without the presence of oxygen; not requiring oxygen."[130] Once you enter your anaerobic zone you have reached a point where you are not able to utilize enough oxygen to keep up with your body's energy demands aerobically. At this point aerobic energy production must be supplemented by anaerobic energy production, which is dependent on a chemical known as creatine phosphate. Although creatine phosphate is capable of producing energy in the absence of oxygen, this source quickly becomes exhausted, therefore utilization of the anaerobic process can only continue for a short period of time. The more dependent you become on anaerobic energy production, the shorter the period of time you can keep up the pace (e.g. sprinting). A great example of a nearly total anaerobic exercise is an Olympic weightlifter attempting a maximum lift, where one attempt lasts only a couple of seconds and results in total exhaustion.

Exercise Type

Exercise type refers to the kind of exercise selected (e.g. jogging, jumping, lifting weights). In this section I will discuss three basic types of exercise: (1) walking, (2) aerobic exercise, and (3) resistance (anaerobic) exercise.

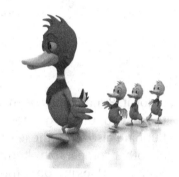

- Walking - Although walking could and should be categorized as an aerobic exercise I have chosen to categorize it separately because in those cases where it does not rise to the level of an aerobic exercise, it doesn't even fit my definition of an exercise. It has been claimed, "walking is a popular and convenient form of exercise that can play an important role in weight management."[131] The operative word is *can*, because walking can have a beneficial effect but frequently doesn't, since its popularity is largely driven by the fact it is convenient and easy. These researchers do point out obese individuals burn more energy during walking than their normal weight counterparts.[132] The same thing is probably true with most other forms of exercise. This occurs because they are moving more weight and consequently doing more work.

    What if you measure your steps with a pedometer? In the absence of dietary intervention, in walking programs where participants used a pedometer to count the number of steps they walked, they lost a moderate amount of weight.[133] An easier way is to forget about the pedometer and just time your walk!

    One thing we know is weight loss resulting from exercise closely parallels improved physical fitness. While "most young adults won't improve their level of fitness by walking,"[134] I think it is safe to conclude they won't find walking to help them lose weight either.

    If on the other hand walking can be raised to the level of an aerobic exercise, beneficial results could be obtained.

- <u>Aerobic Exercise</u> - A multitude of studies have shown belly fat puts the overweight person at an increased risk of several metabolic disorders, including coronary heart disease.[135] Both high-intensity and low-intensity aerobic exercise coupled with a weight loss dietary program has been shown to reduce abdominal fat.[136] "Aerobic exercise training in conjunction to a controlled diet can have positive effects on reducing both total and abdominal fat."[137]

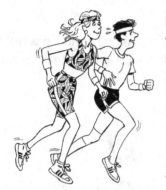

In severely obese adolescents a 90-minute, three day a week program of swimming, gymnastics, walking and recreational team sports coupled with moderate dietary restriction: (1) Improves aerobic and anaerobic fitness markers, (2) reduces the obesity level, and (3) preserves lean muscle mass.[138]

I realize many of us aren't interested in being runners. Furthermore, obese individuals may find it impossible. There is good news for those capable of running who do enjoy it. Running has been shown to be one of the best weight loss exercises, and those who run the greatest distances each week have the lowest body weights.[139] Running also takes the least amount of equipment. If you don't like running there are other comparable alternatives, as long as you have the facilities available to you. Swimming laps in a pool, (not water aerobics), or a good aggressive rowing machine workout can achieve similar results. Think about it, I bet all of the swimmers or rowers that you can think of are lean. If running does appeal to you but you can't run because of your weight, once you've lost weight you might be able to switch to running as a weight maintenance exercise. After you've lost weight you should be able to scale back the amount of running, swimming or rowing you do and still maintain your weight.

Finally, let's go back to walking. As I said earlier, walking can be a good aerobic exercise if it is done properly. Here are some key parameters. You must:

o Keep in mind your goals are to: (1) burn calories, and (2) improve cardio-respiratory fitness,
o Remember the recommended exercise range for accomplishing these goals is 60-80 percent of VO_{2max},
o Determine your desired VO_{2max} range. As discussed earlier in this chapter you can calculate it using this formula:

<u>220 - your age x desired percent = heart rate (beats/minute),</u>

Here's an example for a 50-year old person,
Min heart rate is [220 - 50 x .60 (i.e. 60 percent) = 102 bpm],
Max heart rate is [220 - 50 x .80 (i.e. 80 percent) = 136 bpm],

o Monitor your heart rate so you know you are exercising in your desired range,

o Exercise in your desired range for a *minimum of 20 minutes three or more* times a week in order to achieve cardio-respiratory fitness and begin to lose weight,

o Exercise in your desired range for *longer than 20 minutes five or more* times a week if you want to lose weight quicker.

Many modern aerobic fitness machines (e.g. treadmills, stationary bikes) have two features you will find extremely helpful, these are: (1) a tag displaying the already calculated heart rates for 60 and 80 percent of VO_{2max} for various ages, and (2) a built in heart rate monitor. If you are using older equipment calculate the heart rate targets yourself and purchase a heart rate monitor (approximate cost $50). If you walk at a shopping mall, as your VO_{2max} begins to improve you will probably find it difficult to get your heart rate up to your 80 percent target, that's the reason why a treadmill is so valuable. On the treadmill you can adjust your walking speed and the incline of the track, which will mimic walking uphill. You will probably find in order to hit your 80 percent heart rate target you will probably be walking 3.0-3.5 miles per hour at a six-ten percent incline. **Caveat** - be careful with too steep an incline on the treadmill because it can be hard on your lower back.

- Resistance (Anaerobic) Exercise - If as we saw above, aerobic exercise is so beneficial, isn't that enough? The answer is no. The gradual loss of muscle tissue in adults that don't get adequate exercise results in approximately a five percent decline in metabolic rate every ten years, and interestingly this decrease in metabolism closely parallels a gradual increase in body fat.[140] The reason is lean muscle mass is more metabolically active than fat, so the idea is to gain or at least maintain lean muscle mass in order to keep the metabolic fire burning.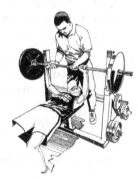

US women between the ages of 25 and 44 tend to gain .5-1 kilogram (1.1-2.2) pounds of bodyweight per year, but twice a week strength training attenuates these fat increases.[141] During moderate caloric restriction, resistance training can help participants increase their muscle strength and preserve fat-free mass.[142] Some encouraged strength training to enhanced lean muscle mass and to promote its continued development.[143] Because of the health related benefits, type 2 diabetics should be encouraged to perform resistance exercise three times a week.[144] Resistance training when coupled with a low-calorie diet and increased protein intake produces a significant loss of fat mass and a gain of lean muscle mass, when compared to a low-calorie diet alone.[145]

Exercise Duration

Exercise duration refers to how long you exercise. Numerous researchers have maintained that, "the benefits of being physically active are available to those who accumulate 30 minutes of moderate-intensity physical activity most days of the week."[146] The generally accepted rule of 30

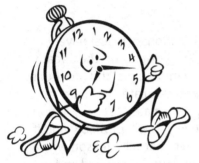

minutes or more of moderate-intensity activity on most days of the week may be sufficient for reducing the health risks associated with chronic disease, but for preventing weight gain or weight regain this guideline could prove highly inadequate.[147] They go on to suggest the average person may need 45-60 minutes per day of moderate-intensity exercise in order to prevent weight gain, and 60-90 minutes of moderate-intensity exercise or 35 minutes of vigorous exercise per day to prevent weight regain after weight loss.[148]

The so-called gold standard of 30 minutes of moderate-intensity physical activity most days of the week, begs the all-important question of what is your goal? Let's take a look some specific goals.

- Cardio-respiratory fitness - If your goal is cardio-respiratory fitness then 30 minutes of aerobic exercise, (maintaining an oxygen consumption rate of between 60-80 percent VO_{2max}), most days of the week should work just fine.

- Weight Loss (Moderate) - If you want moderate weight loss (e.g. a reasonable, sensible weight-loss is about a pound a week), you're routine should change to incorporate three days a week of the cardio-respiratory fitness program suggested above, coupled with an additional two-three days a week of resistant exercise. What this obviously means is the benchmark of 30 minutes of moderate-intensity physical activity most days of the week, just won't cut it.

- Weight Loss (Extreme) - I hope your goal is not extreme weight loss but if it is then you're going to have to do massive amounts of exercise coupled with an exacting dietary plan, in fact this weight-loss effort could become a full-time job. If you've seen what they do on The Biggest Loser TV show you know participants spend several hours each day in the gym, working under the guidance and control of experience personal trainers. This is not only unhealthy but also unnecessary if you are patient and persistent. Think about it, losing a healthy one-pound a week amounts to a reduction in body weight of 52 pounds per year.

- <u>Build Lean Muscle Mass</u> - Although it is outside the scope of this book, if your goal was to build an athletic body (e.g. bodybuilding), your exercise routine would have to be modified even further. Depending on how serious you were you might reduce or eliminate cardio-respiratory work while performing resistance exercises five-six days a week, for one or more hours a day.

Some have gone even further and suggested substantial fitness improvements, (we know fitness improvements closely parallel weight loss), can be obtained with exercise sessions of as little as ten minutes each, with an overall goal of at least two such sessions a day.[149] Study data has demonstrated healthy young men, who accumulated 30 minutes of physical activity in ten three minute bouts, spread throughout the day, were able to lower their triglycerides about the same amount as those who performed the 30 minute exercise routine in one continuous bout.[150] With the continual softening of the recommended guidelines, I bet if we wait long enough some folks will actually be suggesting no exercise is needed. Either way, *I don't believe for one minute, 30 minutes of moderate-intensity physical activity most days of the week, let alone this activity being broken down into smaller chunks, will even get you close to desirable weight loss in a reasonable amount of time.*

Exercise Frequency

Exercise frequency refers to how often the exercise is performed, (e.g. two or three times a week). For older men with type 2 diabetes, progressive resistance training performed only twice a week, can result in "significant improvements in muscle strength, insulin sensitivity, and glucose tolerance and a significant decrease in abdominal fat."[151] I cited this study because I said I would be fair and balanced, but I totally disbelieve this twice a week stuff will do anything of value for reducing abdominal fat, let alone make the significant difference claimed in this study. We know abdominal fat is a big problem because it is so closely related to the diseases 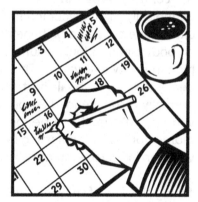 involved in metabolic syndrome and once lost it is quite easily regained. One of the predictors of visceral fat rebound is inconsistency in exercise frequency, or fluctuations in daily exercise regimes.[152]

Even without substantial weight loss, regular exercise is needed to maintain normal glucose balance,[153] and "frequent exercise is more effective than less frequent exercise in improving VO_{2max}."[154] I believe if you are going to err in exercise frequency it is best to exercise more often rather than less often, but remember your body does need time for recovery, so the more severe the exercise regime and the older you are, the more recovery time you need. One study made this all-important finding, "while short-bout exercise has some benefits, they are not as large or as diverse as those seen in the long bout sessions."[155] My study and experience tells me this is a statement worth committing to memory. Here is even better news. Sedentary individuals who become active experience the largest health gains, while active individuals who increase their level of activity do not experience the same gains.[156]

Exercise Intensity

Exercise intensity refers to how hard you exercise (e.g. 50 percent of VO_{2max}, 80 percent of VO_{2max}). Yep, there are still a lot of people advocating that 30 minutes of moderate-intensity physical activity most days of the week is all that is required. But let's look a little deeper. changes in body composition are directly affected by the intensity of exercise training, in fact high-intensity exercise is more effective than low-to-moderate intensity exercise, because it induces secretion of fat processing hormones which facilitate greater post exercise energy expenditure and fat oxidation and it favors a greater negative energy balance.[157] It also reduces fasting insulin levels.[158]

Previously in this chapter I talked about exercising in your desired range for a minimum of 20 minutes three or more times a week in order to achieve cardio-respiratory fitness and to begin to lose weight. This was not intended to imply: (1) you should not vary your exercise intensity because there is no benefit from doing so, or (2) you might hurt yourself if you did. Quite the contrary! **Providing you have medical clearance** to be exercising at higher intensities, periodically varying your intensity is not only one fun way to break the monotony of the same old routine but it can be beneficial, because it "can have a more substantial long-term impact on body composition, presumably because muscle capacity for fat oxidation is boosted by the high-intensity intervals."[159] This means if you are exercising steadily at a given VO_{2max} (e.g. 70 percent), an occasional short spike to 80 percent or higher is just fine. In fact exceeding the normally recommended 80 percent of VO_{2max} by five percent, for short bursts, should cause you no problem. If you perform high intensity intermittent exercise you should experience more improvement in fasting insulin levels and total body fat than you would with little or no variation in exercise intensity.[160]

Taking this line of thinking one step further, scientists demonstrated in male runners a direct relationship exists between age and vigorous exercise, since the need for increased vigorous exercise increases with age because of the tendency for body weight to increase.[161] I would find it hard to believe the same thing doesn't apply equally for women. In fact, endurance training has been shown to improve fatty acid uptake and oxidation in obese people of both sexes.[162] There is a direct relationship between the amount of exercise people get and the amount of weight they lose.[163] This is not surprising since the issue again comes back to one of negative energy balance, if excess weight is to be lost.

Obstacles to Exercise

The following few paragraphs are not intended to be abrasive, offensive or in your face but they will be honest, and hopefully you will respect my honesty even if you don't like what I have to say.

There are as many obstacles to exercise, as there are stars in the sky, and as with the stars some are bigger than others. The two biggest obstacles are *time* and *cost* and you will find most others pale in comparison. Once the obstacles of time and costs are overcome the remaining obstacles should not be showstoppers. The key here is to find ways to overcome these obstacles and not let them turn into excuses. Let's take a look at them separately:

- <u>Time</u> - Unless you don't have to work for a living the time constraints you experience are the same ones the rest of us are facing, and today they are more oppressive than ever before. Our jobs are more time demanding, our family lives are more time demanding and because of time bandits like television and the Internet, our free time is easily sucked up before we realize it. I am very sympathetic and understanding of this problem, primarily because I have to deal with it in my daily life just like you do. Because I don't know your personal situation, you will have to figure out what actions you need to take to come to grips with your own time limitations, but I'm sure if losing weight is important to you, you will be able to figure out how to fit exercise into your schedule. This may be a time when other family members have to bend a little or show a little flexibility in order to help you reach this all-important goal.

- <u>Cost</u> - Unless you are hoping to buy expensive home fitness equipment most of the costs you encounter should be manageable. The biggest costs you will struggle with are a fitness club membership, a personal trainer, or a nutritionist. You will most likely find minor costs like gym shoes, a tennis racket, racquetball court time, etc. won't break you. Again, it's simply a matter of whether you are willing to redirect a small portion of your finances to the important issue of losing weight or whether you just want to complain about how impossible it is.

- In addition to legitimate time and cost constraints there is an endless list of other possible obstacles that can stop you from exercising. Over the years I have heard many of them. In addition to, "I don't have the time to exercise," or "I can't afford to join a fitness center," I have heard other nonsense like; "I'm to old," "I might hurt myself," "I might be sore the next day," "I don't have the energy," and "I don't like to sweat." These apparent obstacles, really aren't obstacles after all, they are simply lame excuses.

Once you've cleared these hurdles, there are some additional considerations that might help you get started. Remember you only need to do a few of them to get results, so adopt those you like the best:

- Join a fitness center,
- Join a fitness center with a friend,
- Hire a personal trainer who will direct and support your effort,
- Avoid loneliness, because "loneliness among middle and older aged adults is an independent risk factor for physical inactivity and increases the likelihood physical activity will be discontinued over time,"[164]
- Join a weight-loss support group,
- Solicit the support of family and friends as your personal support group,
- Start a weight-loss support group (e.g. senior center based, church-based, fitness center based),
- Join a supervised diet and exercise program,[165]
- Join a lifestyle intervention group,[166]
- Focus on the quality of life benefits you will receive,[167]
- Study the next chapter entitled the Psychological Aspects of Weight Loss,
- Refer to the book summary for more details.

If you're still not feeling terribly motivated just do two things: (1) stand in front of your bathroom mirror naked and take a good honest look, and (2) reflect back on the conversations your doctor has had with you about your weight. If these things don't motivate you to take action right now, that's OK, *you can stop reading this book;* just don't give it away because you may decide to refer to it again later.

Summary

The bottom line message here is no weight loss program should be without an aggressive exercise regime. Similarly it's no secret that no matter how good your exercise routine is it will be much better if it incorporates improved food planning.[168] There is however a lot of misconception over what a real exercise program should look like. Here is what you might see If you watch the vast majority of ill-informed, overweight people at most fitness centers. Somewhere along the line they have been led to believe by engaging in some of what I call pinch and tickle physical activities, like: (1) stretching ad infinitum, (2) leisurely walking on the treadmill or casually riding a stationary bike, (3) performing a few wimpy resistance exercises, they will lose weight. Guess what, they won't! The only changes they will experience are that they: (1) get very frustrated, and (2) continue to gain weight. The key here is to keep in mind the distinction I made earlier between physical activity and exercise. Don't be lulled into a false sense of security by thinking that a leisurely walk around the park, shopping mall or golf course meets the requirements of an aggressive exercise regime. It doesn't and it will not get you the result you want!

As discussed previously, exercise brings numerous benefits besides just weight-loss. Exercise can help you with:

- Fat oxidation,
- Chronic disease prevention and/or abatement, including:
  - Heart disease,
  - Cancer,
  - Diabetes,
  - Brain function (e.g. dementia, Alzheimer's, Parkinson's),
  - Bone density,
  - Inflammation,
- Accrued psychological benefits (e.g. mood elevation, minimized depression).

In attempting to create an exercise plan, here are the questions you must answer:

- Exercise Type -
  - Do you want aerobic or anaerobic exercise?
  - What specific exercises?
- Exercise Duration - How long will your exercise sessions be?
- Exercise Frequency - How many exercise sessions per week will you have?
- Exercise Intensity - How hard should you exercise (e.g. percent of VO_{2max})?

Before you begin an exercise routine you need to clear away any obstacles that will put the brakes on your effort, the biggest of which are time and cost. If there are obstacles you can't deal effectively with, in the long run they may prevent you from developing, implementing and maintaining a routine that works for you. To help you overcome obstacles you may need to engage the services of a professional (e.g. psychologist, lifestyle coach, personal trainer). Think about how challenging the obstacles might be for an obese, physically disabled person, living in a difficult social environment. One solution that has had success is to develop a weekly phone-based coaching system, coupled with monthly in-person exercise support group sessions.[169] If you are creative the solutions to your exercise obstacles may not be as far out of reach as they may seem.

An otherwise good intervention might still fail if it is one created by someone else and then forced on you. Here are a couple of potential obstacles to consider:

- Any sensible approach to solving your weight loss problem must involve you in the design and evaluation of the intervention selected.[170]
- In order to sustain an exercise program for the long haul, you must have exercises: (1) you enjoy, or at least can tolerate, (2) you are capable of doing, and (3) that add to your sense of autonomy and self-determination.[171]

One big unanswered question is, if I need a personal trainer how would I select one? Here are a few simple considerations that might help you, when interviewing a potential personal trainer:

- Rule number one is to take a close look at the personal trainer and determine if they are overweight, many are. If they are overweight, that's a clue perhaps they don't know what they are doing. You might want to interview a few others.

- Get some references from other people they are working with in order to find out if they feel they are getting the expected benefits.

- Find out how they plan to help you evaluate your nutritional needs:

    o   If nutrition is not an important part of the service they offer, their help will take you down a dead-end street, because it has been shown repeatedly exercise alone will have a minimal impact on weight loss unless it is combined with an energy restricted diet.[172] Any approach that focuses on a combination of dietary change and increase exercise is more effective than either behavior alone.[173]

    o   If the personal trainer doesn't know anything about nutrition do they have a nutritionist they recommend? If not that sounds like a problem.

Once you have lost weight the next critical step is to address long-term weight maintenance. Relatively high levels of exercise contribute to sustained weight loss.[174] Additionally, it has been shown more exercise may be needed to prevent weight regain than to prevent weight gain in the first place,[175] and "exercise is perhaps the best predictor of weight maintenance."[176] In the next chapter you will see just how important it is for you to resolve any current psychological problems that might impede your weight-loss effort. It is also extremely important to resolve these issues before you move into the maintenance phase of your program, if you are to have long-term success.[177]

Here is an interesting fact I offer to give you encouragement. As you saw in the chapter on genetics our personal genetics may not be, or need not be as controlling as many of us have previously thought them to be. A person's family history of obesity does not necessarily put them at a disadvantage in their response to increased exercise, despite strong genetic factors regulating fat mass.[178] Don't let the old idea that just because you come from an obese family, you must be obese, control your thinking. It is really an outdated model that has been disproven many times and will only serve to hold you back.

Endnotes

1. United States Department of Agriculture, Inside the pyramid, http://www.mypyramid.gov/pyramid/physical_activity.html
2. World Health Organization, Physical activity, http://www.who.int/topics/physical_activity/en/
3. S. Branth, A. Sjodin, A. Forslund, L. Hambraeus, U. Holmback, "Minor changes in blood lipids after 6 weeks of high-volume low-intensity physical activity with strict energy balance control," *Euro J. App Physiol* 96 (2006) 315-321.
4. J.S. Volek, J.L. VanHeest, C.F. Forsythe, "Diet and exercise for weight loss: a review of current issues," *Sports Med* 35 (2005) 1-9.
5. A.C. Tsai, A. Sandretto, Y.C. Chung, "Dieting is more effective in reducing weight but exercise is more effective in reducing fat during the early phase of a weight-reducing program in healthy humans," *J Nutr Biochem* 14 (2003) 541-549.
6. S.G. Aldana, "*The culprit & the cure*," (Mapleton, UT: *Maple Mountain Press*, 2005) 142.
7. T. Matsuo, T. Okura, Y. Nakata, N. Yabushita, S. Numao, H. Sasai, K. Tanaka, "The influence of physical activity-induced energy expenditure on the variance in body weight change among individuals during a diet intervention," *Obes Res Clin Prac* 1 (2007) 109-117.
8. M. Driskell, S. Dyment, L. Mauriello, P. Castle, K. Sherman, "Relationships among multiple behaviors for childhood and adolescent obesity prevention," *Prev Med* 46 (2008) 209-215.
9. D.M. Okay, P.V. Jackson, M. Marcinkiewicz, M.N. Papino, "Exercise and obesity," *Prim Care* 36 (2009) 379-393.
10. F.M. Cachelin, R.H. Striegel-Moore, K.D. Brownell, "Beliefs about weight gain and attitudes toward relapse in a sample of women and men with obesity," *Obes Res* 6 (1998) 231-237.
11. T. Matsuo, T. Okura, Y. Nakata, N. Yabushita, S. Numao, H. Sasai, K. Tanaka, "The influence of physical activity-induced energy expenditure on the variance in body weight change among individuals during a diet intervention," *Obes Res Clin Prac* 1 (2007) 109-117.
12. M.G. Enig, "*Know Your Fats*," (Silver Spring, MD: Bethesda Press 2000) 264.
13. F.G.S. Toledo, S. Watkins, D.E. Kelley, "Changes induced by physical activity and weight loss in the morphology of intermyofibrillar mitochondria in obese men and women," *J. Clin Endocrin Metab* 91 (2006) 3224-3227.
14. K. Hansen, T. Shriver, D. Schoeller, "The effects of exercise on the storage and oxidation of dietary fat," *Sports Med* 5 (2005) 363-373.
15. Ibid.
16. J.R. Berggren, K.E. Boyle, W.H. Chapman, J.A. Houmard, "Skeletal muscle lipid oxidation and obesity: influence of weight loss and exercise," *Am J Physiol Endo Metab* 294 (2008) E726-E732.
17. R.N. Cortright, K.M. Sandhoff, J.L. Basilio, J.R. Berggren, R.C. Hickner, M.W. Hulver, G.L. Dohm, J.A. Houmard, "Skeletal muscle fat oxidation is increased in African-American and white women after 10 days of endurance exercise training," *Obesity* 14 (2006) 1201-1210.
18. J.R. Berggren, M.W. Hulver, G.L. Dohm, J.A. Houmard, "Weight loss and exercise: implications for muscle lipid metabolism and insulin action," *Med Sci Sports Exer* 36 (2004) 1191-1195.
19. U.S. National Library of Medicine, National Institutes of Health, http://www.ncbi.nlm.nih.gov/pubmed/15212756
20. M.C. Venables, A.E. Jeukendrup, "Endurance training and obesity: effect on substrate metabolism and insulin sensitivity," *Med Sci Sports Exer* 495-502.

21.　Ibid.

22.　United States Centers for Disease Control and Prevention, Leading Causes of Death, http://www.cdc.gov/nchs/FASTATS/local.htm

23.　D.M. Okay, P.V. Jackson, M. Marcinkiewicz, M.N. Papino, "Exercise and obesity," *Prim Care* 36 (2009) 379-393.

24.　K. Melzer, B. Kayser, C. Pichard, "Physical activity: the health benefits outweigh the risks," *Curr Opin Clin Nutr Metab Care* 7 (2004) 641-647.

25.　L.H. Kuller, L.S. Kinzel, K.K. Pettee, A.M. Kriska, L.R. Simkin-Silverman, M.B. Conroy, F. Averbach, W.S. Pappert, B.D. Johnson, "Lifestyle intervention and coronary heart disease risk factor changes over 18 months in postmenopausal women: the women on the move through activity and nutrition (WOMAN Study) clinical trial," *J Women's Health* 15 (2006) 962-974.

26.　S. Lee, J.L. Kuk, P.T. Katzmarzyk, S.N. Blair, T.S. Church, R. Ross, "Cardiorespiratory fitness attenuates metabolic risk independent of abdominal subcutaneous and visceral fat in men," *Diabetes Care* 28 (2005) 895-901.

27.　K.J. Stewart, A.C. Bacher, K. Turner, J.G. Lim, P.S. Hees, E.P. Shapiro, M.T. Tayback, P. Ouyang, "Exercise and risk factors associated with metabolic syndrome in older adults," *Am J Prev Med* 28 (2005) 9-18.

28.　K. Samaras, P.J. Kelly, M.N. Chiano, T.D. Spector, L.V. Campbell, "Genetic and environmental influences on total-body and central abdominal fat:: the effect of physical activity in female twins," *Ann Intern Med* 130 (1999) 873-882.

29.　M.S. Faith, K.R. Fontaine, L.J. Cheskin, D.B. Allison, "Behavioral approaches to the problems of obesity," Behav Mod 24 (2000) 459-493.

30.　T. Reinehr, K. Brylak, U. Alexy, M. Kersting, W. Andler, "Predictors of success in outpatient training in obese children and adolescents," *Intl J Obes* 27 (2003) 1087-1092.

31.　T.S. Church, M.J. LaMonte, C.E. Barlow, S.N. Blair, "Cardiorespiratory fitness and body mass index as predictors of cardiovascular disease mortality among men with diabetes," *Arch Intern Med* 165 (2005) 2114-2120.

32.　R. Jankauskiene, K. Kardelis, S. Pajaujiene, "Body weight satisfaction and weight loss attempts in fitness activity involved women," *J Sports Med Phy Fit* 45 (2005) 537-546.

33.　T.L. Mitchell, L.W. Gibbons, S,M. Devers, C.P. Earnest, "Effects of cardiorespiratory fitness on health care utilization," Med Sci Sports Exer (2004) 2088-2092

34.　M.S. Faith, K.R. Fontaine, L.J. Cheskin, D.B. Allison, "Behavioral approaches to the problems of obesity," Behav Mod 24 (2000) 459-493.

35.　J.J. Annesi, J.L. Unruh, "Relations of exercise, self appraisal, mood changes and weight loss in obese women: testing propositions based on Baker and Brownell's (2000) model," *Am J Med Sci* 335 (2008) 198-204.

36.　F.J. Penedo, J.R. Dahn, "Exercise and well-being: a review of mental and physical health benefits associated with physical activity," *Curr Opin Psych* 18 (2005) 189-193.

37.　M. Kiernan, A.C. King, M.L. Stefanick, J.D. Killen, "Men gain additional psychological benefits by adding exercise to a weight-loss program," *Obes Res* 9 (2001) 770-777.

38.　"The reality of the runners high," UPMC Sports Medicine, University of Pittsburg Schools of the Health Sciences, Pittsburg, PA http://www.upmc.com/healthatoz/pages/HealthLibrary.aspx?chunkiid=13764

39.　"Endorphin," *Dorland's Illustrated Medical Dictionary*, 30th ed: 615.

40. A. Ramel, C. Pumberger, A.J. Martinez, M. Kiely, N.M. Bandarra, I. Thorsdottir, "Cardiovascular risk factors in young, overweight, and obese European adults and associations with physical activity and omega-3 Index," *Nutr Res* 29 (2009) 305-312.

41. "Endothelium," *Dorland's Illustrated Medical Dictionary*, 30th ed: 616.

42. A.A. Meyer, G. Kendt, U. Lenschow, P. Schull-Werner, W. Kienast, "Improvement of early vascular changes and cardiovascular risk factors in obese children after a six-month exercise program," *J Am College Cardiol* 48 (2006) 1865-1870.

43. P. Palatini, P. Visentin, F. Dorigatti, C. Guarnier, M. Santonastaso, S. Cozzio, F. Pegoraro, A. Bortolazzi, O. Vriz, L. Mos, "Regular physical activity prevents development of left ventricular hyper trophy in hypertension," *Euro Heart J* 30 (2009) 225-232.

44. "Left Ventricular Hypertrophy," MayoClinic.com, http://www.mayoclinic.com/health/left-venticular-hypertrophy/DS00680

45. Ibid.

46. L.A. Gondoni, A.M. Titon, F. Nibbio, G. Caetani, G. Augello, O. Mian, C. Tuzzi, E. Averna, C. Parisio, A. Liuzzi, "Short-term effects of a hypocaloric diet and a physical activity programme on weight loss and exercise capacity in obese subjects with chronic ischaemic heart disease: a study in everyday practice," *Acta Cardiol* 63 (2008) 153-159.

47. P.A. Ades, P.D. Savage, M.J. Toth, J. Harvey-Bernio, D,J, Schneider, J.Y. Bunn, M.C. Audelin, M. Ludlow, "High-calorie-expenditure exercise: a new approach to cardiac rehabilitation for overweight coronary patients," *Circulation* 119 (2009) 2671-2678.

48. "Inflammation, Heart Disease and Stroke: The Role of C-Reactive Protein," American Heart Association http://www.americanheart.org/presenter.jhtml?identifier=4648

49. Ibid.

50. T.J. Marcell, K.A. McAuley, T. Traustadottir, P.D. Reaven, "Exercise training is not associated with improved levels of C-reactive protein or adiponectin," *Metab Clin Exp* 54 (2005) 533-541.

51. S.Y. Jae, B. Fernhall, K.S. Heffernan, M. Jeong, E.M. Chun, J. Sung, S.H. Lee, Y.J. Lim, W.H. Park, "Effects of lifestyle modifications on C-reactive protein: contribution of weight loss and improved aerobic capacity," *Metab Clin Exp* 55 (2006) 825-831.

52. G.D. Brinkworth, M. Noakes, J.D. Buckley, P.M. Clifton, "Weight loss improves heart rate recovery in overweight and obese men with features of the metabolic syndrome," *Am Heart J* 152 (2006) 693.e1-693.e6.

53. Y. Goldberg, M. Boaz, Z. Matas, I. Goldberg, M. Shargorodsky, "Weight loss induced by nutritional and exercise intervention decreases arterial stiffness in obese subjects," *Clin Nutr* 28 (2009) 21-25.

54. G.A. Kelley, K.S. Kelley, Z.V. Tran, "Aerobic exercise, lipids and lipoproteins in overweight and obese adults: a meta-analysis of randomized controlled trials," *Intl J Obes* 29 (2005) 881-893.

55. A.K. Yancey, A.J. Tomiyama, "Physical activity as primary prevention to address cancer disparities," *Sem Oncol Nurs* 23 (2007) 253-263.

56. K.L. Campbell, A. McTiernan, "Exercise and biomarkers for cancer prevention studies," *J Nutr* 137 (2007) 161S-169S.

57. K.L. Campbell, A. McTiernan, "Exercise and biomarkers for cancer prevention studies," *J Nutr* 137 (2007) 161S-169S.

58. H.J. Freedman, "Risk of gastrointestinal malignancies and mechanisms of cancer development with obesity and its treatment," *Best Prac Res Clin Gastro* 18 (2004) 1167-1175.

59. F. Bianchini, R. Kaaks, H. Vainio, "Overweight, obesity, and cancer risk," *Lancet Oncol* 3 (2002) 565-574.

60. W.C. Buschemeyer III, S.J. Freedland, "Obesity and prostate cancer: epidemiology and clinical implications," *Euro Urol* 52 (2007) 331-343.

61. A.R. Carmichael, T. Bates, "Obesity and breast cancer: a review of the literature," *Breast* 13 (2004) 85-92.

62. Ibid.

63. H. Kuhl, "Breast cancer risk in the WHI study: the problem of obesity," *Maturitas* 51 (2005) 83-97.

64. M. Wenten, F.D. Gilliland, K. Baumbartner, J.M. Samet, "Associations of weight, weight change, and body mass with breast cancer risk in Hispanic and non-Hispanic white women," *Ann Epidemiol* 12 (2002) 435-444.

65. D.J.P. Barker, P.D. Winter, C. Osmond, D.I.W. Phillips, H.Y. Sultan, "Weight gain in infancy and cancer of the ovary," *Lancet* 345 (1995) 1087-1088.

66. A.K. Yancey, A.J. Tomiyama, "Physical activity as primary prevention to address cancer disparities," *Sem Oncol Nurs* 23 (2007) 253-263.

67. P.A. Balch, *"Prescription for Nutritional Healing,"* 4th ed, (Ney York, NY: Avery, 2006) 359.

68. G.D. Zuidema, L. Schlossberg, *"The Johns Hopkins Atlas of Human Functional Anatomy,"* 4th ed, (Baltimore & London: The Johns Hopkins University Press, 1997) 79.

69. E.J. Applegate, *"The Anatomy & Physiology Learning System,"* 2nd ed, (Philadelphia, PA: Saunders, 2000) 222.

70. Ibid.

71. S.E. Black, E. Mitchell, P.S. Freedson, S.R. Chipkin, B. Braun, "Improved insulin action following short-term exercise training: role of energy and carbohydrate balance," *J App Physiol* 99 (2005) 2285-2293.

72. K. Anthony, L.J. Reed, J.T. Dunn, E. Bingham, D. Hopkins, P.K. Marsden, S.A. Amiel, "Attenuation of insulin-evoked responses in brain networks controlling appetite and reward in insulin resistance," *Diabetes* 55 (2006) 2986-2992.

73. C. Carver, "Insulin treatment and the problem of weight gain in type 2 diabetes," *Dia Ed* 32 (2006) 910-917.

74. A.S. Ryan, B.J. Nicklas, D.M. Berman, "Aerobic exercise is necessary to improve glucose utilization with moderate weight loss in women," *Obesity* 14 (2006) 1064-1072.

75. E. Klimcakova, J. Polak, C. Moro, J. Hejnova, M. Majercik, N. Viguerie, M. Berlan, D. Langin, V. Stich, "Dynamic strength training improves insulin sensitivity without altering plasma levels and gene expression of adipokines in subcutaneous adipose tissue in obese men," *J Clin Endocrin Metab* 91 (2006) 5107-5112.

76. V.B. O'Leary, C.M. Marchetti, R.J. Krishnan, B.P. Stetzer, F. Gonzalez, J.P. Kirwan, "Exercise-induced reversal of insulin resistance in obese elderly is associated with reduced visceral fat," *J App Physiol* 100 (2006) 1584-1589.

77. I. Giannopoulou, L.L. Ploutz-Snyder, R. Carhart, R.S. Weinstock, B. Fernhall, S. Goulopoulou, J.A. Kanaley, "Exercise is required for visceral fat loss in postmenopausal women with type 2 diabetes," *J Clin Endocrin Metab* 90 (2005) 1511-1518.

78. R.D. Telford, "Low physical activity and obesity: causes of chronic disease or simply predictors," *Med Sci Sports Exer* 39 (2007) 1233-1240.

79. E.P. Weiss, S.B. Racette, D.T. Villareal, L. Fontana, K. Steger-May, K.B. Schechtman, S. Klein, J. O'Holloszy, "Improvements in glucose tolerance and insulin action induced by increasing energy expenditure or decreasing energy intake: a randomized controlled trial," *Am J Clin Nutr* 84 (2006) 1033-1042.

80.   S.E. Black, E. Mitchell, P.S. Freedson, S.R. Chipkin, B. Braun, "Improved insulin action following short-term exercise training: role of energy and carbohydrate balance," *J App Physiol* 99 (2005) 2285-2293.

81.   H. Yokoyama, K. Mori, M. Emoto, T. Araki, M. Teranura, K. Mochizuki, T. Tashiro, K. Motozuka, Y. Inoue, Y. Nishizawa, "Non-oxidative glucose disposal is reduced and type 2 diabetes, but can be restored by aerobic exercise," *Dia Obes Metab* 10 (2008) 400-407.

82.   S.J. Lee, J.L. Kuk, L.E. Davidson, R. Hudson, K. Kilpatrick, T.E. graham, R. Ross, "Exercise without weight loss is an effective strategy for obesity reduction in obese individuals with and without type 2 diabetes," *J App Physiol* 99 (2005) 1220-1225.

83.   "Comorbid," *Dorland's Illustrated Medical Dictionary*, 30th ed: 397.

84.   M.F. McCarthy, "Optimizing exercise for fat loss," *Med Hypotheses* 44 (1995) 325-330.

85.   T.P.J. Solomon, S.N. Sistrun, R.K. Krishnan, L.F. Del Aguila, C.M. Marchetti, S.M. O'Carroll, V.B. O'Leary, J.P. Kirwan, "Exercise and diet enhance fat oxidation and reduce insulin resistance in older obese adults," *J App Physiol* 104 (2008) 1313-1319.

86.   J.J. Annesi, "Relations of mood with body mass index changes in severely obese women enrolled in a supported physical activity treatment," *Obes Facts* 1 (2008) 88-92.

87.   C.H. Hillman, K.I. Erickson, A.F. Kramer, "Be smart, exercise your heart: exercise effects on brain and cognition," *Nat Rev Neuroscience* 9 (2008) 58-65.

88.   L.S. Evangelista, L.V. Doering, T. Lennie, D.K. Moser, M.A. Hamilton, G.C. Fonarow, K. Dracup, "Usefulness of a home-based exercise program for overweight and obese patients with advanced heart failure," *Am J Cardiol* 97 (2008) 886-890.

89.   R.K. Dishman, H-R Berthoud, F.W. Booth, C.W. Cotman, V.R. Edgerton, M.R. Fleshner, S.C. Gandevia, F. Gomez- Pinilla, B.N. Greenwood, C.H. Hillman, A.F. Kramer, B.E. Levin, T.H. Moran, A.A. Russo-Neustadt, J.D. Salamone, J.D. Van Hoomissen, C.E. Wade, D.A. York, M.J. Zigmond, "Neurobiology of exercise," Obesity 14 (2006) 345-356.

90.   "Dementia," *Dorland's Illustrated Medical Dictionary*, 30th ed: 486.

91.   Ibid.

92.   "Atrophy," *Dorland's Illustrated Medical Dictionary*, 30th ed: 175.

93.   W. Jagust, "What can imaging revealed about obesity and the brain?" *Curr Alzheimer Res* 4 (2007) 135-139.

94.   Ibid.

95.   K.J. Stewart, A.C. Bacher, P.S. Hees, M. Tayback, P. Ouyang, S. J. de Beur, "Exercise effects on bone mineral density: relationships to changes in fitness and fatness," *Am J Prev Med* 28 (2005) 453-460.

96.   A. Vainionpaa, R. Korpelainen, H. Sievanen, E. Vihriala, J. Leppaluoto, T. Jamsa, "Effect of impact exercise and it's intensity on bone geometry at weight-bearing tibia and femur," *Bone* 40 (2007) 604-611.

97.   K.J. Stewart, A.C. Bacher, P.S. Hees, M. Tayback, P. Ouyang, S. J. de Beur, "Exercise effects on bone mineral density: relationships to changes in fitness and fatness," *Am J Prev Med* 28 (2005) 453-460.

98.   National Osteoporosis Foundation, Prevention exercise for health bones, http://www.nof.org/prevention/exercise.htm

99.   N.E. Silverman, B.J. Nicklas, A.S. Ryan, "Addition of aerobic exercise to a weight loss program increases BMD with an associated reduction in inflammation in overweight postmenopausal women," *Calcif Tissue Int* 84 (2009) 257-265.

100. The University of Arizona, Bone Builders, http://ag.arizona.edu/maricopa/fcs/bb/exercise.html
101. N.E. Silverman, B.J. Nicklas, A.S. Ryan, "Addition of aerobic exercise to a weight loss program increases BMD with an associated reduction in inflammation in overweight postmenopausal women," *Calcif Tissue Int* 84 (2009) 257-265.
102. A. Vainionpaa, R. Korpelainen, H. Sievanen, E. Vihriala, J. Leppaluoto, T. Jamsa, "Effect of impact exercise and it's intensity on bone geometry at weight-bearing tibia and femur," *Bone* 40 (2007) 604-611.
103. Ibid.
104. P.S. Hinton, R.S. Rector, T.R. Thomas, "Weight-bearing aerobic exercise increases markers of bone formation during short-term weight loss in overweight and obese men and women," *Metab Clin Exp* 55 (2006) 1616-1618.
105. K.J. Stewart, A.C. Bacher, P.S. Hees, M. Tayback, P. Ouyang, S. J. de Beur, "Exercise effects on bone mineral density: relationships to changes in fitness and fatness," *Am J Prev Med* 28 (2005) 453-460.
106. NASA exploration systems mission directorate education outreach, Weak in the knees - the quest for a cure, http://www.weboflife.nasa.gov/currentResearch/currentResearchGeneralArchives/weakKnees.htm
107. UC Newsroom, Astronaut's on International Space Station lose alarming amounts of hip bone strength, http://www.universityofcalifornia.edu/news/article/19371
108. K. Hind, M. Burrows, "Weight-bearing exercise and bone mineral accrual in children and adolescents: a review of controlled trials," *Bone* 40 (2007) 14-27.
109. Q. Wang, M. Alen, P. Nicholson, H. Suominen, A. Koistinen, H. Kroger, S. Cheng, "Weight-bearing, muscle loading and bone mineral accrual in pubertal girls: a 2-year longitudinal study," *Bone* 40 (2007) 1196-1202.
110. R.A. Bush, "Female high-school varsity athletics: an opportunity to improve bone mineral density," *J Sci Med Sport* 12 (2009) 366-370.
111. Ibid.
112. R. Rizzoli, M.L. Bianchi, M. Garabedian, H.A. McKay, L.A. Moreno, "Maximizing bone mineral mass gain during growth for the prevention of fractures in the adolescents and the elderly," *Bone* (2009) 1-12.
113. R.W. Braith, R.M. Mills, M.A. Welch, J.W. Keller, M.L. Pollock, "Resistance exercise training restores bone mineral density in heart transplant recipients," *J Am Coll Cardiol* 28 (1998) 1471-1477.
114. "Inflammation," *Dorland's Illustrated Medical Dictionary*, 30th ed: 930.
115. Cleveland Clinic, Inflammation: what you need to know, http://my.clevelandclinic.org/symptoms/Inflammation/hic_Inflammation_What_You_Need_To_Know.aspx
116. N. Perricone, *"The Perricone prescription,"* (New York, NY: *HarperCollins Publishers, Inc.,* 2002) 17.
117. B.J. Nicklas, W. Ambrosius, S.P. Messier, G.D. Miller, B. Penninx, R.F. Loeser, S. Palla, E. Bleecker, M. Pahor, "Diet-induced weight loss, exercise, and chronic inflammation in older, obese adults: a randomized controlled clinical trial." *Am J Clin Nutr* 79 (2004) 544-551.
118. J.K. Wegge, C.K. Roberts, T.H. Ngo, R.J. Barnard, "Effect of diet and exercise intervention on inflammatory and adhesion molecules in postmenopausal women on hormone replacement therapy and at risk for coronary artery disease," *Metabolism* 53 (2004) 377-381.
119. Ibid.

120. T. You, D.M. Berman, A.S. Ryan, B.J. Nicklas, "Effects of hypocaloric diet and exercise training on inflammation and adipocyte lipolysis in obese postmenopausal women," *J Clin Endocrin Metab* 89 (2004) 1739-1746.

121. I. Giannopoulou, B. Fernhall, R. Carhart, R.S. Weinstock, T. Baynard, A. Figueroa, J.A. Kanaley, "Effects of diet and/or exercise on the adipocytokine and inflammatory cytokine levels of postmenopausal women with type 2 diabetes," *Metab Clin Exp* 54 (2005) 866-875.

122. C.J.K. Hammett, H. Prapavessis, J.C. Baldi, N. Varo, U. Schoenbeck, R. Ameratunga, J.K. French, H.D. White, R.A.H. Stewart, "Effects of exercise training on 5 inflammatory markers associated with cardiovascular risk," *Am Heart J* 151 (2006) 367.e7-367.e16.

123. J.M. Bruun, J.W. Helge, B. Richelsen, B. Stallknecht, "Diet and exercise reduce low-grade inflammation and macrophage infiltration in adipose tissue but not in skeletal muscle in several obese subjects," *Am J Physiol Endocrin Metab* 290 (2006) E961-E967.

124. N.E. Silverman, B.J. Nicklas, A.S. Ryan, "Addition of aerobic exercise to a weight loss program increases BMD, with an associated reduction in inflammation in overweight postmenopausal women," *Calcif Tissue Int* 84 (2009) 257-265.

125. P.T. Williams, "The relationships of vigorous exercise, alcohol, and adiposity to low and high high-density lipoprotein-cholesterol levels," *Metabolism* 53 (2004) 700-709.

126. A. Weltman, J.Y. Weltman, D.D. Watson-Winfield, K. Frick, J. Patrie, P. Kok, D.M. Keenan, G.A. Gaesser, J.D. Veldhuis, "Effects of continuous versus intermittent exercise, obesity, and gender on growth hormone secretion," *J Clin Endocrin Metab* 93 (2008) 4711-4720.

127. B. Bruner, K. Chad, D. Chizen, "Effects of exercise and nutritional counseling in women with polycystic ovary syndrome," *App Physiol Nutr Metab* 31 (2006) 384-391.

128. "*Ace personal trainer manual-American Council on Exercise*," 3rd ed (San Diego, CA: *American Council on Exercise*, 2003) 9.

129. Ibid., 543.

130. Ibid., 543.

131. R.C. Browning, E.A. Baker, J.A. Herron, R. Kram, "Effects of obesity and sex on the energetic cost and preferred speed of walking," *J App Physiol* 100 (2006) 390-398.

132. Ibid.

133. C.R. Richardson, T.L. Newton, J.J. Abraham, A. Sen, M. Jimbo, A.M. Swartz, "A meta-analysis of pedometer-based walking interventions and weight loss," *Ann Fam Med* 77 (2008) 69-77.

134. S.G. Aldana, "*The culprit & the cure*," (Mapleton, UT: *Maple Mountain Press*, 2005) 161.

135. T. Okura, Y. Nakata, D.J. Lee, K. Ohkawara, K. Tanaka, "Effects of aerobic exercise and obesity phenotype on abdominal fat reduction in response to weight loss," *Intl J Obes* 29 (2005) 1259-1266.

136. T. You, K.M. Murphy, M.F. Lyles, J.L. Demons, L. Lenchik, B.J. Nicklas, "Addition of aerobic exercise to dietary weight loss preferentially reduces abdominal adipocyte size," *Intl J Obes* 30 (2006) 1211-1216.

137. T. Okura, Y. Nakata, D.J. Lee, K. Ohkawara, K. Tanaka, "Effects of aerobic exercise and obesity phenotype on abdominal fat reduction in response to weight loss," *Intl J Obes* 29 (2005) 1259-1266.

138. H.H. Dao, M.L. Frelut, G. Peres, P. Bourgeois, J. Navarro, "Effects of a multidisciplinary weight loss intervention on anaerobic and aerobic aptitudes in severely obese adolescents," *Intl J Obes* 28 (2004) 870-878.

139. P.T. Williams, "Vigorous exercise and the population distribution of body weight," *Intl J Obes* 28 (2004) 120-128.

140. *"Ace personal trainer manual-American Council on Exercise,"* 3rd ed (San Diego, CA: *American Council on Exercise*, 2003) 248.

141. K.H. Schmitz, P.J. Hannan, S.D. Stovitz, C.J. Bryan, M. Warren, M.D. Jensen, "Strength training and adiposity in premenopausal women: strong, healthy, and empowered study," *Am J Clin Nutr* 86 (2007) 566-572.

142. W.W. Campbell, M.D. Haub, R.R. Wolfe, A.A. Ferrando, D.H. Sullivan, J.W. Apolzan, H.B. Iglay, "Resistance training preserves fat-free mass without impacting changes in protein metabolism after weight loss in older women," *Obesity* 17 (2009) 1332-1339.

143. J.S. Volek, J.L. VanHeest, C.F. Forsythe, "Diet and exercise for weight loss: a review of current issues," *Sports Med* 35 (2005) 1-9.

144. R.J. Sigal, G.P. Kenny, D.H. Wasserman, C. Castaneda-Sceppa, R.D. White, Physical activity / exercise and type 2 diabetes," *Diabetes Care* 29 (2006) 1433-1438.

145. R.H. Demling, L. DeSanti, "Effect of a hypocaloric diet, increased protein intake and resistance training on lean muscle mass gains and fat mass loss in overweight police officers," *Ann Nutr Metab* 44 (2000) 21-29.

146. S.G. Aldana, *"The culprit & the cure,"* (Mapleton, UT: *Maple Mountain Press*, 2005) 141.

147. L. Di Pietro, J. Dziura, S.N. Blair, "estimated change in physical activity level (PAL) and prediction of 5-year weight change in men: the Aerobics Center longitudinal study," *Intl J Obes* 28 (2004) 1541-1547.

148. Ibid.

149. *"Ace personal trainer manual-American Council on Exercise,"* 3rd ed (San Diego, CA: *American Council on Exercise*, 2003) 13.

150. M. Miyashita, S.F. Burns, D.J. Stensel, "Exercise and postprandial lipemia: effect of continuous compared with intermittent activity patterns," *Am J Clin Nutr* 83 (2006) 24-29.

151. J. Ibanez, M. Izquierdo, I. Arguelles, L. Forga, J.L. Larrion, M. Garcia-Unciti, F. Idoate, E.M. Gorostiaga, "Twice-weekly progressive resistance training decreases abdominal fat and improves insulin sensitivity in older men with type 2 diabetes," *Diabetes Care* 28 (2005) 662-667.

152. R. Koga, M. Tanaka, H. Tsuda, K. Imai, S. Abe, T. Masuda, M. Iwamoto, E. Nakazono, T. Kamohara, T. Sakata, "Daily exercise fluctuations and dietary patterns during training predict visceral fat regain in obese women," *Am J Med Sci* 336 (2008) 450-457.

153. N.G. Boule, S.J. Weisnagel, T.A. Lakka, A. Tremblay, R.N. Bergman, T. Rankinen, A.S. Leon, J.S. Skinner, J.H. Wilmore, D.C. Rao, C. Bouchard, "Effects of exercise training on glucose homeostasis," *Diabetes Care* 28 (2005) 108-114.

154. G.E. Duncan, M.G. Perri, S.D. Anton, M.C. Limacher, A.D. Martin, D.T. Lowenthal, E. Arning, T. Bottiglieri, P.W. Stacpoole, "Effects of exercise on emerging and traditional cardiovascular risk factors," *Prev Med* 39 (2004) 894-902.

155. K.B. Osei-Tutu, P.D. Campagna, "The effects of short- versus long-bout exercise on mood, VO_{2max}, and percent body fat," *Prev Med* 40 (2005) 92-98.

156. Ibid.

157. B.A. Irving, C.K. Davis, D.W. Brock, J.Y. Weltman, D. Swift, E.J. Barrett, G.A. Gaesser, A. Weltman, "Effect of exercise training intensity on abdominal visceral fat and body composition," *Med Sci Sports Exer* 40 (2008) 1863-1872.

158. G.E. Duncan, M.G. Perri, S.D. Anton, M.C. Limacher, A.D. Martin, D.T. Lowenthal, E. Arning, T. Bottiglieri, P.W. Stacpoole, "Effects of exercise on emerging and traditional cardiovascular risk factors," *Prev Med* 39 (2004) 894-902.

159. B. Bahadori, M.F. McCarty, J. Barroso-Aranda, J.C. Gustin, F. Contreras, "A "mini-fast with exercise" protocol for fat loss," *Med Hypotheses* 73 (2009) 619-622.

160. E.G. Trapp, D.J. Chisholm, J. Freund, S.H. Boutcher, "The effects of high-intensity intermittent exercise training on fat loss and fasting insulin levels of young women," *Intl J Obes* 32 (2008) 684-691.

161. P.T. Williams, R.R. Pate, "Cross-sectional relationships of exercise and age to adiposity in 60,617 male runners," *Med Sci Sports Exer* 37 (2005) 1329-1337.

162. C.R. Bruce, A.B. Thrush, V.A. Mertz, V. Bezaire, A. Chabowski, G.J.F. Heigenhauser, D.J. Dyck, "Endurance training in obese humans improves glucose tolerance and mitochondrial fatty acid oxidation and alders muscle lipid content," *Am J Physiol Endocrin Metab* 291 (2006) E99-E107.

163. C.A. Slentz, B.D. Duscha, J.L. Johnson, K. Ketchum, L.B. Aiken, G.P. Samsa, J.A. Houmard, C.W. Bales, W.E. Kraus, "Effects of the amount of exercise on body weight, body composition, and measures of central obesity," *Arch Int Med* 164 (2004) 31-39.

164. L.C. Hawkley, R.A. Thisted, J.T. Cacioppo, "Loneliness predicts reduced physical activity: cross-sectional and longitudinal analysis," *Health Psych* 28 (2009) 354-363.

165. S.L. Volpe, H. Kobusingye, S. Bailur, E. Stanek, "Effect of diet and exercise on body composition, energy intake in leptin levels in overweight women and men," *J Am Coll Nutr* 27 (2008) 185-208.

166. R.C. Colley, A.P. Hills, T.M. O'Moore-Sullivan, I.J. Hickman, J.B. Prins, N.M. Byrne, "Variability in adherence to an unsupervised exercise prescription in obese women," *Intl J Obes* 32 (2008) 837-844.

167. J.L. Huberty, L.B. Ransdell, C. Sidman, J.A. Flohr, B. Shultz, O. Grosshans, L. Durrant, "Explaining long-term exercise adherence in women who complete a structured exercise program," *Res Qtly Exer Sport* 79 (2008) 374-384.

168. J.G. Alves, C.R. Gale, N. Mutrie, J.B. Correia, G.D. Batty, "A 6-month exercise intervention among inactive and overweight favela-residing women in Brazil: the Caranguejo exercise trial," *Am J Pub Health* 99 (2009) 76-80.

169. J.H. Rimmer, A. Rauworth, E. Wang, P.S. Heckerling, B.S. Gerber, "A randomized controlled trial to increase physical activity and reduce obesity in a predominantly African American group of women with mobility disabilities and severe obesity," *Prev Med* 48 (2009) 473-479.

170. S.L. Thomas, J. Hyde, A. Karunaratne, R. Kausman, P.A. Komesaroff, "They all work…when you stick to them: a qualitative investigation of dieting, weight loss, and physical exercise, in obese individuals," *Nutr J* 7 (2008) 1-7.

171. P.J. Teixeira, S.B. Going, L.B. Houtkooper, E.C. Cussler, L.L. Metcalfe, R.M. Blew. L.B. Sardinha, T.G. Lohman," Exercise motivation, eating, and body image variables as predictors of weight control," *Med Sci Sports Exer* 38 (2006) 179-188.

172. C. Kerksick, A. Thomas, B. Campbell, L. Taylor, C. Wilborn, B. Marcello, M. Roberts, E. Pfau, M. Grimstvedt, J. Opusunju, T. Magrans-Courtney, C. Rasmussen, R. Wilson, R.B. Kreider, "Effects of a popular exercise and weight loss program on weight loss, body composition, energy expenditure and helped in obese women," *Nutr Metab* 6 (2009) 1-17.

173. C.L. Dunn, P.J. Hannan, R.W. Jeffery, N.E. Sherwood, N.P. Pronk, R. Boyle, "The comparative and cumulative effects of a dietary restriction and exercise on weight loss," *Intl J Obes* 30 (2006) 112-121.

174. J.M. Jakicic, B.H. Marcus, W. Lang, C. Janney, "Effect of exercise on 24-month weight loss maintenance in overweight women," *Arch Int Med* 168 (2008) 1550-1559.

175. S. Phelan, M. Roberts, W. Lang, R.R. Wing, "Empirical evaluation of physical activity recommendations for weight control in women," *Med Sci Sports Exer* 39 (2007) 1832-1836.
176. J.E. Donnelly, B. Smith, D.J. Jacobsen, E. Kirk, K. DuBose, M. Hyder, B. Bailey, R. Washburn, "The role of exercise for weight loss and maintenance," *Best Prac Res Clin Gastroent* 18 (2004) 1009-1029.
177. N. Villanova, F. Pasqui, S. Burzacchini, G. Forlani, R. Manini, A. Suppini, N. Melchionda, G. Marchesini, "A physical activity program to reinforce weight maintenance following a behavior program in overweight / obese subjects," *Intl J Obes* 30 (2006) 697-703.
178. K. Samaras, P.J. Kelly, M.N. Chiano, T.D. Spector, L.V. Campbell, "Genetic and environmental influences on total-body and central abdominal fat:: the effect of physical activity in female twins," *Ann Intern Med* 30 (1999) 873-882.

5   Psychological Aspects of Weight Loss

For most people the strongest driving force for a weight loss program is their appearance. "Body image dissatisfaction (BID) has been identified as the most consistent psychosocial consequence of obesity."[1] This obsession with body appearance, as it relates to weight loss, has led researchers to focus primarily on girls and to neglect boys. The majority of the studies have either not found significant levels of body image dissatisfaction for males or have excluded them all together as being not important enough for study. While study data makes clear that both males and females consider obesity unacceptable, boys are frequently dissatisfied with being too thin.[2] We have been programmed by all forms of advertising to believe beauty must be attained at all cost. Less frequently health issues prompt individuals to attempt weight loss. As previously stated weight loss and health improvement are inseparable, so whatever the real motivating factor is for weight loss, both the appearance and health goals can and must be accomplished at the same time.

There is a large body of psychological study data that will be discussed in the following sections, but before I do that let's take a look at how obesity and psychology might be intertwined. There is evidence demonstrating an increased risk of mental and psychological disorders in obese individuals.[3] These mental disorders are usually a dysregulation of the body's stress systems. The different relationships between obesity and mental disorders suggest a complex etiological pathway,[4] (etiology is the causes or origin of a disease or disorder). Multiple or simultaneously occurring mental disorders in obese individuals are associated with an increased use of the healthcare system and a lower quality of life.[5] Some have attempted to explain being overweight and depressed, especially among the highly educated, may be the result of poor health.[6]

There have been conflicting findings as to whether or not emotional disorders caused by obesity are confined to women. Some studies have found only women are affected by obesity related emotional disorders.[7] Additional studies have demonstrated overweight women report a lower quality of life because of their obesity, they are less likely to experience enjoyment in pleasurable experiences and activities and they are often targets of public ridicule and discrimination.[8] In plain words "obese women appear to internalize the negative perceptions toward obesity held by society and to devaluate themselves."[9] Young overweight and obese women are at particular risk for developing a depressive disorder. Merwe argues both drugs and psychotherapy should be adopted as part of the clinical treatment strategy.[10] "Health professional delivered, individual information-based weight control programs are the most popular among young adult women. Tailoring the content and delivery mode of weight management programs to match consumer preferences may enhance program participation and adherence."[11]

It has been suggested that there is no sex difference in the association between obesity and either mood or anxiety disorders.[12] Two reasons have been suggested as to why there seem to be less obesity related mood or anxiety disorders in men, either: (1) they have fewer emotional disorders, or (2) they just report fewer of them. Statistically it may appear women are the only sex having obesity induced emotional difficulties while in fact that may be an inaccurate conclusion.

Additionally, "body image dissatisfaction and disordered eating problems are common among children and adolescents. A variety of factors are associated with the development of these problems including social reinforcement, conflictual family relationships, low self-esteem and among girls, early puberty."[13] A dual pathway model has been suggested for understanding the causes of body dissatisfaction and eating disorders in girls. The first pathway is the *Restraint Pathway*, which "involves internalization of social ideals about beauty and thinness."[14] These ideals lead to "dieting behavior in response to the discrepancy between the individual's actual body shape and the ideal body shape promoted by society."[15] The second pathway is the *Interpersonal Vulnerability Pathway*, which begins with inadequate parental nurturing, leading to disturbances in self-image and social functioning. "Body image dissatisfaction and disordered eating then arises in response to feelings of ineffectiveness."[16] While disordered eating and body dissatisfaction can arise from either pathway they most often arise as a result of the combination of both.

As disturbing as it may seem, there is evidence suggesting temperament traits can contribute to the accumulation of body fat in childhood. For example, "negative mood has been found to predict increased weight gain in infants between six and twelve months old."[17] "It has been shown children with high levels of aggressiveness and impulsivity are likely to engage in risky lifestyles, including smoking and alcohol abuse as adults. Furthermore, it is known that impatience and aggressiveness are risk factors for excess caloric intake and a sedentary lifestyle."[18] Finally, these health-related behaviors have been associated with abdominal body fat.[19]

One of the major missing links in many weight loss programs is the search to find what really created the overweight condition in the first place. Often it is a deep-seated and difficult to identify psychological struggle. Without finding this link and taking the necessary steps to correct it, diets and exercise are destined to failure. Many people struggle with a variety of psychological issues having a direct impact on their body weight. Some have failed relationships, others have excessive family or job stress, still others have self-esteem issues and the list goes on and on. The goal of this chapter is to help you: (1) understand the role psychological dysfunction can have in obesity, (2) find the resources necessary to solve this dilemma, and (3) resolve the underlying issues. In determining your readiness for a weight-loss program one question needs an honest answer. Is this the right time to attempt weight loss? It may take professional help to resolve any underlying issues.

As you tackle weight loss it will quickly become evident setting proper goals is critical to the success of any weight loss endeavor. First, unrealistic weight loss goals undermine the effort. Goals aimed at losing a defined amount of weight are generally far less effective than goals directed towards monitoring of body weight, weight control behaviors, dietary habits and physical activity.[20] Given the high rates of attrition and noncompliance in weight loss programs, it seems imperative health care professionals understand the disparities between beliefs and behaviors.[21]

How the Brain Affects Weight Loss

The brain is an extremely complex organ. Eating disorders are one of the problems that originate there. It is unlikely eating disorders are the result of abnormalities in only a specific area of the brain. It is more realistic to believe several components of the brain play an integrated role in eating disorders.[22] There is a lot more on eating disorders later in this chapter.

"The brain activates an energy-on-demand system that directly couples cerebral supply with cerebral need."[23] This system initiates one or more of three different behaviors. They are:

- "Allocation Behavior (i.e. allocation of energy from body to brain),"[24]
- "Ingestive Behavior (intake of energy from the immediate environment),"[25]
- "Exploratory Behavior (foraging in the distant environment)."[26]

All three behaviors ensure a continuous energy supply to the brain. Disruption of this energy supply is vital to the development of obesity.[27] "If the brain fails to receive sufficient energy from the peripheral body, it compensates for the undersupply by increasing energy intake from the immediate environment, leaving the body with a surplus."[28] In the long run the results are obesity.

Frequently it is thought the metabolic process takes place in a variety of different places in the body. In reality metabolism does not go on independently in different organs or tissues, but rather takes place in a coordinated and regulated manner throughout the body. Regulation of the metabolic process requires a vast amount of communication between the various organs and tissues, all of which is orchestrated by the brain and central nervous system. The brain obtains a variety of metabolic information from the organs and tissues, where that information is integrated, processed and then transmitted back, as regulatory signals necessary for controlling the metabolic process. "In addition to its role in digestion and the absorption of nutrients, the gut has an important role in regulating energy homeostasis. Neural and hormonal signals from the gut transmit information to specific areas of the brain...regarding energy status."[29] "Disturbance of this coordinated control system may be implicated in the development of metabolic disorders, such as obesity."[30]

The hypothalamus is the area of the brain most critical to the regulation of food intake and metabolism, with many nuclei interconnecting the different parts of the hypothalamus. Appetite is then regulated by an intricate system of signals that interact with one another in order to modulate the response to nutrient intake.[31]

Existing simultaneously in the brain are two different types of tissues, which are referred to as *Gray Matter* and *White Matter*. The gray matter in the brain appears to correlate positively with the various abilities and skills we possess, while the speed with which we process information is governed by the white matter.[32] In computer terminology, the various compartments of gray matter in our brains represent a group of computers, while our white matter represents the networking cables connecting the computers. The volume of white matter in the brains of obese individuals is greater than it is in lean individuals and it has been shown as the volume of white matter increases so does the risk of cognitive decline; for example, as we gain weight the risks increase for acquiring Alzheimer's disease and Parkinson's disease.[33] We also experience atrophy of the temporal lobes of the brain and smaller hippocampal volumes as we age. Increased body fat has also been shown to have detrimental effects on brain integrity and function. Obesity is also relevant because studies have found worse learning, declining memory and executive functioning in obese older adults and alterations in brain form and structure in overweight young adults.[34]

The mechanisms underlying these complex relationships are not well understood, but one possible link between obesity and dementing diseases is the development of insulin resistance and/or diabetes, which ultimately affect cognition.[35] To complicate matters further, higher leptin levels typically accompany obesity and are correlated with less gray matter in the brain than had previously been implicated in obesity.[36] Also a significant negative correlation exists between BMI and the volume of gray matter in the brains of men, but not in women.[37]

The sensations of hunger or fullness originate in the central nervous system. The hypothalamus and brainstem are critical regions of the brain that receive messages from a variety of sources. The gastrointestinal tract is one of those message sources. It plays a vital role in the regulation of food intake and energy balance. "Signals from the gastrointestinal tract generally function to limit ingestion in the interest of efficient digestion. These signals may be released into the bloodstream or may activate afferent neurons that carry information to the brain and its cognitive centres [sic], which regulates food intake."[38] The main appetite-stimulating hormone produced in the gastrointestinal tract is grehlin. Researchers claim it may not be long before drugs are available that counteract this hormone and trick the brain into believing we are full, even though less than sufficient calories have been consumed.[39]

Another source of messages to the brain and central nervous system is the eyes. Evidence suggests there are regions of the brain that perform a food reward function.[40] In obese individuals visual stimulation with food activates regions in the brain related to reward anticipation and learning. In addition, high calorie food images activate regions of the brain associated with the processing of taste, motivation and functioning of the emotions and memory. These results suggest apart from the physiological need to eat, the obese person may in fact be driven to eat by visual stimuli alone.[41] In fact it has been shown simply thinking about food can activate specific brain areas known to be involved in appetite control.[42] Even without real food, food cues that have been previously identified with specific foods may stimulate a hunger response.[43]

The hormone and neurotransmitter dopamine modulates reward circuitry and motivational processing and is known to regulate food intake. Ironically, the obese individual is similar to a drug addict because both show significantly reduced dopamine receptor availability, which is negatively correlated with BMI.[44] The action of dopamine is based on the satisfaction of food properties, such as, food palatability[45] and fat content.[46] It has also been shown high calorie foods tend to activate the emotional responses of obese people more than they do lean people. "Overeating in obese individuals is triggered by an exaggerated reactivity to stimuli associated with high-calorie foods."[47]

The bottom line is individual differences and rewards may lead to over consumption of certain foods relative to what the body truly requires. It has been suggested some people may experience an exaggerated pleasure seeking response to palatable foods, and since those foods are more satisfying than others, they are eaten in greater amounts for longer periods of time. In addition some people may not be able to experience pleasure from food and therefore tend to over eat in an attempt to reach satisfaction. Other individuals may have a diminished ability to resist the motivation to eat when they are full which may promote an unbalanced eating pattern. And last of all, some people may choose highly palatable, energy dense foods out of habit, which ultimately promotes over consumption and an excessive caloric intake.[48]

The consumption of certain foods has been shown to be an activity that reinforces the brain.[49] This makes a lot of sense intuitively sense sweets, for example, taste good and are reinforcing. Generally individuals who find food to be a highly reinforcing item may consume more food during eating than those who do not get the same reinforcing satisfaction. "Obese individuals may find food more reinforcing and may be more motivated to eat than normal weight individuals."[50] "The same brain areas associated with alcohol and drug addiction may be related to food cravings as well since there are many overlaps in characteristics of these cravings."[51]

There is a variety of lesser known but potentially very important brain to bodyweight related topics, some or all of which could be helpful in a weight loss program. Here are some important ones:

- There is synergy between central obesity and hypertension as they relate to cognition. The control of central obesity and hypertension in young and middle aged adults may be advantageous in helping maintain sound cognitive function later in life.[52]

- Emotions play an important part in body weight regulation. Research data reveals positive emotions tend to drive people to consume healthy foods and negative emotions tend to drive unhealthy food consumption. Additionally, meals eaten by people experiencing positive or negative moods are generally larger than the same meals eaten during a neutral mood.[53] "Certain moods such as anger or joy have been found to have a greater influence on eating than sadness or fear."[54] Simply put "mood affects food cravings and the amount and type of food consumed."[55]

- In some parts of the world, India for example, marijuana has been used as a treatment for the loss of appetite and to overcome hunger pangs. It was determined an endocannabinoid system within the body exists to serve a variety of purposes. One of those purposes is to participate in the process of energy balance beginning with the stimulation of food intake, passing through the stage of intestinal absorption and ending with the energy storage and energy conservation. This system appears to maximize the intake of high-energy foods and redirect energy balance towards fat metabolism in the fat tissue. If this system becomes dysfunctional it can lead the body into a number of metabolic disorders, one of them being obesity.[56]

- Leptin is a hormone produced in the fat cells that reports nutritional information to the brain. A high-level of triglycerides, usually a factor in obesity, has been found to play an active role in leptin resistance. Triglycerides may impair the movement of leptin across the blood brain barrier. By lowering triglycerides the related cognitive impairment can be improved and oxidative stress on the brain can be reduced.[57]

- The vagas nerve is one of 12 cranial nerves that carry information back-and-forth between the brain and major organs of the body. The vagas nerve has long been linked to neurological systems associated with hunger and satiety and it plays a central role in the short-term regulation of food intake.[58] There is evidence in humans stimulation of the vagas nerve can be used to impact eating behavior and weight loss.[59]

- There is one little known but rapidly emerging technology referred to as *Mind Technology*. The purpose of mind technology devices is to stimulate the brain in a way that challenges it to function optimally. They work by using light, sound, motion, electrical energy, and in some cases silence, to stimulate the brain. Among their many claims are they have the potential to reduce stress, produce deep relaxation, boost IQ, enhance creativity, accelerate learning, increased memory, increased sexual pleasure, produce peak performance states, eliminate substance abuse, overcome depression and anxiety, alleviate pain, boost immune function and change or eliminate unwanted habits and attitudes. If a lot of our overeating or unwanted eating behaviors are the result of a desire to relieve anxiety or stress, which we will discuss later, then the use of mind technology to stimulate the brain's natural reward system may be extremely beneficial in controlling body weight.[60]

Stress

The topic of stress as it relates to overweight or obesity is an interesting one. "Chronic stress has been associated with an accumulation of excess body fat, particularly in the abdominal region in humans."[61] There is a lot of acceptance among the general population that weight gain, oftentimes a large weight gain, especially around the midsection, is part of the aging process. Some researchers agree with that idea, describing visceral obesity (i.e. fat that accumulates around internal organs, especially the abdomen) as a Civilization Syndrome.[62]

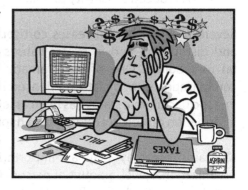

In addition, whenever the topic of stress comes up, in weight loss conversations among psychological researchers, the following conversations usually do as well.

The first is about the function and affect of the *hypothalamic-pituitary-adrenal (HPA) axis*. Whenever a physical or psychological stress impinges upon the body the hypothalamus produces a hormone called corticotrophin releasing factor (CRF), discussed in more detail in the chapter on hormones. CRF in turn stimulates the pituitary gland to produce adrenocorticotropic hormone (ACTH). ACTH in turn stimulates the adrenals to produce cortisol.

The HPA axis determines most of the long-term effects of stressors. Each of us has our own specific combination of heredity factors, personality characteristics, life experience and coping ability, all of which results in the meaning we attach to any event. People suffering from anxiety, depression, a low standard of living, a low level of education or are unemployed are more likely to become the victim of frequent challenges of the HPA axis.[63] "Subjects with increased visceral fat accumulation are frequently characterized as anxious or depressed and they often consume rather large amounts of alcohol, tobacco and drugs."[64] The primary factor in this chain of negative metabolic events is an excess excitement of the HPA axis, resulting from a defeatist approach to psychosocial stress.[65]

The second is about the hormone cortisol, which is produced by the adrenals, and involved in the response to stress. It is often referred to as the *Stress Hormone*, because it is secreted in higher levels during the body's *Fight or Flight Response* to stress and is responsible for several stress related changes in the body. Whenever the adrenals dump cortisol into the bloodstream, the body experiences:

- A quick burst of energy,
- Heightened memory functions,
- Increased immunity,
- A reduced sensitivity to pain.

Severe mental stress increases cortisol. Cortisol regulates fat tissue differentiation, function and distribution and in excess causes abdominal obesity. It also exerts chronic effects on fat metabolism. One of the dramatic effects cortisol has on humans is the characteristic centralization of body fat experienced in Cushing Syndrome.[66] Finally, perceived stress from a low socioeconomic status has been associated with an elevated cortisol level. For more detailed information on cortisol refer to the chapter on hormones.[67]

Mental stress may play an important role in obesity. For example, job-related stress, organizational level, amount of personal control and imbalances between effort and reward all correlate negatively with BMI.[68] However, other studies claim the opposite. High busyness but low control over the job and low busyness with high control over the job were found to increase weight gain, thus concluding both job busyness and control over ones job are independent risk factors for weight gain.[69] There may be a "bi-directional effect of work related stress on BMI among men. While stress seems to result in weight gain among overweight and obese male employees, weight loss is more likely among their lean colleagues."[70] Similarly "stressful situations can impair reproductive axis function, by reducing…sex hormones, particularly androgens, can regulate adipose tissue development…and lean muscle tissue growth."[71] As a result, "age associated decreases of sex hormones in humans are a risk factor for obesity in the elderly. Taken together these data suggest that stress and sex hormones are important in influencing the metabolic profile of an organism."[72] In addition, stressful situations frequently promote disturbed eating behavior in obese individuals.[73] Finally, poor cardiovascular recovery from mental stress is an indicator of an increase in abdominal obesity in men and women.[74]

"In the face of adversity, poor coping skills may lead to a rise in stress, which in turn may result in a reduction in dietary restraint, forming a spiral relationship and ultimately leading to weight gain."[75] "Traditional behavioral interventions include cognitive restructuring, stress management techniques, self-monitoring and social support."[76] Since we cannot avoid stressors entirely, our ability to effectively deal with them moderates the effect these stresses have on weight gain. Simultaneously improving our coping skills and reducing our caloric intake enhances our chance of success.[77]

One body weight related behavior that is definitely affected by stress is eating behavior.[78] "When stressed some individuals increase their food consumption, which can lead to obesity and all the health problems associated with it. Other individuals decrease their intake when stressed producing other adverse health effects."[79] Stress also has an effect on health by affecting which foods people choose to eat. When people are stressed they tend to overeat foods they normally would avoid for weight control or health reasons. Stress causes people to lose the control they usually exert to prevent themselves from eating food they believe is fattening or unhealthy.[80]

When people are stressed they tend to eat high caloric, sweet and fatty snack foods.[81] In fact research has found cravings for sweet foods are often associated with depression.[82] People who are depressed or under stress frequently over eat high caloric snack foods in an attempt to feel better. In addition, people who attempt to decrease their caloric intake during stressful situations show an increased interest in junk food.[83] It is interesting to note that, "eating a snack has no effect on how much is consumed in a subsequent meal,"[84] as a result total caloric intake often rises when a lot of snacks are consumed. Ironically, the consumption of fat in the diet decreases anxiety related behavior and helps the person recover from stress.[85] The problem is fat has a higher number of calories per gram than either protein or carbohydrates and as a result over consumption can easily lead to weight gain.

Stressful situations can cause some people to eat what has been referred to as comfort foods. The consumption of comfort food by men is motivated by positive emotions, whereas the consumption of comfort food by women is motivated by negative emotions. Women frequently find consumption of comfort foods alleviates their negative emotions but may also produce guilt. Age may also play a part in the use of comfort foods. Elderly individuals find the positive benefits that come from eating comfort foods, provides a particularly powerful trigger for their use. While on the other hand younger participants tend to report more intense negative emotions prior to the use of comfort foods. As discussed above, foods high in sugar and fat are best for relieving negative effects whereas low-calorie foods increase positive emotions.[86]

Restrained eating is the conscious effort made by people to restrict their food intake to control their body weight. "Restrained eaters tend to increase and unrestrained eaters tend to decrease their food intake when stressed."[87] "Behavioral and physiological data suggest that restrained eating may be a risk factor for vulnerability to weight gain."[88]

Consider how stress vis-à-vis weight gain relates to various individuals. A high level of stress predicts major weight gain in men. A low level of life satisfaction and a highly neurotic personality tend to be risk factors for weight gain in older women. High levels of extroverted behavior are related to a decreased risk of major weight gain in young men. Interestingly, these findings tend to weaken over time.[89] The "parents of children recently diagnosed with cancer reported significant psychological distress and experienced weight gains over three months compared to weight stability in non-stressed parents."[90]

Visceral fat has been shown to be a contributor to stress, which indicates visceral fat accumulation represents a physiological adaptation to stress. Although the available literature does not make it clear which comes first, obesity or stress, obesity treatment should include stress management strategies if one is to be successful with weight management.[91]

Depression

Depression as it relates to overweight and obesity is a controversial topic. A lot of literature discusses whether or not obesity and depression have a direct relationship. While there is no simple connection between obesity and either depression or anxiety,[92] there are statistics demonstrating people suffering from depression are as much as 60 percent more likely to be obese than their non-depressed counterparts.[93] Because there is conflicting evidence as to whether or not obesity causes depression, that may be the 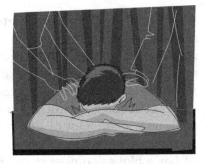 reason why there are no psychosomatic diseases listed among the conditions identified in the metabolic syndrome, discussed in the introduction.

There are some important terms discussed in the literature I want you to be familiar with. The researchers talk about, *adjustment disorder*, *depressed mood*, *depression* and *major depressive disorder (MDD)*. Here is what they mean.

The symptoms of adjustment disorder and depressed mood are normally one and the same. They usually begin in response to some specific stressful situation. The symptoms are usually milder than they are in other forms of clinical depression; nevertheless they are severe enough they interfere with a person's ability to function normally. The symptoms only last a short time after the stressful situation ends, usually disappearing within a few months. A person may be suffering from adjustment disorder or a depressed mood if the depressed state is in excess of what the average person might have experienced. They may have simply overreacted to the circumstances. A person suffering from these symptoms may or may not require treatment. It should be noted that drugs, alcohol and medications also cause a depressed mood.

Depression is often referred to as *major depression, unipolar depression, clinical depression* or simply *depression*. It is a mental disorder frequently characterized by a low mood, loss of interest in a person's usual activities and a diminished ability to experience pleasure. One study team defines depression, "as a mental state characterized by feelings of sadness, loneliness, despair, low self-esteem and self-reproach, is greater among women than men."[94] A person suffering from depression frequently requires a clinical diagnosis and treatment.

Arguments "In Favor of" a Relationship Between Obesity and Depression

Many studies purport to find a relationship between obesity and depression.[95] One of the most recent and comprehensive reviews of obesity vis-à-vis depression provides a compelling argument for the potentially reciprocal relationship between the two.[96] Some say there is definitely a relationship between obesity and depression, but the form of the association may be different between males and females.[97] The relationship between depression and obesity is dependent on gender, age and race. Here is some interesting data:

- Young obese women are more likely to be depressed than young non-obese women,
- Young overweight but not obese men are more likely to be depressed than non-overweight and non-obese men,
- Young obese Hispanic women have been shown to be more prone to depression than non-obese women in general.[98]

Studies lend support to the hypothesis that there are shared factors between recurrent depression, obesity and a variety of other physical disorders (e.g. asthma, thyroid disease). One example, elevated cortisol is a frequent finding in depression and it may be a link between obesity and depression.[99] A computerized tomography scan has been used to analyze the abdomens of patients suffering from depression, with the result being they showed an elevated level of visceral fat accumulation.[100] An association also exists between elevated levels of total body weight and depression,[101] consequently "the obese appear to be at risk for depression."[102] People with extreme obesity are at increased risk of depression and impaired health related quality of life.[103] In fact these individuals have a 1.5 fold increase in the risk of depression compared with persons of average weight, which could not be accounted for by differences in age, education, health or dieting history.[104] In both black and white adolescent girls, depression appears to be a predictor of obesity and elevated BMI.[105]

Theories have been offered to explain the relationship between obesity and mental health, particularly depression. They include the possible role of psychological, sociological and biological factors. Research has suggested two possible theories. The first theory called the "*Reflected Self-Appraisal Perspective*, argues that the stigma toward and devaluation of the obese may cause overweight individuals to suffer lower self-esteem, have more negative self-images, think others dislike them and have higher levels of depression."[106] The second theory called the "*Fitting the Norms of Appearance Perspective*, argues that for those who are obese fitting the norm for weight is stressful because dieting is stressful rather than obesity per se."[107] This of course could be the case because so often a dietary approach to weight loss is unsuccessful.

Some researchers subscribe to the theory obesity might be related to depression through the consumption of nutrients that could affect depression, since the consumption of carbohydrates appears to affect depression.[108] A supporting study compared a low protein high carbohydrate (LPHC) diet to a high-protein low carbohydrate (HPLC) diet. The results clearly showed the high-protein low carbohydrate diet related closely to improvement in depression and self-esteem.[109]

Arguments "Against" a Relationship Between Obesity and Depression

Although there are a variety of studies that claim there is no relationship between obesity and depression, little is known about that relationship. Gilmore studied this relationship but failed to clearly show a significant relationship between weight and depression except among overweight and obese former smokers.[110]

An interesting concept is that of *Cynical Hostility*. The word cynical as it is used in the research literature means a lack of confidence in or bitterness with other people. One study noted high levels of depression predict weight gain and weight loss, while evaluation for cynical hostility did not demonstrate any weight change. It was also felt that even though depressive symptoms predicted the possibility of either weight gain or weight loss, an evaluation and understanding of mood may be important among persons who are interested in losing weight or preventing obesity.[111] Other experts disagreed, finding education moderates a positive association of cynical hostility in obesity among women but not among men; in fact cynical hostility was not even observed among highly educated women. "A successful educational career includes rewards and feelings of success that may create stronger self-esteem, protecting obese well-educated individuals from the psychological consequences of negative views towards obese persons."[112] Depression and cynical hostility are generally regarded as psychological factors that are influenced by a host of other factors, with obesity being only one of them.

Another interesting hypothesis is called the *Jolly Fat Hypothesis*. One of the early proponents of the Jolly Fat Hypothesis was German physicist Ernest Kretschmer. In 1931 he suggested heavy people are jolly, friendly and gregarious suggesting a greater BMI is associated with a reduced risk of major psychiatric disturbances, but in contradiction he found his schizophrenic patients were tall and thin rather than obese.[113] Other findings suggest, "(BMI) measured in middle age is inversely associated with the risk of subsequent hospital admissions for psychosis and depression/anxiety."[114] A higher (BMI) in postmenopausal women with lower education has been associated with decreased depressive symptoms.[115]

There are still other relationships between obesity and depression. One of those is diet. Being on a diet can tend to worsen mood in a couple of ways: (1) as mentioned earlier excess consumption of carbohydrates can add to a depressed mood, and (2) the simple act of restricting calories has been associated with irritability.[116] A negative relationship between obesity and depression can occur when psychotropic drugs are taken for depression because of an elevated risk of weight gain.[117] Antidepressants cause weight gain, especially tri-cyclic antidepressants, monoamine-oxidase inhibitors, and selective serotonin reuptake inhibitors.[118]

Here's an outlandish thought. "There is consistent evidence…that people with dementia are more likely to have had earlier depression."[119] If there is a cause and effect relationship between obesity and depression it is reasonable to believe in cases of long-term obesity, with related depression, the obesity could be the driving force for the depression.

It is known that part of the aging process is the development of inflammation in the body. There is a growing body of evidence linking depressive symptoms with the inflammatory process.[120] It stands to reason if depressive symptoms can result from obesity then by reversing the obesity we should be able to reduce the inflammation and perhaps slow the aging process.

It has also been shown C-reactive protein is one of the biological markers used for diagnosing and monitoring coronary heart disease. There is increasing evidence fat tissue releases various proteins and cytokines that may be an important factor in determining the risk of coronary heart disease. In addition, the levels of C-reactive protein concentrations and cytokines are significantly related to obesity. Anxiety and a depressed mood are also related to high levels of protein and increased cytokine secretion.[121] What this tells us is obesity is one of the drivers for an abnormally high level of C-reactive protein and a larger than normal amount of pro-inflammatory markers, all resulting in a depressed mood and increased risk of coronary heart disease.

No evaluation of depression would be complete without a brief discussion about the impact it has on suicide. "Mental illness, particularly depression has been linked to obesity,"[122] even though the association between obesity and suicide shows limited supporting study data. On the other hand (Class III) obesity is significantly associated with attempted suicide and when compared to the general population extremely obese individuals demonstrate a significantly increased risk for attempted suicide.[123] However, a higher BMI is strongly associated with a lower risk of suicide mortality among men.[124] Notice the subtle distinction between the choice of the words (attempted suicide) and (suicide mortality) in these two studies.

There is also an interesting body of evidence dealing with how obesity in pre-menopausal and postmenopausal women relates to depression. It has been shown female adolescent obesity is associated with an increased risk of major depressive disorder and other anxiety disorders.[125] In fact, the risk is about four times greater, but the same does not hold true for boys.[126] It isn't surprising females in Western society would be more vulnerable than males to the psychosocial consequences of obesity given the great social pressure they are under to remain thin.[127] "Adolescent females at any weight tend to have greater body dissatisfaction and to rate their body image lower than do adolescent males."[128] A depressed mood is associated with an increase in visceral abdominal fat in overweight pre-menopausal women.[129] As far as postmenopausal women are concerned, depression contributes to an accumulation of abdominal fat.[130]

Finally, "it is important to evaluate and treat depression in persons who seek medical treatment for severe obesity and it may be that routine screening for depression should be promoted as the standard of care for these patients."[131] Some go further claiming one in two people who registered for a dietary treatment program showed some symptoms of depression. "These symptomatic participants were more concerned about shape, weight and eating; had a more restrained eating style; lower self-esteem; and a higher BMI than non-depressed participants."[132] "Obesity and the related conditions overweight and abdominal obesity, are common problems in persons seeking treatment for certain mood disorders, especially childhood-onset major depression and bipolar disorder."[133]

Eating Disorders

The subject of eating disorders is a fairly large and encompassing topic that is comprised of many psychological factors. Even though eating disorders often result in weight loss, they are devastating to personal health, which obviously makes them undesirable. I will discuss them here so you will know the dominant signs. There are a variety of eating disorders, although they are different, they have related patterns. "A combination of interpersonal and weight related problems, together with dieting behavior, constitutes the main risk factor for the emergence of eating disorders."[134]

The main characteristics of the two most prevalent eating disorders, anorexia and bulimia are: (1) dysfunctional patterns of eating behavior and weight regulation, (2) unusual attitudes toward weight and shape, and (3) abnormal perceptions of body shape.[135] There are a number of specific factors that appear to be necessary for the development of an eating disorder:

- "It is difficult to imagine developing an ED without the presence of body dissatisfaction, although the majority of individuals who are dissatisfied with their bodies will never go on to develop an ED."[136]
- Depression, anxiety and a low self-esteem are also recognized as important factors in eating disorders.
- Environmental stressors and distortions of reality, like obsessive thinking seem to be factors.
- Maladjusted personality features like a need for control have been suggested as necessary components for an eating disorder.[137]

"Both men and women frequently attempt to change the shape of their bodies,"[138] although the pursuit of the ideal body shape, has proven to be an elusive target because it changes over time. Also, the pursuit of the ideal body shape appears to be related to outbreaks of eating disorders. Studies have shown the desired female shape has changed from the hourglass shape to a less curvaceous shape with a smaller bust and hips. In addition, body shape changes vary from one culture to another. Slimness has been associated with a variety of personality traits, such as, self-control, elegance, social attractiveness and youth, while on the other hand obesity has been associated with feelings of isolation, depression, failure and unattractiveness.[139] In the West our idea of the perfect female body is frequently the professional model or actress. In 1990 Wolf estimated the average model to be 23 percent lighter than the average North American woman.[140] We have become so crazed over the perfect body one study demonstrated females exposed to pictures of thin, ideal models developed the symptoms of depression, stress, guilt, shame, insecurity and body dissatisfaction.[141] Although the preference is for a thin, slim female body the healthiest female body shape is one that has a low waist to hip ratio (WHR).[142]

On the other hand women prefer men with a tapering 'V' look, and tend to dislike a pear shaped man.[143] People from lower socio-economic countries rate fuller figures higher than they do thin figures, confirming the idea people in poorer countries admire obesity probably because it is a sign of success and economic status.[144] In most Western countries people believe obesity is unhealthy and unattractive, and since women are more conscious about health and physical appearance than men are, they diet and exercise more in order to achieve their desired body shape.[145]

Overweight and obesity are a growing problem for adolescents. As a matter of fact, adolescence and early adult-hood are the peak risk periods for the development of an eating disorder, especially among girls.[146] It has been estimated that 1 in 200 young women develop anorexia,[147] and an additional one-three percent develop bulimia.[148] The path that leads to an eating disorder among adolescent girls often proceeds through the following defined steps: (1) increasing body size, (2) increasing body dissatisfaction, (3) increasing risk of the eating disorder.[149] If mother had an eating disorder, it is a risk factor for preadolescent and young adult females to start purging[150] and there is "strong evidence for a genetic component to binge eating."[151] "Overweight adolescents are often dissatisfied with their weight and frequently turn to unhealthy methods in their pursuit of weight loss, ultimately putting them at even greater risk for developing an eating disorder and increased adiposity."[152]

Young people who overeat are at a greater risk for suicidal thoughts and behaviors than those who do not overeat: 28.6 percent of girls and 27.8 percent of boys who met the criteria for binge eating syndrome reported they had attempted suicide compared with 9.8 percent of girls and 4.9 percent of boys who do not overeat.[153] In Canada, "disordered eating attitudes and behaviors were present in over 27% of girls aged 12-18 and were seen to increase gradually throughout adolescence."[154] The Canadian study even went so far as to suggest all girls be screened for eating disorders before they enter middle school and targeted for appropriate interventions.[155]

Finally, there is support for the idea that a genetic tendency exists for developing an eating disorder; there is more discussion of this topic in the chapter on genetics.[156] Possible candidates for such an eating disorder are those people who: (1) lose weight easily, (2) vomit easily, (3) react abnormally to starvation, and (4) demonstrate a failure of proper responses to overeating, such as feeling full.[157] Also, people who insist on engaging in rigid dieting are more likely to report symptoms of an eating disorder.[158]

How can these kids be helped? Eating disorders among children are frequently of long duration and depending upon the severity of the situation relapse easily if they are not properly dealt with. Often professional help is needed in order to achieve an acceptable outcome. Health care professionals and families need to advocate for medical and mental health services for children and adolescents suffering from eating disorders.[159] Results of clinical observations suggest asking kids in a sensitive way whether they are satisfied with their weight or their attempts to lose weight could provide an opportunity to discuss with them healthy weight ranges, healthy eating and an appropriate activity level for them. The obvious aim is to decrease the number of kids who might develop a disordered eating pattern without disrupting their self-esteem.[160]

It has been documented depressive symptoms commonly coexist with eating disorders and the prevalence of a coexistent mood disorder among women with bulimia has been estimated at 24-33 percent.[161] Women with eating disorders experience high levels of depression but their depression is different from the depression experienced by depressed women who have no eating disorder, and rehabilitative treatment for these women needs to focus on helping them to get passed the point of feeling responsible for the bad events in their lives.[162]

"Gay and bisexual men have a higher prevalence of eating disorders than heterosexual men."[163] Conversely, lesbian and bisexual women are comparable to heterosexual women in the amount of eating disorders experienced. Younger gay, lesbian and bisexual men and women, 18-29 years old, are more likely to have subclinical bulimia compared with their older counterparts, 30-59 years old. Black and Latino gay, lesbian and bisexuals have about the same prevalence of eating disorders as their white counterparts.[164]

There are also some predictive factors that can help determine if a person will be prone to an eating disorder later in life. Eating conflicts, struggles with food, and unpleasant meals during childhood have been shown to increase the risk of what has been termed a relaxed definition of anorexia in adolescents and young adults and eating too little during childhood has been shown to be suggestive of a future diagnosis of bulimia.[165] The *Transdiagnostic Theory* of eating disorders is based on the idea that "perfectionism is a proximal risk factor for the development of overvaluation of the importance of weight and shape,"[166] and therefore, precedes the development of eating disorder symptoms. Some researchers have made the argument that appropriate studies have not clearly determined the role of perfectionism with respect to diagnosing an eating disorder.[167] Frequently, trained health professionals attempt to make a determination as to whether a person is at risk of an eating disorder by an eating disorder examination interview or an eating disorder examination questionnaire.[168] Performance of the questionnaire has been extensively studied both in isolation and comparison with the interview. The findings indicate that in many respects the questionnaire is a reasonable substitute for the interview.[169]

Scientists have attempted to evaluate patient satisfaction with the treatment they received for their eating disorders. One study concluded "after 36 months 38% of the patients were highly satisfied with the treatment while 39% were satisfied and 23% were unsatisfied."[170] The study concluded that although the researchers were successful in helping patients who were receptive to strategies focused on support and control of eating problems, they were not as successful with those patients who had a large number of interpersonal problems and who were not as focused on their symptoms of disordered eating.[171]

Here are the generally recognized eating disorders in detail.

Anorexia Nervosa

Anorexia Nervosa is an eating disorder "characterized by refusal to maintain a normal, minimal bodyweight, intense fear of gaining weight or becoming obese and a disturbance of body image resulting in a feeling of being fat or having fat in certain areas, even when the body is extremely emaciated."[172] In anorexia the pursuit of weight loss is successful and a very low weight is achieved, primarily the result of a severe and selective restriction of food intake. In some patients the restriction of food intake is driven by a desire for self-punishment.[173] Anorexia is divided into two subtypes. First is "a *Restricting Type* in which weight loss is achieved primarily through diet or exercise,"[174] and it includes a subcategory called anorexia athletica, characterized by "abnormal exercise patterns, including the desire to exercise while injured and compulsive exercise beyond the normal training regimens."[175] Second is "a *Binge Eating/ Purging Type* in which binge eating and purging behavior also occurs regularly."[176] The latter type resembles bulimia excepted anorexics exhibit the characteristic underweight condition. The most typical and obvious symptom of anorexia is a body weight that is 15 percent below the normal weight. Although anorexia has increased in both sexes between 1935 in 1958,[177] it occurs most frequently in adolescent females, between15 and 19 years old.[178]

Anorexia is characterized by a cluster of psychological traits including, "emotional restraint, avoidance of novelty, anxious worry and self-doubt, weight and shape related anxiety, compliancy, obsessionality, rigidity, over control, perfectionism and perseverance in the face of non-reward."[179] "Patients with anorexia nervosa have more negative self-beliefs than dieters,"[180] and it has been suggested, "anorexics may feel guilty about the indulgent act of eating, and this serves to exacerbate feelings of self negation."[181] Anorexics also suffered from: "symptoms of depression and anxiety disorders, irritability…impaired concentration, loss of sexual appetite… typically these features get worse as weight is lost."[182] In addition, when questioned, anorexic "patients have also identified the importance of social institutions such as school, family and the media in contributing to their illness."[183] Common symptoms of anorexia include: an absence of menstrual period, constipation, abdominal pain, and intolerance of cold, lethargy, anxious energy, fatigue and headaches.[184]

Additional medical complications can occur in kids before any real evidence of significant weight loss appears. Of particular importance is the potential for permanent growth retardation.[185] "Anorexia nervosa…is associated with the highest mortality rate of any mental disorder."[186]

The research on treatment for anorexia is rather skimpy; however, four possible approaches have been suggested: (1) help the patient understand they need immediate help, (2) help them develop a program of weight restoration, (3) address the patient's out of proportion concern for their shape and weight, their eating habits and their general psychological well being, and (4) use compulsory treatment, whenever that becomes necessary.[187] "Family therapy is recognized as one of the most effective treatment modalities in adolescent anorexia nervosa."[188] Anorexia is a difficult disease, which places complex and extraordinary demands on the family, therefore, the smartest family therapists do not attempt to completely revamp the family with a one-size-fits-all approach, rather they attempt to blend the different personalities, into a style and level of functioning that supports the anorexic in their effort to rid themselves of the disease.[189] On the other hand drug treatment does not have an established place in the management of anorexia, since no drug has been shown to be of value in promoting reasonable weight gain.[190] Good prognosis for recovery from anorexia has been associated with a variety of variables including: (1) shorter duration of illness, (2) higher social class, and (3) younger onset.[191] Unfortunately some studies suggest the prognosis for recovery of childhood anorexia is rather poor,[192] especially for children under age 11.[193]

Bulimia Nervosa

Bulimia Nervosa is an eating disorder characterized "by episodic binge eating usually followed by behavior designed to negate the excessive caloric intake, most commonly purging behaviors such as self-induced vomiting or laxative abuse…excessive exercise or fasting."[194] "In contrast to persons with anorexia nervosa, patients with bulimia nervosa tend to be somewhat older, more socially inclined, have less obsessive characteristics and do not exhibit extreme weight loss."[195] Individuals with bulimia tend to be of average weight. Bulimia occurs most frequently in adolescent females. As a matter of fact, "eating disorders, such as bulimia nervosa, have been found to be up to ten times more common among women than men."[196] Common symptoms include: irregular menses, abdominal pain, lethargy, fatigue, headaches, depression, swelling of the hands and feet, bloating, parathyroid gland enlargement and erosion of the enamel on the teeth.[197] "Perceived control, low assertiveness, low self-esteem and self-directed hostility are characteristics of anorectics [sic] and bulimics that differentiate them from obese and non-obese individuals."[198] Women may be more well informed about the causes and risk factors for bulimia, in particular the significance of low self-esteem, than their male counterparts.[199]

Bulimia is characterized by a cluster of psychological traits including, "thrill seeking and excitability, affective instability and impulsivity, and a tendency towards dysphoria (i.e. a state of feeling not well or unhappy) in response to rejection or non-reward."[200] The main feature distinguishing bulimia from anorexia is attempts to restrict food intake are followed by repeated binges. In most cases of bulimia binge eating is followed by periods of self-induced vomiting or laxative misuse. The combination of under eating coupled with binge eating results in a fairly normal body weight.[201] Some researchers believe dietary restraint increases the likelihood of binge eating in bulimia.[202] There appear to be a couple of alternative explanations for the correlation between dieting and bulimia. "First, binge eating may cause dietary restraint. It is possible that people who binge eat attempt to avoid consequent weight gain, by dieting. Second, it may be that both of these processes are operating and that restraint and bulimic pathology are reciprocally related."[203]

Here may be one reason why women are more affected by bulimia than men. Fluctuation in bulimia symptoms appear to be related to two hormonal phenomena: (1) the hormones released during the menstrual cycle, and (2) cortisol secretion. The hormones released during the menstrual cycle influence the severity of bulimic symptoms and the severity of those symptoms increases the secretion of cortisol. In addition to the hormonal stress caused by the symptoms of bulimia, a woman may experience psychological stress because of the increased frequency of her binging, which in turn could increase cortisol secretion.[204] In addition, "repeated purging causes dehydration and electrolyte imbalances,"[205] which have been shown to lead to increased cortisol secretion.[206] Once it was believed there is a correlation between binging and cortisol, but in fact it may be a correlation between purging and cortisol.

Unlike anorexia, life-threatening, "medical complications are rare in bulimia...but, trauma to the gastro-intestinal tract, fluid and electrolyte imbalance and renal dysfunction can occur."[207] Another problem is the adverse dental effects resulting from vomiting, due to the concentration of stomach acid passing through the mouth.[208]

Unlike the treatment options for people with anorexia, the treatment options for patients with bulimia appear to be much better. The most effective treatment is cognitive behavior therapy that focuses on modifying the specific behaviors and ways of thinking that are causing the patients eating disorder.[209] Another fairly effective treatment for the bulimic is the use of antidepressant drugs, which frequently "result in a rapid decline in the frequency of binge eating and purging and an improvement in mood."[210] It is interesting to note combining cognitive behavioral therapy with antidepressant drugs does not give a better result than just the cognitive behavioral therapy alone.[211] Unlike anorexia, there appear to be few consistent predictors of outcome,[212] other than possibly low self-esteem.[213] Finally, if there is any good news about bulimia, it is that some data suggests women may tend to grow out of it as they age.[214]

Binge-Eating Disorder

"Binge eating was described as far back as the time of Hippocrates, who called it bulimia (ox hunger) and viewed it as a sick form of hunger."[215] The first proposal of this type of disordered eating as a syndrome came in 1959 when Stunkard described the Binge Eating Disorder

Syndrome.[216] "Between 20% and 46% of all obese patients, seeking treatment, report moderate to severe problems with binge eating,"[217] and these binge eating obese eaters experience more severe psychological problems than do obese non-binge eaters.[218] The first feature underlying binge eating is "eating, in a discrete period of time…an amount that is definitely larger than most individuals would eat under similar circumstances."[219] "The second core feature is experiencing a loss of control over eating during this period of time, as if one cannot either stop eating or limit the quantity that one eats."[220] Binge eating often consists of eating large amounts of food when one is not hungry.

While men and women suffering from binge eating disorder are most often overweight there are few other visible signs.[221] There are a few known risk factors for example, restrained eating and dieting behavior is associated with a tendency to binge eat,[222] but it isn't clear as to whether dieting precedes binge eating or binge eating precedes dieting.[223] Women with binge eating disorder experience "high levels of family tension at meal times, frequent arguments between parents, low parental affection, and limited contact with parents…parental high expectations… frequent criticism…and parental ill health."[224] Other possible risk factors for binge eating are a tendency toward perfectionism, parents who suffer from high rates of psychological problems, frequent separation of the child from the parent and a parenting style where there is minimal affection but a lot of control exerted,[225] and a high consumption of junk food.[226]

Finally, children seem to be presented with special problems with dysfunctional eating behavior vis-à-vis dieting. It has been reported that "children as young as eight years old engage in dieting behaviors."[227] Evidence demonstrates among obese youngsters seeking treatment, 20 percent have experienced loss of control over their eating. Additionally these youngsters demonstrated symptoms of depression and have more concerns about eating, bodyweight and body shape, than their lean counterparts.[228] Emotional upset with feelings of loss of control over eating is the single most dominant psychological disturbance of binge eating.[229] Childhood teasing about weight and size, especially among females, is a significant predictor for binge eating.[230] Obviously, "binge eating is a risk factor for obesity during adolescence."[231]

Among the predictors of binge eating are, excessive dieting, pressure to be thin, overvaluation of appearance, body dissatisfaction, emotional eating, low self-esteem, and a weak social support system.[232] Binge eating has also been associated with much higher rates of, depression, panic disorder, phobias, and alcohol dependence.[233] Obese women with binge eating disorder have been shown to be more neurotic and also suffer from what are called neurovegetative symptoms (e.g. insomnia, agitation, retardation, obsessive-compulsive traits).[234]

There are basically three types of treatment programs for binge eating disorder, they are: (1) psychotherapy, (2) pharmacotherapy, and (3) weight reduction programs.[235] Psychological treatments involve two types of therapy. First, is cognitive behavioral therapy where participants meet in groups and focus on the eating disturbance and associated attitudes about eating, body shape and body weight. This form of therapy has been shown to reduce binge eating more than

50 percent.[236] Second is interpersonal therapy, also known as behavioral weight loss therapy where individuals focus on altering behaviors that have lead to obesity. Interpersonal therapy has shown a reduction of over 70 percent in binge eating.[237] Pharmacotherapy has also been used to reduce binge eating. Stunkard & Allison found a combination of the drugs phentermine and fluoxetine completely eliminated binge eating.[238] Stunkard & Allison also came to the surprising conclusion, "weight loss programs that ignore the issue of binge eating may perform as effectively as those designed solely to reduce binge eating."[239]

Night Eating Syndrome

Stunkard first used the term night eating syndrome in 1955.[240] "The core characteristics of this syndrome included: morning anorexia (lack of appetite in the morning), evening hyperphagia (over eating in the evening), emotional distress and insomnia."[241] Later on in 1996 Stunkard et al added to these characteristics by specifying that more than 50 percent of the daily calories were consumed after 7 PM.[242] Stunkard's initial definition has been tinkered with over the years. For example, there have been a variety of cutoff times suggested (e.g. 6 PM, 8 PM or after the evening meal), and the amount of food consumed has been altered (e.g. 25 percent, 50 percent or simply a large amount).[243] Those with night eating syndrome are "less adherent with diet, exercise and glucose monitoring and more likely to be depressed, to report childhood maltreatment histories, to have nonsecure attachment styles, and to report eating in response to anger, sadness, loneliness, worry and being upset…and more likely to be obese…and to have two or more diabetes complications."[244] Night eating syndrome patients also report their mood is the lowest in the morning.[245] It is interesting to note, when looking at childhood maltreatment histories, individuals with binge eating disorder reported strikingly higher emotional neglect, whereas people with night eating syndrome complained of more physical neglect.[246]

To complicate matters other researchers have further expanded the night eating syndrome features. One study revealed "two features were most predictive of a diagnosis of night eating syndrome, namely eating 25% or more of the daily total caloric intake after the evening meal and experiencing awakenings with nocturnal ingestions at least half of the time."[247] Simply put "the night eating syndrome is an eating disorder characterized by a phase delay in the circadian pattern of eating, manifested by: (1) evening hyperphagia [over eating in the evening], (2) awakenings accompanied by nocturnal ingestions, or (3) both".[248]

Night eating syndrome differs from binge eating disorder in two ways. First is the far greater frequency of nighttime awakenings and second is in the smaller amount of the food ingested at those times. Stunkard & Allison suggest during night awakenings the quantity of food ingested is a modest 270 calories per awakening, in the case of night eating syndrome, as compared to the approximately 1300 calories ingested during binge eating sessions.[249] In addition people suffering with night eating syndrome do not appear to suffer to the same degree from the diet and body image distortions that are commonly seen in people with binge eating disorder[250] and the prevalence of night eating syndrome seems to increase with the severity of obesity. Both binge eating disorder and night eating syndrome "share other clinical characteristics such as eating in response to negative affect, eating until uncomfortably full, eating alone and corresponding feelings of depression or guilt after an overeating episode."[251] Night eating, sometimes referred to as nocturnal snacking, occurs most frequently among men and is characterized by a time-delayed pattern of eating relative to sleep, where most food is consumed in the evening and night.[252]

If you study the subject of night eating syndrome beyond what is covered in this chapter you may see a couple of less talked about variations of this subject you need to be aware of. There are two types of night eating syndrome described in some of the literature on sleep disorders. One is called Night Eating/Drinking Syndrome (NEDS) and the other is called Nocturnal Sleep Related Eating Disorder (NSRED). "(NEDS) involves frequent and recurrent awakenings to eat and/or drink and normal sleep onset following the ingestion of the desired foods."[253] The distinctions between night eating syndrome and NEDS appear to be largely dependent upon whether the author used the word night or nocturnal in describing the period of over eating. On the other hand NSRED relates to the extent of consciousness during the night eating. Wow! What a play on words. Let's make it simple. For our purposes if the eating takes place after dinner and constitutes more than 30-40 percent of the day's caloric intake, I will refer to its as night eating syndrome and I don't care whether the person doing the eating is conscious or unconscious. The result is the same.

One group vulnerable to night eating syndrome are psychiatric patients. Experts have demonstrated a pattern of "substance use disorder was more likely to occur among patients with night eating syndrome (30.6%) than among those without the syndrome (8.3%)…Alcohol was the most commonly abused substance for patients both with night eating syndrome (46.7%) and without (66.7%)."[254]

Similar to the treatment protocol for binge eating disorder the most effective treatment for night eating syndrome appears to be the class of antidepressants known as selective serotonin reuptake inhibitors (SSRI's).[255]

Self Esteem

We cannot ignore the fact that our self-esteem is affected by how we view an overweight condition. Self-esteem plays a major role in how an individual views their body and/or weight status. One of the difficulties in addressing this issue is we often perceive our situation to be something quite different from reality, and "weight perceptions rather than actual weight status are significantly associated with psychological distress."[256]

One expert proposed the *Social Comparison Theory*.[257] His theory holds:

- Individuals are driven to evaluate their own opinions and abilities,
- Without objective criteria, individuals make a social comparison, and
- These comparisons are made with other people of similar circumstance.[258]

Social comparison theory still remains one of the most reliable theories of body comparison. It is still a "powerful predictor of body-image evaluation and body image investment among male and female adolescence."[259] There is a tendency for individuals to make a self-evaluation of attractiveness by comparing their physical appearance to models in magazine advertisements,[260] and actors in movies and on TV.

It is interesting to see how high-achieving overweight women view themselves and their bodies. Research on eating disorders "suggests a link between achievement and how women feel about their bodies. Eating disorders are more common in women from higher socioeconomic status backgrounds."[261] European American women experience more eating disorders than African-American women, but interestingly there appears to be little or no difference in body dissatisfaction, self-esteem, or disparities between ideal and actual weight, when all the study participants are from the middle or upper class. Furthermore, high achieving college women from middle to high-class socio-economic backgrounds seem to maintain a heightened concern about their weight and as a result are at high risk for eating disorders.[262] It is no surprise to find out there is a lot of body dissatisfaction among achievement-oriented women in general.[263]

There is a social stigmatization experienced by overweight individuals. People make negative assumptions about overweight people (e.g. having low expectations of the individual), and there are also physical barriers and social rejection because of being overweight.[264] "Obese children and adolescents are subjected to social rejection, discrimination and negative stereotyping."[265] Body dissatisfaction begins at an early age. "Body dissatisfaction in children is not a random phenomenon, or a whim of fashion. Body dissatisfaction, especially desire to be thinner, may be the result of a long development."[266] Early in life children become painfully aware of generally recognized social standards regarding the ideal, preferable slim body size and shape. Body image disturbances and obesity in children and adolescents occur much more frequently today than they did in the past. The two most important goals for helping kids are to: (1) support their development of a positive self-image, and (2) help them prevent excess weight gain.[267]

Overweight girls show concerns about weight, body shape, eating and physical appearance and attempt to control their diets much more than their average weight friends. Overweight girls show significantly lower ratings of self-esteem as well. All this lends support to the idea overweight girls may be at increased risk of developing an eating disorder since each of the identified factors have been shown to be risk factors for the later development of an eating disorder.[168] There is however, some research data that tends to mitigate this idea. A concern for slimness is only one of the major life concerns for adolescent girls; ranking behind "academic success, intelligence and physical attractiveness, but it has the most detrimental consequences for them."[169] Interventions attempting to improve the well being of adolescent girls would be best if they targeted those girls with a big concern for slimness and helped them decrease the importance of slimness and increase the maintenance of a healthy body weight.[270]

The critical point to remember is low self-esteem has been reported in a number of studies to be associated with adolescent obesity. One followed adolescents into adulthood and showed the importance of dealing with "known risk factors, such as, reduction of sedentary behaviors and reduction of unhealthy eating patterns (consumption of carbonated drinks and takeaway foods, dieting) in the prevention of the persistence of obesity from childhood into adult life."[271] Even if it's not the most important factor, it remains a fact that "individuals with obesity have a high prevalence of body dissatisfaction."[272] Obesity in children as young as 11, has been shown to have a clear and measurable impact on their self-esteem. These obese kids often have "lower perceived athletic competence, physical appearance and global self-worth."[273] Also, girls in particular had lower self-perception when it came to social acceptance.[274] Mental health professionals need to help obese children build their self-esteem in order to help them lead full lives regardless of their body weight.[275]

As mentioned previously in the section on depression, the comparison of a low protein high carbohydrate (LPHC) diet to a high-protein low carbohydrate (HPLC) diet, clearly showed the HPLC diet was closely associated with improvement in ratings of depression and self esteem. Dieting has been shown to worsen mood since it is understood that caloric restriction is associated with irritability.[276] Depending on the individual's experience, dieting may either improve or worsen mood. The actual experience of losing weight may increase a person's self-esteem, which in turn could have a positive effect on mood and help reduce depressive symptoms.[277]

The self-esteem side of body image dissatisfaction varies across different groups. Women are generally far more dissatisfied with their body image than men are. African-American women usually exhibit less body image dissatisfaction than Caucasian women. The level of body image dissatisfaction of Asian and Hispanic American individuals, acclimated to the American culture, is similar to those of Caucasian Americans.[278] Frequently obese women attempt to conceal their obesity by "camouflaging their bodies with clothing, changing their posture or body movements, avoiding looking at their bodies, and becoming upset when thinking about their appearance,"[279] and a number of them admit being embarrassed in social situations, such as work or parties.[280]

Two separate bodies of research are developing on the relationship between obesity and body image. "The first group is looking primarily at changes in body image that accompany weight-loss. The second group is looking more specifically at changes in body image, through the use of psychotherapy, often independent of weight loss."[281] While at the present time it doesn't appear either one has the complete and correct approach it is very likely in the long run changing the body and the body image simultaneously may lead to better results.[282]

Behavior Changes

The most important reasons men and women give for weight gain is: (1) a lack of exercise, and (2) they just enjoyed eating; and interestingly when it came to what men and women considered a reasonable weight loss, men thought a loss of 17 percent of their current weight would be reasonable, whereas women thought 29 percent would be reasonable.[283] Given the high rates of attrition and noncompliance in weight-loss programs, resolution of the disparities between beliefs and behaviors seems necessary.[284] "Although many are able to maintain at least two thirds of their weight loss for more than 1 year, the vast majority (over 80%) regain to their pre-treatment weight, if not more, within three years after formal treatment has ended."[285]

Research demonstrates that behavioral treatment programs provide a very good approach for producing significant weight loss,[286] since human beings have the inherent ability to control their conduct. "Health-compromising behaviors can be overcome by self-regulatory efforts and health-enhancing behaviors can be adopted instead."[287] "After a person develops an inclination toward adopting a particular health behavior, the good intention has to be transformed into detailed instructions on how to perform the desired action...once an action is initiated it needs to be maintained." [288] Good intentions are more likely to be translated into reality when people develop action plans and prepare strategies for attacking the specific task. A good action plan needs to define the specifics of when, where and how the objective will be accomplished.[289]

Our children and adolescents are a group in great need of weight related behavioral change. "Overweight children and adolescents are at risk for physical health problems and psychological vulnerabilities."[290] "Of greatest concern is the probability of childhood obesity persisting into adulthood increases from 20% at age four to 80% by adolescents."[291] "Evidence exists for the clustering of behavioral risks among adolescents...80% of 11 to 15 year-olds had multiple risk factors related to diet and physical activity,"[292] and "11 to 15 year-olds who engaged in the most sedentary behavior also engaged in lower levels of physical activity and fruit and vegetable consumption."[293] A declining level of fruit and vegetable consumption is the most prevalent health risk factor among our kids. "The percentage of students eating fruit declined from about 65% in ES [elementary school] to 37% in MS [middle school], while vegetable consumption decreased from 56% to about 42%."[294]

"Children in the United States spend an estimated 75% of the day being inactive."[295] Sedentary activities, like watching TV and videos have been shown to promote higher bodyweight in children and adolescents, however, evidence does suggest simply trying to reduce TV and video viewing time, may not be a successful method of losing weight and keeping it off. The most successful strategies utilize a combination of reducing: (1) overall sedentary behavior, and (2) caloric intake.[296] Furthermore, the level of adolescent physical activity tends to decrease with increasing age. "As adolescents move into their teenage years, they likely increase the time that they spend engaging in multiple sedentary behaviors that compete with physical activities,"[297] and minority boys are more likely to become more sedentary than white boys, and boys become more sedentary than girls.[298] This leads to the logical conclusion that exercise is an important part of any effective obesity treatment. It is important to establish active lifestyles early in children, since active children are more likely to become active adults.[299]

Although it is not the goal of this book to turn you into a psychologist, there are several basic behavior change models psychologist refer to in the research literature, you should least be aware of. Of these models, the following two are the most discussed, highly recognized and understandable:

- Transtheoretical Model - The transtheoretical model has been successful in changing behaviors associated with obesity and is the most commonly cited model. "Specifically it has been used with dietary fat reduction, increasing fruit and vegetable intake, and increasing exercise."[300] The transtheoretical model relies heavily on the idea that behavioral change occurs in stages,[301] however, the number of stages required for successful change is the subject of a substantial amount of dispute.[302] "The most common set of stages include:
  o Pre-contemplation - Not thinking about change or suppressing thoughts of change,
  o Contemplation - Considering change but taking no action,
  o Planning or Preparation - Anticipating making efforts to change and considering what behavior one will do,
  o Action - Actually engaging in efforts to change,
  o Maintenance - Expending effort to retain the changes made during action."[303]

  The transtheoretical model uses the identified process steps to promote an overall change in motivation and/or behavior to help the person advance through the stages of change.[304]

- Health Belief Model - The primary motivation to change within the health belief model is the level of perceived threat or risk of a specific condition and the primary resource for the change is the belief one has the power to produce the necessary result.[305] The health belief model factors include a persons:
  o Perceived susceptibility - The perception of the risk for contracting an illness,
  o Perceived severity - The perception of the personal impact of contracting the illness,

- Perceived benefits - The perception of the good things that could happen from undertaking the behaviors especially in regard to reducing the threat of the illness,
- Perceived barriers - The perception of the difficulty in performing the behaviors and the negative things that could happen from performing those behaviors,
- Self-Efficacy - The person's belief or level of confidence he or she can perform the behaviors.

One of the main features of most of the behavior change models is the significance of the individual's beliefs. Through the application of these models the participant frequently sees a shift in their beliefs. Two terms that are often used within the context of beliefs are:

- Self-efficacy, which is defined as "an individual's belief in his or her ability to perform and succeed in challenging situations."[306] Self-efficacy has been tied to performance of health behaviors and thus is frequently offered by researchers as an important feature of the behavior change process.[307]

- Health Locus of Control, which is defined as "the individuals beliefs in the possibility to influence one's own health by adjusting various aspects of his or her own individual behavior."[308] The understanding that we control our life circumstances rather than them controlling us has long been believed to be beneficial to positive mental and physical health. The belief we can produce the desired result ourselves is contingent on our acceptance of responsibility for the problem and its solution.[309]

Respondents in one study who believed they had control over health related parameters were shown to be more likely to have healthy lifestyles, while obese and overweight individuals showed a psychological lack of belief in the possibility of influencing their own health.[310] Health related beliefs play an important role for children as well. "The processes that lead to childhood obesity can be traced back to early elementary school years when children are developing their beliefs about health behaviors."[311] Young children's negative reactions to other children who exercise encourages a childhood pattern that tends to reduce their physical activity levels and thus leads to adolescent weight gain. Strategies directed at changing the way children view themselves can result in their adopting more healthful habits.[312] While some researchers have cautioned high expectations for control over health could be detrimental in some circumstances,[313] research has offered very little solid evidence of any negative consequences for physical and mental health.[314]

In order to defeat obesity, behavior modification is an absolute necessity. Two of the most important behaviors that need adjustment are:

- Food planning,

- Exercise,
  - Resistance training,
  - Aerobic exercise,
  - Lifestyle activity.

To accomplish needed behavior changes in your effort to lose weight, you must implement successful behavior change strategies. Your choices may consist of any or all of the following strategies:[315]

- Goal Setting - Goal setting involves establishing specific, measurable, achievable, realistic, timed objectives. Goal setting is an effective tool for managing progress by ensuring you are clearly aware of what you expect from yourself. Goals provide a sense of direction and purpose. Goal setting requires motivation since you need to understand why you want to achieve the goal. Some examples of good weight loss goals are to: (1) reduce caloric intake by 500 calories per day, over the next two weeks, (2) reduce intake of nonessential dietary fat by 15 percent over the next four weeks, etc. Emphasis should be on short-term goals you can reasonably achieve, (e.g. one goal might be to lose one-two pounds per week).[316] The goal of weight loss should not focus on weight loss alone, which is often aimed at appearance, but should focus on weight management, directed at achieving the best body weight possible for overall health.[317]

- Self-Monitoring - Self-monitoring is the process of regulating your own behavior. This technique identifies and records various trends of weight loss, which will aid in your understanding of situations or emotions that may be a threat to adherence to your goals.[318]

- Stimulus Control - A specific stimulus increases the probability of a behavior because of your history of that behavior being reinforced in the presence of the stimulus. In plain words stimulus control is simply learning to pay attention to the things you identify that give you information about the effectiveness of your behavior. It might also be thought of as the identification of environmental cues associated with the behavior you desire, (e.g. laying out your exercise clothes the night before a workout).[319]

- Behavioral Contracting - A behavioral contract is a written statement of how you intend to behave, spelling out your detailed expectations. As a positive reinforcement tool it provides structure for self-management by indicating the consequences for failure, and the time limitations for accomplishment.

- Cognitive Restructuring - Cognitive restructuring is the process of refuting behavioral distortions or simply faulty thinking, and replacing your irrational counterfactual beliefs with more accurate and beneficial ones. This theory holds your own unrealistic beliefs are directly responsible for generating dysfunctional emotions and the resultant behaviors, and humans can rid themselves of such emotions and their effects by dismantling the beliefs that are counter productive.

- Stress Management - Stress management utilizes techniques intended to equip you with effective coping mechanisms for dealing with psychological stress. These techniques become effective when you use them to cope with or alter stressful situations, (e.g. muscle relaxation and meditation to reduce your stress level).

- Social Support - Social support is the physical and/or emotional comfort given to you by your family, friends, coworkers or others. It results from knowing you are part of a community of people who love and care for you and value what you think. For social support to be effective you must understand it and believe it to be supportive. Numerous studies have shown people with higher levels of support do better in weight loss programs.[320]

- Financial Incentives - Financial incentives are used as rewards to give you positive reinforcement, for the completion of a specific goal (e.g. you may buy a lottery ticket after losing five pounds).

- Lapse Prevention - Since lapses are a natural part of the weight-loss process, you must anticipate events that might cause a lapse to occur and then devise strategies to cope with them.[321]

Changes in lifestyle involve utilizing behavior modification principles to make changes in diet and exercise patterns, which are the foundation upon which successful obesity treatments rest. It is true drug and surgical treatments may augment a weight loss or weight maintenance effort, but obese patients always have to make some alterations in their lifestyle in order to experience long-term success.[322] A big shift in thinking about weight management is needed to decrease the high prevalence of obesity. Of great concern are the negative outcomes that are frequently associated with dieting and the use of unhealthy weight loss behaviors.[323] Interventions are needed that aim at preventing the onset of obesity and eating disorders by promoting healthy eating and exercise as ongoing lifestyle behaviors.[324]

The "criteria that lead people to initiate a change in their behavior are different from those that lead them to maintain that behavior."[325]

- Behavior Initiation - People attempt to change their behavior when their outcome expectations are perceived to be more favorable than those provided by their current behavior.[326] The more optimistic people are about: (1) the possible results, and (2) their ability to obtain those results, the more willing they are to get into action.

Because the process of behavioral initiation is oriented toward obtaining a favorable result in the future, it is thought of as a self-regulatory system in which people progress toward their goals by reducing the difference between the current state and the desired state.[327]

- Behavior Maintenance - The decision to maintain an adopted pattern of behavior is based on people's satisfaction with the results they obtain from a current pattern of behavior. "The guiding premise is that people will maintain a change in behavior only if they are satisfied with what they have accomplished."[328]

The *Health at Every Size Approach* encourages people to accept their body weight and to rely on their body signals to support positive health behaviors that help regulate their weight. It is claimed that health at every size group participants tend to show sustained improvements in many health behaviors and attitudes as well as many health risk indicators associated with obesity, including total cholesterol, LDL cholesterol, elevated blood pressure, depression and self esteem. In short, it suggests reducing diet related behavior but makes no mention of exercise. It counts exclusively on listening to our body's signals to tell us what to do. Although it makes for interesting dialog, I believe it's deeply flawed in two ways. First, it fails to address the question as to specifically how we might go about listening to our body's signals. If we knew how to listen we would have been doing it all along. Second, it makes the incorrect assumption we are powerless to alter our size within reason.

Many weight-loss programs today are fairly effective at short-term weight-loss, but they often fail to help the participant keep the weight off. Long-term strategies for effective weight-loss maintenance are still needed. The design of a successful maintenance program must focus on a healthy lifestyle rather than weight-loss per se. Researchers report that weight that was initially lost during a 6-month weight loss program, was gained back over the next 18 months, after the face-to-face contact with the program leader ended. Participants failed to keep the weight off, even though the transtheoretical model criteria provided promise that long-term maintenance and treatment induced weight loss should have been successful.[329]

Finally, how much does the general public trust the scientific experts? "Trust can be understood as a state of vulnerability based on positive expectations of the intentions or behavior of another person."[330] Since experts play a critical role in the interpretation and dissemination of information to the public,[331] "an improved understanding of public trust in scientific experts on obesity is necessary for improving obesity related risk communication."[332] It has been speculated as to why there may be a low level of trust in scientific experts. Among the reasons are: (1) the potential financial conflicts of interest involving scientific experts, (2) instances where scientific research is found to be incorrect, and (3) general uncertainties about science or disagreements among scientists.[333] It has been suggested that white females, with higher levels of education, and Democratic Party affiliation might experience higher levels of trust in scientific experts.[334]

Summary

I hope you have become much more aware of the significant contribution your psychological condition makes in your ability to control your body weight. Tests prove that when behavior therapy, drug therapy or exercise, are added to a weight loss diet, maximum weight loss is achieved with the addition of the behavior therapy.[335] It isn't by accident this chapter turned out to be one the largest in this book. During the course of my research it became evident that the psychological contribution to obesity can be far greater than I first imagined. Unfortunately for those of you struggling with a weight problem, the psychological underpinnings of sensible and effective weight management are so pervasive and intertwined they are seldom understood or satisfactorily explored by health, exercise and nutrition professionals. This usually results in a less than desirable result.

An interest in weight loss is frequently an egocentric situation, driven by body image considerations rather than real health concerns. This situation is not something strictly experienced in the adult population but is commonly seen among children and adolescents as well. To add to the already difficult growth period that adolescents are experiencing, being "overweight is associated with poorer quality of life in adolescents."[336] To make matters worse even a baby's habitual negative mood may be a predictor of weight gain. Supported by the data presented earlier, you should now recognize psychological dysfunction can be a real contributor to obesity.

We have all known for a long time the brain controls the body, but it is amazing when we consider the depth of brain's role in the functioning of our metabolic processes. The brain receives signals not only from sight, hearing, smell, touch and taste, but the signals it receives from the hormones circulating in our blood stream, may be even more powerful. All the information the brain gathers from the various organs of the body is processed and used later in its control function, over those same organs.

Stress is a fact of life in today's developed societies. Stress is hard to avoid and in some instances and at certain times it has been shown to be beneficial to humans. However, the amount of stress people are under today goes far beyond anything ever thought to be beneficial to the body, and in fact there is an abundance of research demonstrating excess stress can wreak havoc with the body in a number of ways. One of those ways is it can cause weight gain (e.g. increased cortisol production and overeating). The data suggests properly applied stress reduction techniques could be a friend of many people trying to lose weight.

Depression and its relationship to weight gain is an interesting yet somewhat controversial topic. On one hand there is study data claiming depression causes weight gain and on the other there is data, claiming depression does not cause weight gain. My research unearthed a lot more data in favor of depression causing weight gain and that data appears to be strong. Studies report, "adults with current depression or a lifetime diagnosis of depression or anxiety were significantly more likely than those without each diagnosis to smoke, to be obese, to be physically inactive, to binge drink and drink heavily."[337] I also examined the linkage between other mental health issues and weight gain (e.g. dementia and eating disorders). The obvious conclusion is, if there is an underlying mental health issue, it must be addressed for a weight-loss program to be optimized.

A discussion of psychologically based weight related concerns would not be complete without consideration of eating disorders. Eating disorders need to be understood because of the: (1) tremendous potential they have for the destruction of health, and (2) importance of your being able to recognize them. While anorexia actually causes weight loss, it can be life threatening and has no place in your weight loss plan. Both binge eating disorder and night eating syndrome are of particular importance because they typically result in weight gain. Here is a short summary of the major eating disorders.

Anorexia Nervosa
Anorexia is an eating disorder where the person has such an extreme fear of gaining weight they refuse to eat, resulting in an abnormally low body weight.

Bulimia Nervosa
Bulimia is an eating disorder where the person binges and then purges their system, usually by either self-induced vomiting or the abuse of laxatives. Often this person appears to be of normal weight, making the situation more difficult to detect.

Binge Eating Disorder
Binge eating often consists of eating a large amount of food, in a relatively short period of time, frequently when one is not hungry, accompanied by a perceived loss of control. If the focus is on psychological well being and not on dieting the results might be more positive and longer lasting than what might be expected with dieting alone approaches, since caloric restriction is an important determinant of binge eating.[338]

Night Eating Syndrome
Night eaters usually eat the majority of their daily caloric intake after 7 PM.

Self-esteem plays a big role in how we view our bodies and our weight situation. Psychological distress is associated with our weight perception rather than with our actual weight. People often make negative assumptions about overweight people tending to drive their self-esteem down.

Presently, two separate bodies of research are developing on the relationship between obesity and body image. The first group is looking primarily at changes in body image that accompany weight-loss, with investigators focusing on how changes to the physical body influence the body image. A second group is looking more at changes in body image, through the use of psychotherapy, independent of weight loss. The focus of course is attempting to change the body image without changing the body. If results are what you want, it seems obvious while the researchers are fooling around with competing theories the best approach is to try to change both the body and the body image simultaneously.

Finally, working hand-in-hand with the physical act of changing the body is the psychological principle of behavior change. If you want to change your weight status you need to adopt new behaviors. "Eating and exercise behaviours [sic] and physiological factors…are 'direct' influences on weight while other psychological and environmental factors must be considered 'indirect' influences exerting their effects through behaviour [sic] or physiology."[339] It has been suggested, "obesity is not a problem of defective physiological regulation, but is an environmental and societal problem and therefore, must be approached through environmental and social solutions."[340] We can choose our environments or they can be chosen for us. In some cases, our food and/or exercise environments may be predetermined by the culture, community or family we live in.[341] "There is general agreement that a contributor to the obesity epidemic is an… environment that encourages over eating and discourages physical activity."[342] Most everything we do, to control our weight will ultimately rest upon the foundation of behavior change.

Although this chapter is about the psychological aspects of weight loss I don't want to over-emphasize that issue. Don't be misled into believing if you find a weakness in some psychological aspect of your life and fix it your weight problem will go away. Focusing on a single weight loss strategy alone often results in disappointment. One group of experts concluded by saying, "we recognize that better results may be obtained by including a focus on food choice and activity as well as psychological input."[343]

Given the extent of your overweight condition it may be a mistake to begin an exercise or nutrition program without first dealing with a psychological problem. If you are 50, 75, 100 or more pounds overweight, that could be an indicator of psychological dysfunction, which may need to be explored first in your weight loss effort. If you take the time to think about it rationally and honestly you will be able to make sound decisions that best fit your needs.

The most important point to take from this chapter is if you believe an emotional disorder could be contributing to your over-weight condition, you need to address that issue in order to optimize your chances of success with your overall weight loss program. I hope you now have the knowledge to recognize the problem and the possibilities.

Endnotes

1. P.E. Matz, M.S. Faith, G.D. Foster, T. Fallon, A. Wadden, "Correlates of body image dissatisfaction among overweight women seeking weight loss," *J Consult Clin Psych* 70 (2002) 1040-1044.
2. M. Kostanski, A. Fisher, E. Gullone, " Current conceptualization of body image dissatisfaction: have we got it wrong," *J Child Psych & Psych* 45 (2004) 1317-1325.

3. M.A. Friedman, K.D. Brownell, "Psychological correlates of obesity: moving to the next research generation," *Psych Bull* 117 (1995) 3-20.
4. "Etiology," *Dorland's Illustrated Medical Dictionary*, 30th ed: 647.
5. H. Baumeister, M. Harter, "Mental disorders in patients with obesity in comparison with healthy probands," *Int'l J Obes* 31 (2007) 1155-1164.
6. J.M. Siegel, A.K. Yancey, W.J. McCarthy, "Overweight and depressive symptoms among African-American women," *Prev Med* 31 (2000) 232-240.
7. K.M. Scott, R. Bruffaerts, G.E. Simon, J. Alonso, M. Angermeyer, G. de Girolamo, K. Demyttenaere, I. Gasquet, J.M. Haro, E. Karam R.C. Kessler, D. Levinson, M.E. Medina-Mora, M.A. Oakley-Browne, J. Ormel, J.P. Villa, H. Uda, M. Von Korff, "Obesity and mental disorders in the general population: results from the world mental health surveys," *Int'l J Obes* 32 (2008) 192-200.
8. S. Kasen, P. Cohen, H. Chen, A. Must, "Obesity and psychopathology in women: a three decade prospect of study," *Int'l J Obes* 32 (2008) 558-566.
9. Ibid.
10. M.T. Vander Merwe, "Psychological correlates of obesity in women," *Int'l J Obes* 31 (2007) S14-S18.
11. D. Crawford, K. Ball, "What help do young women want in their efforts to control their weight? Implications for program development," *Nutr & Diet* 64 (2007) 99-104.
12. K.M. Scott, R. Bruffaerts, G.E. Simon, J. Alonso, M. Angermeyer, G. de Girolamo, K. Demyttenaere, I. Gasquet, J.M. Haro, E. Karam R.C. Kessler, D. Levinson, M.E. Medina-Mora, M.A. Oakley-Browne, J. Ormel, J.P. Villa, H. Uda, M. Von Korff, "Obesity and mental disorders in the general population: results from the world mental health surveys," *Int'l J Obes* 32 (2008) 192-200.
13. H.L. Littleton, T. Ollendick, "Negative body image and disordered eating behavior in children and adolescents: what places youth at risk and how can these problems be prevented," *Clin Child& Fam Psych Rev* 6 (2003) 51-66.
14. Ibid.
15. Ibid.
16. Ibid.
17. L. Pulkki-Raback, M. Elovainio, M. Kivimaki, O.T. Raitakari, L. Keltikangas-Jarvinen, "Temperament in childhood predicts body mass in adulthood: the cardiovascular risk in young Finns study, *Health Psych* 24 (2005) 307-315.
18. Ibid.
19. Ibid.
20. R.W. Jeffery, A. Drewnowski, L.H. Epstein, et al, "Long-term maintenance of weight loss: current status," *Health Psych* 19 (2000) 5-16.
21. F.M. Cachelin, R.H. Striegel-Moore, K.D. Brownell, "Beliefs about weight gain and attitudes toward relapse in a sample of women and men with obesity," *Obes Res* 6 (1998) 231-237.
22. A. Peters, L. Pellerin, M.F. Dallman, K.M. Oltmanns, U. Schweiger, J. Born, H.L. Fehm, " Causes of obesity: looking beyond the hypothalamus," *Prog in Neurobio* 81 (2007) 61-68.
23. Ibid.
24. Ibid.
25. Ibid.
26. Ibid.
27. Ibid.
28. Ibid.
29. W.S. Dhillo, "Appetite regulation: an overview," *Thyroid* 17 92007) 433-445.

30. T. Yamada, H. Katagiri, "Avenues of communication between the brain and tissues/organs involved in energy homeostasis," *Endocrin J* 54 (2007) 497-505.

31. E. Valassi, M. Sacchi, F. Cavagnini, "Neuroendocrine control of food intake," *Nutr Met Cardio Dis* 18 (2008) 158-168.

32. F. McPherson, *"The Memory Key"* (Franklin Lakes, NJ: The Career Press, 2000).

33. L.T. Haltia, A. Viljanen, R. Parkkola, N. Kemppainen, J.O. Rinne, P. Nuutila, V. Kaasinen, "Brain white matter expansion in human obesity and the recovering effect of dieting," *J Clin Endocrinol Metab* 92 (2007) 3278-3284.

34. S. Gazdzinski, J. Kornak, M.W. Weiner, D.J. Meyerhoff, D.R. Nat, "Body mass index and magnetic resonance markers of brain integrity in adults," *Ann Neurol* 63 (2008) 652-657.

35. L.T. Haltia, A. Viljanen, R. Parkkola, N. Kemppainen, J.O. Rinne, P. Nuutila, V. Kaasinen, "Brain white matter expansion in human obesity and the recovering effect of dieting," *J Clin Endocrinol Metab* 92 (2007) 3278-3284.

36. N. Pannacciulli, D.S.N.T. Le, K. Chen, E.M. Reiman, J Krakoff, "Relationships between plasma leptin concentrations and human brain structure: a voxel based morphometric study," *Neurosci Letters* 412 (2007) 248-253.

37. Y. Taki, S. Kinomura, K. Sato, K. Inoue, R. Goto, K. Okada, S. Uchida, R. Kawashima, H. Fukuda, "Relationship between body mass index and gray matter volume in 1428 healthy individuals," *Obesity* 16 (2008) 119-124.

38. R. Capasso, A.A. Izzo, "Gastrointestinal regulation of food intake: General aspects and focus on anadamide and oleoyletanolamide," *J Neuroendocrinol* 20 (2008) 39-46.

39. H.R. Berthoud, "Vagal and hormonal gut-brain communication from satiation is satisfaction," *Neurogastroenterol Motil* 20 (2008) 64-72.

40. W.S. Dhillo, "Appetite regulation: an overview," *Thyroid* 17 92007) 433-445.

41. Y. Rothemund, C. Preuschhof, G. Bohner, H.C. Bauknecht, R. Klingebiel, H. Flor, B.F. Klapp, "Differential activation of the dorsal striatum by high-calorie visual food stimuli in obese individuals," *NeuroImage* 37 (2007) 410-421.

42. L.E. Stoeckel, R.E. Weller, E.W. Cook III, D.B. Twieg, R.C. Knowlton, J.E. Cox, "Widespread reward-system activation in obese women in response to pictures of high-calorie foods," *NeuroImage* 41 (2008) 636-647.

43. T.L. Davidson, "Pavlovian occasion setting: a link between physiological change and appetite behavior," *Appetite* 35 (2000) 271-272.

44. Y. Rothemund, C. Preuschhof, G. Bohner, H.C. Bauknecht, R. Klingebiel, H. Flor, B.F. Klapp, "Differential activation of the dorsal striatum by high-calorie visual food stimuli in obese individuals," *NeuroImage* 37 (2007) 410-421.

45. P. Martel, M. Fantino, "Mesolimbic dopaminergic system activity as a function of food reward: a microdialysis study," *Pharmacol Biochem Behav* 53 (1996) 221-226.

46. I.E. De Araujo, E.T. Rolls, "Representation in the human brain of food texture and oral fat," *J Neurosci* 24 (2004) 3086-3093.

47. L.E. Stoeckel, R.E. Weller, E.W. Cool III, D.B. Twieg, R.C. Knowlton, J.E. Cox, "Widespread reward-system activation in obese women in response to pictures of high-calorie foods," *NeuroImage* 41 (2008) 636-647.

48. G. Finlayson, N. King, J.E. Blundell, "Liking vs wanting food: importance for human appetite control and weight regulation," *Neurosci Biobehav Rev* 31 (2007) 987-1002.

49. R.A. Wise, "Role of brain dopamine and food reward and reinforcement," *Philosoph Transact Royal Soc* 361 (2006) 1149-1158.

50. L.H. Epstein, J.L. Temple, B.J. Neaderhiser, R.J. Salis, R.W. Erbe, J.J. Leddy, "Food reinforcement, the dopamine D_2 receptor genotype and energy intake in obese and nonobese humans," Behav Neurosci 121 (2007) 877-886.

51. J.S. Bodenlos, S. Kose, J.J. Borckardt, Z. Nahas, D. Shaw, P.M. O'Neil, M.S. George, "Vagas nerve stimulation acutely alters food craving in adults with depression," *Appetite* 48 (2007) 145-153.

52. P.A. Wolf, A. Beiser, M.F. Elias, R. Au, R.S. Vasan, S. Seshadri, "Relation of obesity to cognitive function: importance of central obesity and synergistic influence of concomitant hypertension, The Framingham Heart Study," *Cur Alzheimer Res* 4 (2007) 111-116.

53. J.S. Bodenlos, S. Kose, J.J. Borckardt, Z. Nahas, D. Shaw, P.M. O'Neil, M.S. George, "Vagas nerve stimulation acutely alters food craving in adults with depression," *Appetite* 48 (2007) 145-153.

54. Ibid.

55. Ibid.

56. I. Matias, L. Cristino, V. Di Marzo, "Endocannabinoids: some like it fat (and sweet too)," *J Neuroendocrinol* 20 (2008) 100-109.

57. S.A. Farr, K.A. Yamada, D.A. Butterfield, H.M. Abdul, L. Xu, N.E. Miller, W.A. Banks, J.E. Morley, "Obesity and hypertriglyceridemia produce cognitive impairment," *Endocrinol* 149 (2008) 2628-2636.

58. J.S. Bodenlos, S. Kose, J.J. Borckardt, Z. Nahas, D. Shaw, P.M. O'Neil, M.S. George, "Vagas nerve stimulation acutely alters food craving in adults with depression," *Appetite* 48 (2007) 145-153.

59. Ibid.

60. M. Hutchison, *Mega brain power: transform your life with mine machines and brain nutrients,* (New York, NY: Hyperion, 1994) 4-6.

61. M.B. Solomon, M.T. Foster, T.J. Bartness, K.L. Huhman, "Social defeat and footshock increase body mass and adiposity in male Syrian hamsters," *Am J Physiology - Reg Integr Comp Physiology* 292 (2007) R283-R290.

62. V. Drapeau, F. Therrien, D. Richard, A. Tremblay, "Is visceral obesity a physiological adaptation to stress," *Panminerva Med* 45 (2003) 189-195.

63. R. Rosmond, "Role of stress in the pathogenesis of the metabolic syndrome," *Psychoneuroendocrinol* 30 (2005) 1-10.

64. J. Marniemi, E. Kronholm, S. Aunola, T. Toikka, C.E. Mattlar, M. Koskenvuo, T. Ronnemaa, "Visceral fat and psychosocial stress in identical twins discordant for obesity," *J Int Med* 251 (2002) 35-43.

65. Ibid.

66. R. Rosmond, "Role of stress in the pathogenesis of the metabolic syndrome," *Psychoneuroendocrinol* 30 (2005) 1-10.

67. R. Rosmond, P. Bjorntorp, "Occupational status, cortisol secretory pattern, and visceral obesity in middle-aged men," *Obes Res* 8 (2000) 445-450.

68. A. Kouvonen, M. Kivimaki, S.J. Cox, T. Cox, J. Vahtera, "Relationship between work stress and body mass index among 45,810 female and male employees," *Psych Med* 67 (2005) 577-583.

69. D. Overgaard, M. Gamborg, F. Gyntelberg, B.L. Heitmann, "Psychological workload is associated with weight gain between 1993 and 1999: analyses based on the Danish Nurse Cohort Study," *Int'l J Obes* 28 (2004) 1072-1081.

70. M. Kivimaki, J. Head, K.E. Ferrie, M.J. Shipley, E. Brunner, J. Vahtera, M.G. Marmot, "Work stress, weight gain and weight loss: evidence for bidirectional effects of job strain on body mass index and the Whitehall II study," *Int'l J Obes* 30 (2006) 982-987.

71. M.M.N. Nguyen, K.L.K. Tamashiro, S.J. Melhorn, L.Y. Ma, S.R. Gardner, R.R, Sakai, "Androgenic influences on behavior, body weight and body composition in a model of chronic social stress," *Endocrinol* 148 (2007) 6145-6156.

72. Ibid.

73. K. Laederach-Hoffamn, S. Kupferschmid, L. Mussgay, "Links between body mass index, total body fat, cholesterol, high density lipoprotein and insulin sensitivity in patients with obesity related to depression, anger and anxiety," *Int'l J Eat Disord* 32 (2002) 58-71.

74. A. Serlachius, M. Hamer, J. Wardle, "Stress and weight change in university students in the United Kingdom," *Psych Behav* 92 (2007) 548-553.

75. C. Roberts, N. Troop, F. Connan, J. Treasure, I.C. Campbell, "The effects of stress on body weight:: biological and psychological predictors of change in BMI," *Obesity* 15 (2007) 3045-3055.

76. A.D. Ozier, O.W. Kendrick, J.D. Leeper, L.L. Knol, M. Perko, J. Burnham, "Overweight and obesity are associated with the emotion and stress-related eating as measured by the eating and appraisal due to emotions and stress questionnaire," *J Am Diet Assn* 108 (2008) 49-56.

77. C. Roberts, N. Troop, F. Connan, J. Treasure, I.C. Campbell, "The effects of stress on body weight:: biological and psychological predictors of change in BMI," *Obesity* 15 (2007) 3045-3055.

78. D.A. Zellner, S. Loaiza, Z. Gonzalez, J. Pita, J. Morales, D. Pecora, A. Wolf, "Food selection changes under stress," *Psych Behav* 87 (2006) 789-793.

79. Ibid.

80. Ibid.

81. S.L. Teegarden, T.L. Bale, Effects of stress on dietary preference and intake are dependent on access and stress sensitivity," *Psych Behav* 93 (2008) 713-723.

82. N. Pecoraro, F. Reyes, F. Gomez, A. Bhargave, M.F. Dallman, "Chronic stress promotes palatable feeding which reduces signs of stress: feedforward and feedback effects of chronic stress," Endocrinol 145 (2004) 3754-3762.

83. S.L. Teegarden, T.L. Bale, Effects of stress on dietary preference and intake are dependent on access and stress sensitivity," *Psych Behav* 93 (2008) 713-723.

84. D.A. Zellner, S. Loaiza, Z. Gonzalez, J. Pita, J. Morales, D. Pecora, A. Wolf, "Food selection changes under stress," *Psych Behav* 87 (2006) 789-793.

85. N. Pecoraro, F. Reyes, F. Gomez, A. Bhargave, M.F. Dallman, "Chronic stress promotes palatable feeding which reduces signs of stress: feedforward and feedback effects of chronic stress," Endocrinol 145 (2004) 3754-3762.

86. L. Dube, J.L. LeBel, J. Lu, "Affect asymmetry and comfort food consumption," *Psych Behav* 86 (2005) 559-567.

87. M.R. Lowe, T.V.E. Kral, "Stress-induced eating in restrained eaters may not be caused by stress or restraint," *Appetite* 46 (2006) 16-21.

88. Ibid.

89. M. Korkeila, J. Kaprio, A. Rissanen, M. Koskenvuo, T.I.A. Sorensen, "Predictors of major weight gain in adult Finns: stress, life satisfaction and personality traits," *Int'l J Obes* 22 (1998) 949-957.

90. A.W. Smith, A. Baum, R.R. Wing, "Stress and weight gain in parents of cancer patients," *Int'l J Obes* 29 (2005) 244-250.

91. V. Drapeau, F. Therrien, D. Richard, A. Tremblay, "Is visceral obesity a physiological adaptation to stress," *Panminerva Med* 45 (2003) 189-195.

92. M.S. Faith, P.E. Matz, M.A. Jorge, "Obesity-depression associations in the population," *J Psych Res* 53 (2002) 935-942.

93. T.W. Strine, A.H. Mokdad, S.R. Dube, L.S. Balluz, O. Gonzalez, J.T. Berry, R. Manderscheid, K. Kroenke, "The association of depression and anxiety with obesity and unhealthy behaviors among community-dwelling US adults," *Gen Hosp Psych* 30 (2008) 127-137.

94. E. Johnston, S. Johnson, P. McCleod, M. Johnston, "The relation of body mass index to depressive symptoms," *Can J Pub Health* 95 (2004) 179-183.

95. J.I. Hrabosky, J.J. Thomas, "Elucidating the relationship between obesity and depression: recommendations for future research," *Clin Psych Sci Prac* 15 (2008) 28-34.

96. Ibid.

97. A. Dragan, N. Akhtar-Danesh, "Relation between body mass index and depression: a structural equation modeling-approach," *BMC Med Res Method* 7 (2007) http://www.biomedcentral.com/1471-2288/7/17.

98. M. Heo, A. Pietrobelli, K.R. Fontaine, J.A. Sirey, M.S. Faith, "Depressive mood and obesity in US adults: comparison and moderation by sex age and race," *Int'l J Obes* 30 (2006) 513-519.

99. A. Farmer, A. Korszun, M.J. Owen, N. Craddock, L. Jones, I. Jones, J. Gray, R.J. Williamson, P. McGuffin, "Medical disorders in people with recurrent depression," *Brit J Psych* 192 (2008) 351-355.

100. A.C. Ahlberg, T. Ljung, R. Rosmond, B. McEwen, G. Holm, H.O. Akesson, P. Bjorntorp, "Depression and anxiety symptoms in relation to anthropometry and metabolism in men," *Psych Res* 112 (2002) 101-110.

101. C. Dong, L.E. Sanchez, R.A. Price, "Relationship of obesity to depression: a family-based study," *Int'l J Obes* 28 (2004) 790-795.

102. R.E. Roberts, S. Deleger, W.J. Strawbridge, G.A. Kaplan, " Prospective association between obesity and depression: evidence from the Alameda County study," *Int'l J Obes* 27 (2003) 514-521.

103. R.L. Kolotkin, R.D. Crosby, G.R. Williams, "Health related quality of life varies among obese subgroups," *Obes Res* 10 (2002) 748-756.

104. C.U. Onyike, R.M. Crum, H.B. Lee, C.G. Lyketsos, W.W. Eaton, "Is obesity associated with major depression? Results from the third national health and nutrition examination survey," *Am J Epidermiol* 158 (2003) 1139-1147.

105. D.L. Franko, R.H. Striegel-Moore, D. Thompson, G.B. Schreiber, S.R. Daniels, "Does adolescent depression predict obesity in black and white young adult women?" *Psych Med* 35 (2005) 1505-1513.

106. R.E. Roberts, G.A. Kaplan, S.J. Shema, W.J. Strawbridge, "Are the obese at greater risk for depression," *Am J Epidermiol* 152 (2000) 163-170.

107. Ibid.

108. Ibid.

109. C. Galletly, L. Moran, M. Noakes, P. Clifton, L. Tomlinson, R. Norman, "Psychological benefits of a high-protein low-carbohydrate diet in obese women with polycystic ovary syndrome - a pilot study," *Appetite* 49 (2007) 590-593.

110. J. Gilmore, "Body mass index and health," *Health Rep* 11 (1999) 1-43.

111. A. Haukkala, A. Uutela, V. Salomaa, " Depressive symptoms, cynical hostility and weight change: a three-year follow-up among middle-aged men and women," *Int'l J Behav Med* 8 (2001) 116-133.
112. A. Haukkala, A. Uutela, "Cynical hostility, depression and obesity: a moderating role of education and gender," *Int'l J Eat Disord* 27 (2000) 106-109.
113. D.A. Lawlor, C.L. Hart, D.J. Hole, D. Grunnell, G.D. Smith, "Body mass index in middle life and future risk of hospital admission for psychosis or depression: findings from the Renfrew/Paisley study," *Psych Med* 37 (2007) 1151-1161.
114. Ibid.
115. J. Grazyna, A. Ziomkiewicz, M. Gorkiewicz, A. Pajak, "Body mass, depressive symptoms and menopausal status: an examination of the Jolly Fat Hypothesis," *Women's Health Issues* 15 (2005) 145-151.
116. K. Laederach-Hoffamn, S. Kupferschmid, L. Mussgay, "Links between body mass index, total body fat, cholesterol, high density lipoprotein and insulin sensitivity in patients with obesity related to depression, anger and anxiety," *Int'l J Eat Disord* 32 (2002) 58-71.
117. P.S. Chen, Y.K. Yang, T.L. Yeh, I-H Lee, W.J. Yao, N.T. Chiu, R.B. Lu, "Correlation between body mass index and striatal dopamine transporter availability in healthy volunteers - a SPECT study," *NeuroImage* 40 (2008) 275-279.
118. S. Markowitz, M.A. Friedman, S.M. Arent, "Understanding the relationship between obesity and depression: causal mechanisms and implications for treatment," *Clin Psychol Sci Prac* 15 (2008) 1-20.
119. C. Brayne, L. Gao, F. Matthews, "Challenges in the epidemiological investigation of the relationships between physical activity, obesity, diabetes, dementia and depression," *Neurobio Aging* 26S (2005) S6-S10.
120. K-H. Ladwig, B. Marten-Mittag, H. Lowel, A. Doring, W. Koenig, "The influence of depressive mood on the association of CRP and obesity in 3205 middle aged healthy men," *Brain Behav Immun* 17 (2003) 268-275.
121. Ibid.
122. C. Dong, W-D Li, D. Li, R.A. Price, "Extreme obesity is associated with attempted suicides: results from a family study," *Int'l J Obes* 30 (2006) 388-390.
123. Ibid.
124. K.J. Mukamal, I. Kawachi, M. Miller, E.B. Rimm, "Body mass index and risk of suicide among men," *Arch Intern Med* 167 (2007) 468-475.
125. S.E. Anderson, P. Cohen, E.N. Naumova, P.F. Jacques, A. Must, "Adolescent obesity and risk for subsequent major depressive disorder and anxiety disorder: prospective evidence," *Pyschosom Med* 69 (2007) 740-747.
126. Ibid.
127. Ibid.
128. Ibid.
129. E.S. Lee, Y.H. Kim, S-H Beck, S. Lee, S.W. Oh, "Depressive mood and abdominal fat distribution in overweight premenopausal women," *Obes Res* 13 (2005) 320-325.
130. B. Weber-Hamann, F. Hentschel, A. Kniest, M. Deuschle, M. Colla, F. Lederbogen, I. Heuser, "Hypercortisolemic depression is associated with increased intra-abdominal fat," *Physosom Med* 64 (2002) 274-277.

131. C.U. Onyike, R.M. Crum, H.B. Lee, C.G. Lyketsos, W.W. Eaton, "Is obesity associated with major depression? Results from the third national health and nutrition examination survey," *Am J Epidemiol* 158 (2003) 1139-1147.
132. M.Q. Werrij, S. Mulkens, H.J. Hospers, A. Jansen, "Overweight and obesity: the significance of a depressed mood," *Patient Ed & Coun* 62 (2006) 126-131.
133. S. McElroy, R. Kotwal, S. Malhotra, E.B. Nelson, P.E. Keck, Jr., C.B. Nemeroff, "Are mood disorders and obesity related: a review for the mental health professional," *J. Clin Psych* 65 (2004) 634-651.
134. L. Nevonen, A.G. Broberg, "The emergence of eating disorders: an exploratory study," *Euro Eat Disord Rev* 8 (2000) 279-292.
135. K.L. Klump, W.H. Kaye, M. Strober, "The evolving genetic foundations of eating disorders," *Psych Clin North Am* 24 (2001) 215-225.
136. J. Polivy, C.P. Herman, "Causes of eating disorders," *Ann Rev Psych* 53 (2002) 187-213.
137. Ibid.
138. A. Furnham, R. Nordling, "Cross-cultural differences in preferences for specific male and female body shapes," *Person Indiv Diff* 25 (1998) 635-648.
139. Ibid.
140. N. Wolf, "The beauty myth," (Chatto and Windus: London 1990).
141. E. Stice, H.E. Shaw, "Adverse effects of the media portrayed thin-ideal on women and linkages to bulimic symptomatology," *J Soc Clin Psych* 13 (1994) 288-308.
142. A. Furnham, R. Nordling, "Cross-cultural differences in preferences for specific male and female body shapes," *Person Indiv Diff* 25 (1998) 635-648.
143. Ibid.
144. Ibid.
145. Ibid.
146. P.K. Keel, M.G. Baxter, T.F. Heatherton, T.E. Joiner, Jr., "A 20-year longitudinal study of body weight, dieting, and eating disorder symptoms," *J Abnormal Psych* 116 (2007) 423-432.
147. C.M. Bulik, P.F. Sullivan, F. Tozzi, H. Furberg, P. Lichetenstein, N.L. Pederson, "Prevalence, heritability and prospective risk factors for anorexia nervosa," *Arch Gen Psych* 63 (2006) 305-312.
148. J. Gusella, J. Goodwin, E. van Roosmalen, "I want to lose weight: early risk for disordered eating," *Paediatr Child Health* 13 (2008) 105-110.
149. W.C. Lynch, D.P. Heil, E. Wagner, M.D. Havens, "Body dissatisfaction mediates the association between body mass index and risky weight control behaviors among white and native American adolescent girls," *Appetite* 51 (2008) 210-213.
150. C.M. Bulik, P.F. Sullivan, F. Tozzi, H. Furberg, P. Lichetenstein, N.L. Pederson, "Prevalence, heritability and prospective risk factors for anorexia nervosa," *Arch Gen Psych* 63 (2006) 305-312.
151. A.E. Field, K.M. Javaras, P. Aneja, N. Kitos, C.A. Camargo, C.B. Taylor, N.M. Laird, "Family, peer and media predictors of becoming eating disordered," *Arch Ped Adolesc Med* 162 (2008) 574-579.
152. A.C. Doyle, D. le Grange, A. Goldschmidt, D.E. Wilfley, "Psychosocial and physical impairment in overweight adolescents at high risk for eating disorders," *Obesity* 15 (2007) 145-154.
153. D.M. Ackare, D. Nuemark-Sztainer, M. Story, C. Perry, "Overeating among adolescents: prevalence and associations with weight related characteristics and psychological health," *Pediatrics* 111 (2003) 67-74.

154. J.M. Jones, S. Bennett, M.P. Olmsted, M.L. Lawson, G. Rodin, "Disordered eating attitudes and behaviors in teenage girls: a school-based study," *Can Med Assn J* 4 (2001) 547-552.

155. Ibid.

156. K.L. Klump, W.H. Kaye, M. Strober, "The evolving genetic foundations of eating disorders," *Psych Clin North Am* 24 (2001) 215-225.

157. S.F. Abraham, "Dieting, body weight, body image and self-esteem in young women: doctors dilemmas," *Med J Australia* 178 (2003) 607-611.

158. T.M. Stewart, D.A. Williamson, M.A. White, "Rigid vs flexible dieting: association with the eating disorder symptoms in non-obese women," *Appetite* 38 (2002) 39-44.

159. E.S. Rome, S. Ammerman, D.S. Rosen, R.J. Keller, J. Lock, K.A. Mammel. J. O'Toole, J.M. Rees, M.J. Sanders, S.M. Sawyer, M. Schneider, E. Sigel, T.J. Silber, "Children and adolescents with eating disorders: the state-of-the-art,"*Pediatrics* 111 (2003) 98-108.

160. J. Gusella, J. Goodwin, E. Van Roosmalen, "I want to lose weight: early risk of disordered eating," *Paediatr Child Health* 13 (2008) 105-110.

161. J.L. Mansfield, T. Wade, "Assessing the relevance of the hopelessness theory of depression in women with disordered eating," *Int'l J Eat Disord* 28 (2000) 113-119.

162. J.L. Mansfield, T. Wade, "Assessing the relevance of the hopelessness theory of depression in women with disordered eating," *Int'l J Eat Disord* 28 (2000) 113-119.

163. M.B. Feldman, I.H. Meyer, "Eating disorders in diverse lesbian, gay and bisexual populations," *Int'l J Eat Disord* 40 (2007) 218-226.

164. Ibid.

165. L.A. Kolter, P. Cohen, M. Davies, D.S. Pine, B.T. Walsh, "Longitudinal relationships between childhood, adolescent and adult eating disorders," *J Am Acad Child Adol Psych* 40 (2001) 1434-1440.

166. T.D. Wade, C.M. Bulik, "Shared genetic and environmental risk factors between undue influence of body shape and weight on self-evaluation and dimensions of perfectionism," *Psych Med* 37 (2007) 635-644.

167. Ibid.

168. C.G. Fairburn, Z. Cooper, H.A. Doll, B.A. Davies, "Identifying dieters who will develop an eating disorder: a prospective, population-based study," *Am J Psych* 162 (2005) 2249-2255.

169. Ibid.

170. D. Clinton, C. Bjorck, S. Sohlberg, C. Norring, "Patient satisfaction with treatment in eating disorders: cause for complacency or concerned," *Euro Eat Disord Rev* 12 (2004) 240-246.

171. Ibid.

172. "Anorexia," *Dorland's Illustrated Medical Dictionary*, 30th ed: 95.

173. P.J.V. Beaumont, "Clinical presentation of anorexia nervosa and bulimia nervosa," In C.G. Fairburn, K.D. Brownell, *Eating disorders and obesity: a comprehensive handbook*, (2nd ed) (New York, NY: Guildford Press, 2002 162-170).

174. "Anorexia," *Dorland's Illustrated Medical Dictionary*, 30th ed: 95.

175. D. Benardot, *Advanced Sports Nutrition: Fine-tune your food and fluid intake for optimal training and performance*, (Champaign, IL: Human Kinetics, 2006) 230.

176. "Anorexia," *Dorland's Illustrated Medical Dictionary*, 30th ed: 95.

177. C.M. Bulik, P.F. Sullivan, F. Tozzi, H. Furberg, P. Lichtenstein, N.L. Pedersen, "Prevalence, heritability and prospective risk factors for anorexia nervosa," *Arch Gen Psych* 63 (2006) 305-312.

178. Ibid.

179. M. Vervaet, K. Audenaert, C. van Heeringen, "Cognitive and behavioral characteristics are associated with a personality dimensions in patients with eating disorders," *Euro Eat Disord Rev* 11 (2003) 363-378.

180. H. Turner, M. Cooper, "Cognitions and their origins in women with anorexia nervosa, normal dieters and female controls," *Clin Psych & Psychotherapy* 9 (2002) 242-252.

181. J. Burney, H.J. Irwin, "Shame and guilt in women with eating-disorder symptomatology," *J Clin Psych* 56 (2000) 51-61.

182. C.G. Fairburn, P.J. Harrison, "Eating disorders," *Lancet* 361 (2003) 407-416.

183. A. Dignon, A. Beardsmore, S. Spain, A. Kuan, "Why I won't eat:: patient testimony from 15 anorexics concerning the causes of their disorder," *J Health Psych* 11 (2006) 942-956.

184. D.E. Wilfley, C.M. Grillo, "Eating disorders: a woman's health problem in primary care," *Nurse Pract Forum* 5 (1994) 34-45.

185. S. Gowers, R. Bryant-Waugh, "Management of child and adolescent eating disorders: the current evidence base and future directions," *J Child Psych & Psych* 45 (2004) 63-83.

186. C.M. Bulik, P.F. Sullivan, F. Tozzi, H. Furberg, P. Lichtenstein, N.L. Pederson, "Prevalence, heritability and prospective risk factors for anorexia nervosa," *Arch Gen Psych* 63 (2006) 305-312.

187. C.G. Fairburn, P.J. Harrison, "Eating disorders," *Lancet* 361 (2003) 407-416.

188. S. Cook-Darzens, C. Doyen, B. Falissard, M. Christine-Mouren, "Self-perceived family functioning in 40 French families of anorexic adolescents: implications for therapy," *Euro Eat Disord Rev* 13 (2005) 223-236.

189. Ibid.

190. J.E. Mitchell, "Psychopharmacology of eating disorders: current knowledge and future directions," In R. Striegel-Moore, L. Smolak (eds) *Eating disorders: innovative directions in research and practice*," (Washington, DC: American Psychological Association, 2001 197-214).

191. S. Collings, M. King, "Ten year follow-up of 50 patients with bulimia nervosa," *Brit J Psych* 164 (1994) 80-87.

192. E.S. Rome, S.D. Ammerman, D.S. Rosen, R.J. Keller, J. Lock, K.A. Mammel, J. O'Toole, J.M. Rees, M.J. Sanders, S.M. Sawyer, M. Schneider, E. Sigel, T.J. Silber, "Children and adolescents with eating disorders: the state-of-the-art," *Pediatrics* 111 (2003) 98-108.

193. S. Gowers, R. Bryant-Waugh, "Management of child and adolescent eating disorders: the current evidence base and future directions," *J Child Psych & Psych* 45 (2004) 63-83.

194. "Bulimia," *Dorland's Illustrated Medical Dictionary*, 30th ed: 259.

195. Ibid.

196. "*Diagnostic and statistical manual of mental disorders*, 4th ed, (Washington, DC: American Psychiatric Association, 1994).

197. D.E. Wilfley, C.M. Grillo, "Eating disorders: a woman's health problem in primary care," *Nurse Pract Forum* 5 (1994) 34-45.

198. K. Laederach-Hoffman, S. Kupferschmid, L. Mussgay, "Links between body mass index, total body fat, cholesterol, high-density lipoprotein and insulin sensitivity in patients with obesity related to depression, anger and anxiety," *Int'l J Eat Disord* 32 (2002) 58-71.

199. J.M. Mond, P.J. Hay, B. Rodgers, C. Owen, P.J.V. Beumont, "Beliefs of women concerning causes and risk factors for bulimia nervosa," *Aust & New Zeal J Psych* 38 (2004) 463-469.

200. M. Vervaet, K. Audenaert, C. van Heeringen, "Cognitive and behavioral characteristics are associated with a personality dimensions in patients with eating disorders," *Euro Eat Disord Rev* 11 (2003) 363-378.

201. C.G. Fairburn, P.J. Harrison, "Eating disorders," *Lancet* 361 (2003) 407-416.
202. E. Stice, "Relations of restraint and negative affect to bulimic pathology: a longitudinal tests of three competing models," *Int'l J Eat Disord* 23 (1998) 243-260.
203. Ibid.
204. N.A. Lester, P.K. Keel, S.F. Lipson, "Symptom fluctuation in bulimia nervosa: relation to menstrual cycle phase and cortisol levels," *Psych Med* 33 (2003) 51-60.
205. Ibid.
206. Ibid.
207. S. Gowers, R. Bryant-Waugh, "Management of child and adolescent eating disorders: the current evidence base and future directions," *J Child Psych & Psych* 45 (2004) 63-83.
208. Ibid.
209. C.G. Fairburn, M.D. Marcus, G.T. Wilson, "Cognitive behavioral therapy for binge eating and bulimia nervosa: a comprehensive treatment manual," In C.G. Fairburn, G.T. Wilson (eds) *Binge eating nature, assessment and treatment*, (New York, NY: Guilford Press, 1993 361-404.
210. C.G. Fairburn, P.J. Harrison, "Eating disorders," *Lancet* 361 (2003) 407-416.
211. B.T. Walsh, G.T. Wilson, K.L. Loeb, et al, "Medication and psychotherapy in the treatment of the bulimia nervosa," *Am J Psych* 154 (1997) 523-531.
212. S. Gowers, R. Bryant-Waugh, "Management of child and adolescent eating disorders: the current evidence base and future directions," *J Child Psych & Psych* 45 (2004) 63-83.
213. L. Bell, "Does concurrent psychopathology at presentation influence response to treatment for bulimia nervosa," *Eat Weight Disord* 7 (2002) 168-181.
214. P.K. Keel, M.G. Baxter, T.F. Heatherton, T.E. Joiner, Jr., "A 20-year longitudinal study of body weight, dieting, and eating disorder symptoms," *J Abnormal Psych* 116 (2007) 423-432.
215. K.C. Allison, A.J. Stunkard, "Obesity and eating disorders," *Psych Clin North Am* 28 (2005) 55-67.
216. C. Pull, "Binge eating disorder," *Curr Opin Psych* 17 (2004) 43-48.
217. H. Nauta, H. Hospers, A. Jansen, "One-year follow-up effects of two obesity treatments on psychological well-being and weight," *Brit J Health Psych* 6 (2001) 271-284.
218. Ibid.
219. American Psychiatric Association, "Diagnostic and statistical manual of mental disorders," 4th ed, text revision, (Washington, DC: American Psychiatric Association, 2000 p787).
220. K.C. Allison, A.J. Stunkard, "Obesity and eating disorders," *Psych Clin North Am* 28 (2005) 55-67.
221. B. Bruce, D.E. Wilfley, "Binge eating among the overweight population: a serious and prevalent problem," *J Am Diet Assn* 96 (1995) 1-8.
222. J. Wardle, " Dietary restraint and binge eating," *Behav Anal Mod* 4 (1980) 201-209.
223. C.M. Grilo, R.M. Masheb, "Onset of dieting versus binge eating in outpatients with binge eating disorder," *Int'l J Obes Rel Met Disord* 24 (2000) 404-409.
224. R.H. Striegel-Moore, C.G. Fairburn, D.E. Wilfley, K.M. Pike, F.A. Dohm, H.C. Kraemer, "Toward an understanding of risk factors for binge-eating disorder in black and white women: a community-based case control study," *Psych Med* 35 (2005) 907-917.
225. R.C. Kessler, C.G. Davis, K.S. Kendler, "Childhood adversity and adult psychiatric disorder in the US National Comorbidity Survey," *Psych Med* 27 (1997) 1101-1119.
226. M.M. Boggiano, A.I. Artiga, C.E. Pritchett, P.C. Chandler-Laney, M.L. Smith, A.J. Eldredge, "High intake of palatable food predicts binge-eating independent of susceptibility to obesity: an

animal model of lean versus obese binge-eating and obesity with and without binge-eating," *Int'l J Obes* 31 (2007) 1357-1367.

227. M. Tanofsky-Kraff, D. Faden, S.Z. Yanovski, D.E. Wilfley, J.A. Yanovski, "The perceived onset of dieting and loss of control eating behaviors in overweight children," *Int'l J Eat Disord* 38 (2005) 112-122.

228. L. Goossens, C. Braet, V. Decaluwe, "Loss of control over eating in obese youngsters," *Behav Res Ther* 45 (2007) 1-9.

229. S.L. Colles, J.B. Dixon, P.E. O'Brien, "Loss of control is central to psychological disturbance associated with binge eating disorder," *Obesity* 16 (2008) 608-614.

230. C.M. Grilo, R.M. Masheb, "Correlates of body image dissatisfaction in treatment seeking men and women with binge eating disorder," *Int'l J Eat Disord* 38 (2005) 162-166.

231. E. Stice, K. Presnell, D. Spangler, "Risk factors for binge eating onset and adolescent girls: a 2-year prospective investigation," *Health Psych* 21 (2002) 131-138.

232. Ibid.

233. C.M. Bulik, P.F. Sullivan, K.S. Kendler, "Medical and psychiatric morbidity in obese women with and without binge eating," *Int'l J Eat Disord* 32 (2002) 72-78.

234. Ibid.

235. A.J. Stunkard, K.C. Allison, "Two forms of disordered eating and obesity: binge eating and night eating," *Int'l J Obes* 27 (2003) 1-12.

236. Ibid.

237. D.E. Wilfley, W.S. Agras, C.F. Telch, E.M. Rossiter, J.A. Schneider, A.G. Cole, L. Sifford, S.D. Raeburn, " Group cognitive-behavioral therapy and group interpersonal psychotherapy for the nonpurging bulimic individual: a controlled comparison," *J Consult Clin Psych* 61 (1993) 296-305.

238. A.J. Stunkard, K.C. Allison, "Two forms of disordered eating and obesity: binge eating and night eating," *Int'l J Obes* 27 (2003) 1-12.

239. Ibid.

240. M.A. Napolitano, S. Head, M.A. Babyak, J.A. Blumenthal, "Binge eating disorder and night eating syndrome: psychological and behavioral characteristics," *Int'l J Eat Disord* 30 (2001) 193-203.

241. Ibid.

242. J.P. O'Reardon, A. Peshek, K.C. Allison, "Night eating syndrome: diagnosis, epidemiology and management," *CNS Drugs* 19 (2005) 997-1008.

243. K.C. Allison, C.M. Grilo, R.M. Masheb, A.J. Stunkard, "Binge eating disorder and night eating syndrome: a comparative study of disordered eating," *J Consult Clin Psych* 73 (2005) 1107-1115.

244. S.A. Morse, P.S. Ciechanowski, W.J. Katon, I.B. Hirsch, "Isn't this just bedtime snacking: the potential adverse effects of night-eating syndromes on treatment adherence and outcomes in patients with diabetes," *Diabetes Care* 29 (2006) 1800-1804.

245. R.H. Striegel-Moore, F.A. Dohm, J.M. Hook, G.B. Schreiber, P.B. Crawford, S.R. Daniels, "Night eating syndrome in young adult women: prevalence and correlates," *Int'l J Eat Disord* 37 (2005) 200-206.

246. K.C. Allison, C.M. Grilo, R.M. Masheb, A.J. Stunkard, "High self-reported rates of neglect and emotional abuse, by persons with binge eating disorder and night eating syndrome," *Behav Res Ther* 45 (2007) 2874-2883.

247. K.C. Allison, C.M. Grilo, R.M. Masheb, A.J. Stunkard, "Binge eating disorder and night eating syndrome: a comparative study of disordered eating," *J Consult Clin Psych* 73 (2005) 1107-1115.

248. K.C. Allison, A.J. Stunkard, "Obesity and eating disorders," *Psych Clin North Am* 28 (2005) 55-67.

249. A.J. Stunkard, K.C. Allison, "Two forms of disordered eating and obesity: binge eating and night eating," *Int'l J Obes* 27 (2003) 1-12.

250. S.Z. Yanovski, A.J. Stunkard, "Obesity and eating disorders," In: G.A. Bray, C. Bouchard (eds) *Handbook of Obesity* 2nd ed, Marcel Dekker: NY.

251. M.A. Napolitano, S. Head, M.A. Babyak, J.A. Blumenthal, "Binge eating disorder and night eating syndrome: psychological and behavioral characteristics," *Int'l J Eat Disord* 30 (2001) 193-203.

252. S.L. Colles, J.B. Dixon, P.E. O'Brien, "Night eating syndrome and nocturnal snacking: association with obesity, binge eating and psychological distress," *Int'l J Obes* 31 (2007) 1722-1730.

253. A.J. Stunkard, K.C. Allison, "Two forms of disordered eating and obesity: binge eating and night eating," *Int'l J Obes* 27 (2003) 1-12.

254. J.D. Lundgren, K.C. Allison, S. Crow, J.P. O'Reardon, K.C. Berg, J. Galbraith, N.S. Martino, A.J. Stunkard, "Prevalence of night eating syndrome in a psychiatric population," *Am J Psych* 163 (2006) 156-158.

255. J.P. O'Reardon, A. Peshek, K.C. Allison, "Night eating syndrome: diagnosis, epidemiology and management," *CNS Drugs* 19 (2005) 997-1008.

256. E. Atlantis, K. Ball, "Association between weight perception and psychological distress," *Int'l J Obes* 32 (2008) 715-721.

257. L. Festinger, "A theory of social comparison processes," *Human Rel* 7 (1954) 117-140.

258. Ibid.

259. T.G. Morrison, R. Kalin, M.A. Morrison, "Body-image evaluation and body-image investment among adolescents: a test of sociocultural and social comparison theories," *Adolescence* 39 (2004) 571-592.

260. Ibid.

261. S. Jambekar, D.M. Quinn, J. Crocker, "The effects of weight and achievement messages on the self-esteem of women," *Psych Women Qrtly* 25 (2001) 48-56.

262. Ibid.

263. Ibid.

264. K.E. Friedman, S.K. Reichmann, P.R. Costanzo, A. Zelli, J.A. Ashmore, G.J. Musante, "Weight stigmatization and ideological beliefs: relation to psychological functioning in obese adults," *Obes Res* 13 (2005) 907-916.

265. J. Wardle, L. Cooke, "The impact of obesity on psychological well-being," *Best Prac & Res: Clin Endocrin & Metab* 19 (2005) 421-440.

266. S. Angle, S. Keskinen, H. Lapinleimu, H. Helenius, P. Raittinen, T. Ronnemaa, O. Simell, "Weight gain since infancy and prepubertal body dissatisfaction," *Arch Ped Adolesc Med* 159 (2005) 567-571.

267. Ibid.

268. A. Burrows, M. Cooper, "Possible risk factors in the development of eating disorders in overweight pre-adolescent girls," *Int'l J Obes* 26 (2002) 1268-1273.

269. M. Tiggemann, "The impact of adolescent girls' life concerns and leisure activities on body dissatisfaction, disordered eating and self-esteem," *J Clin Psych* 162 (2001) 133-142.

270. Ibid.
271. R.M. Viner, T.J. Cole, "Who changes body mass between adolescence and adulthood: factors predicting change in BMI between 16 year and 30 years in the 1970 British Birth Cohort," *Int'l J Obes* 30 (2006) 1368-1374.
272. R.D. Grave, M. Cuzzolaro, S. Calugi, F. Tomasi, F. Temperilli, G. Marchesini, the QUOVADIS Study Group, "The effect of obesity management on body image in patients seeking treatment at medical centers," *Obesity* 15 (2007) 2320-2327.
273. J. Franklin, G. Denyer, K.S. Steinbeck, I.D. Caterson, A.J. Hill, "Obesity and risk of low self-esteem: a statewide survey of Australian children," *Pediatrics* 118 (2006) 2481-2487.
274. Ibid.
275. JA.J. Zametkin, C.K. Zoon, H.W. Klein, S. Munson, "Psychiatric aspects of child and adolescent obesity: a review of the past 10 years," *J Am Acad Child Adol Psych* 43 (2004) 134-150.
276. K. Laederach-Hoffman, S. Kupferschmid, L. Mussgay, "Links between body mass index, total body fat, cholesterol, high-density lipoprotein and insulin sensitivity in patients with obesity related to depression, anger and anxiety," *Int'l J Eat Disord* 32 (2002) 58-71.
277. S. Markowitz, M.A. Friedman, S.M. Arent, "Understanding the relation between obesity and depression: causal mechanisms and implications for treatment," *Clin Psych: Sci & Pract* 15 (2008) 1-20.
278. D.B. Sarwer, J.K. Thompson, T.F. Cash, "Body image and obesity in adulthood," *Psychiatric Clin N Am* 28 (2005) 69-87.
279. D.B. Sarwer, T.A. Wadden, G.D. Foster, "Assessment of body image dissatisfaction in obese women: specificity, severity and clinical significance," *J Consult Clin Psych* 66(1998) 651-654.
280. Ibid.
281. D.B. Sarwer, J.K. Thompson, T.F. Cash, "Body image and obesity in adulthood," *Psych Clin N Am* 28 (2005) 69-87.
282. Ibid.
283. F.M. Cachelin, R.H. Striegel-Moore, K.D. Brownell, "Beliefs about weight gain and attitudes toward relapse in a sample of women and men with obesity," *Obes Res* 6 (1998) 231-237.
284. R.R. Wing, "Behavior treatment of severe obesity," *Am J Clin Nutr* 55 (1992) 545S-551S.
285. M.S. Faith, K.R. Fontaine, L.J. Cheskin, D.B. Allison, "Behavioral approaches to the problem of obesity," *Behav Mod* 24 (2000) 459-493.
286. M.S. Faith, K.R. Fontaine, L.J. Cheskin, D.B. Allison, "Behavioral approaches to the problem of obesity," *Behav Mod* 24 (2000) 459-493.
287. R. Schwarzer, A. Luszczynska, "How to overcome health-compromising behaviors: the health action process approach," *Euro Psych* 13 (2008) 141-151.
288. Ibid.
289. Ibid.
290. M.M. Driskell, S. Dyment, L. Mauriello, P. Castle, K. Sherman, "Relationships among multiple behaviors for childhood and adolescent obesity prevention," *Prev Med* 46 (2008) 209-215.
291. Ibid.
292. Ibid.
293. Ibid.
294. Ibid.
295. G.J. Norman, B.A. Schmid, J.F. Sallis, K.J. Calfas, K. Patrick, "Psychosocial and environmental correlates of adolescent sedentary behaviors," *Pediatrics* 116 (2005) 908-916.
296. Ibid.

297. Ibid.
298. Ibid.
299. M.M. Driskell, S. Dyment, L. Mauriello, P. Castle, K. Sherman, "Relationships among multiple behaviors for childhood and adolescent obesity prevention," *Prev Med* 46 (2008) 209-215.
300. D. Riebe, B. Blissmer, G. Greene, M. Caldwell, L. Ruggiero, K.M. Stillwell, C.R. Nigg, "Long-term maintenance of exercise and healthy eating behaviors in overweight adults," *Prev Med* 40 (2005) 769-778.
301. T. Baranowski, K.W. Cullen, T. Nicklas, D. Thompson, J. Baranowski, "Are current health behavioral change models helpful in guiding prevention of weight gain efforts," Obes Res 11 (2003) 23S-43S.
302. Ibid.
303. Ibid.
304. D. Riebe, B. Blissmer, G. Greene, M. Caldwell, L. Ruggiero, K.M. Stillwell, C.R. Nigg, "Long-term maintenance of exercise and healthy eating behaviors and overweight adults," *Prev Med* 40 (2005) 769-778.
305. T. Baraanowski, K.W. Cullen, T. Nicklas, D. Thompson, J. Baranowski, "Are current health behavioral change models helpful in guiding prevention of weight gain efforts," Obes Res 11 (2003) 23S-43S.
306. J.A. Linde, A.J. Rothman, A.S. Baldwin, R.W. Jeffery, "The impact of self-efficacy and behavior change and weight change among overweight participants in a weight-loss trial," *Health Psych* 25 (2006) 282-291.
307. Ibid.
308. S.M. Ali, M. Lindstrom, "Socioeconomic, psychosocial, behavioral and psychological determinants of BMI among young women: differing patterns of underweight and overweight obesity," *Euro J Pub Health* 16 (2005) 324-330.
309. T.T. Watt, S.F. Sharp, L. Atkins, "Personal control and disordered eating patterns among college females," *J Applied Soc Psych* 32 (2002) 2502-2512.
310. S.M. Ali, M. Lindstrom, "Socioeconomic, psychosocial, behavioral and psychological determinants of BMI among young women: differing patterns of underweight and overweight obesity," *Euro J Pub Health* 16 (2005) 324-330.
311. S.E. Hampson, J.A. Andrews, M. Peterson, S.C. Duncan, "A cognitive-behavioral mechanism leading to adolescent obesity: children's social images and physical identity," *Ann Behav Med* 34 (2007) 287-294.
312. Ibid.
313. B.R. Strickland, "Internal – external expectancies and health-related behaviors," *J Consult Clin Psych* 46 (1978) 1192-1211.
314. T.T. Watt, S.F. Sharp, L. Atkins, "Personal control and disordered eating patterns among college females," *J Applied Soc Psych* 32 (2002) 2502-2512.
315. W.S.C. Poston, M.L. Hyder, K.K. O'Byrne, J.P. Foreyt, "Where do diets, exercise and behavior modification fit in the treatment of obesity," *Endocrine* 13 (2000) 187-192.
316. Ibid.
317. Institute of Medicine, *"Weighing the options: criteria for evaluating weight management programs,"* Washington, DC: National Academy Press (1995) p 5.
318. W.S.C. Poston, M.L. Hyder, K.K. O'Byrne, J.P. Foreyt, "Where do diets, exercise and behavior modification fit in the treatment of obesity," *Endocrine* 13 (2000) 187-192.
319. Ibid.

320. Ibid.
321. Ibid.
322. Ibid.
323. D. Neumark-Sztainer, M. Wall, M. Story, J. Haines, M. Eisenberg, "Obesity, disordered eating and eating disorders in a longitudinal study of adolescent's: how do dieters fare 5 years later," *J Am Diet Assn* 106 (2006) 559-568.
324. D. Neumark-Sztainer, "Obesity an eating disorder prevention: an integrated approach," Adolesc Med 14 (2003) 159-173.
325. A.J. Rothman, "Toward a theory based analysis of behavioral maintenance," *Health Psych* 19 (2000) 64-69.
326. Ibid.
327. Ibid.
328. Ibid.
329. D. Riebe, B. Blissmer, G. Greene, M. Caldwell, L. Ruggiero, K.M. Stillwell, C.R. Nigg, "Long-term maintenance of exercise and healthy eating behaviors in overweight adults," *Prev Med* 40 (2005) 769-778.
330. S. Bleich, R. Blendon, A. Adams, "Trust in scientific experts on obesity: implications for awareness and behavior change," *Obesity* 15 (2007) 2145-2156.
331. Ibid.
332. Ibid.
333. Ibid.
334. Ibid.
335. A. Avenell, T.J. Brown, M.A. McGee, M.K. Campbell, A.M. Grant, J. Broom. R.T. Jung, W.C.S. Smith, "What interventions should we add to weight reducing diets in adults with obesity? A systematic review of randomized controlled trials of adding drug therapy, exercise, behaviour therapy or combinations of these interventions," *Brit Diet Assoc* 17 (2004) 293-316.
336. E.M. Fallon, M. Tanofsky-Fraff, A. Norman, J.R. McDuffe, E.D. Taylor, M.L. Cohen, D. Young-Hyman, M. Keil, R.L. Kolotkin, J.A. Yanovski, "Health-related quality of life in overweight and nonoverweight black and white adolescents," *J Ped* 147 (2005) 443-450.
337. T.W. Strine, A.H. Mokdad, S.R. Dude, L.S. Balluz, O. Gonzalez, J.T. Berry, R. Manderscheid, K. Kroenke, "The association of depression and anxiety with obesity and unhealthy behaviors among community dwelling US adults," *Gen Hosp Psych* 30 (2008) 127-137.
338. H. Nauta, H. Hospers, A. Jansen, "One-year follow-up effects of two obesity treatments on psychological well-being and weight," *Brit J Health Psych* 6 (2001) 271-284.
339. S.C. Stotland, M. Larocque, "Early treatment response as a predictor of ongoing weight loss in obesity treatment," *Brit J Health Psych* 10 (2005) 601-614.
340. M.R. Lowe, "Self-regulation of energy intake in the prevention and treatment of obesity: is it feasible?" *Obes Res* 11 (2003) 44S-59S.
341. Ibid.
342. C.M. Devine, J.A. Nelson, N. Chin, A. Dozier, I.D. Fernandez, "Pizza is cheaper than salad: assessing workers' views for an environmental food intervention," *Obesity* 15 (2007) 57S-68S.
343. J. Buckroyd, S. Rother, D. Stott, "Weight loss as a primary objective of therapeutic groups for obese women: two preliminary studies," *Brit J Guid & Counsel* 34 (2006) 245-265.

6   The Role of Hormones

The material presented in this chapter is somewhat technical. Every effort has been made to make it as simple and understandable as possible. The following information is offered to support the related discussion. Nothing you read here is intended to suggest that you should attempt to become your own doctor. The material is arranged to provide you with an understanding of what hormones are and the impact they can have on weight loss, followed by a discussion of how to determine your hormone levels and what to do about any that need adjustment.

What are Hormones

One of the most overlooked aspects of weight loss is the role the body's hormones play. Hormones are "chemical substance[s] produced in the body by an organ, cells of an organ or scattered cells having a specific regulatory effect on the activity of an organ or organs."[1] In plain words hormones are chemical messengers produced in one part of the body, transported via the bloodstream, and ultimately used to regulate the activities of a different part of the body. "Numerous circulating peptides and steroids produced in the body influence appetite through their actions on the hypothalamus, the brainstem and the autonomic nervous system. These hormones come from three major sites: fat cells, the gastrointestinal tract and the pancreas."[2]

No one particular hormone has a singular role in appetite control; rather the hormonal system operates with a great degree of redundancy.[3] The specific cells designed to utilize a hormone have receptor sites that recognize the hormone and welcome it into the cell. This arrangement functions as a sort of lock and key mechanism. Once inside the cell the hormone modifies cellular activity. For example, the pancreas produces the hormone insulin, which acts to facilitate the movement of glucose from the blood stream into the cells, where it can be used as a source of energy.

There are over 125 protein and peptide hormones.[4] Every person who lives past 50 usually experiences some kind of decline in hormone production and/or hormone utilization. "It is well known that obesity is accompanied by many hormone changes."[5] In fact, visceral fat is basically an indicator of hormonal disturbance.[6] Hormones virtually control the actions of all the organs and the body's metabolism. Each hormone is unique and the impact it has on the body is unique.

The human body has two systems for self-regulation. They are the endocrine system, discussed here, and the nervous system, discussed later in this chapter, in the section entitled Neurosystem Stimulating Hormones. The endocrine system is characterized by the vast array of hormones that until recently were thought to be produced only by the glands of the endocrine system. This system is made up of a variety of ductless glands that manufacture hormones and dump them into the bloodstream, for use in other parts of the body. The principle glands of the endocrine system are the adrenals, ovaries (in women), pancreas, parathyroid, pineal, pituitary, thymus, thyroid and testes (in men). Recent research has shown that other chemical substances (e.g. cytokines, which are soluble proteins produced by the immune system as well as some non-immune cells), act like hormones and mediate communication between the cells.[7] While cytokines have similar controlling characteristics as classical hormones, they are usually produced outside the endocrine system (e.g. the muscles).[8] The following pages will present evidence that a variety of the hormones can affect weight loss.

Hormones and Weight Loss

Following is a discussion of the hormones that could have an effect on weight loss and a review of current and pertinent scientific research. No attempt has been made to discuss all of the hormones under each of the categories mentioned. Rather this review is intended to include those hormones that could have at least a moderate effect on body weight. Those not discussed have been omitted because:

- Their contribution to overall weight control was not considered significant,
- There was little or no study data upon which to base a sensible discussion,
- There was study data but the resulting disagreement was large enough to cast a doubt on the validity of any single position.

This chapter attempts to discuss the hormones with the largest possible impact on weight loss first and then progresses on to those with an arguably lesser potential.

Thyroid Hormones

The thyroid produces a large group of hormones most of which have an impact on body weight. There are two basic things to understand about thyroid function.

First, an over-active thyroid is a *hyperthyroid*. Hyperthyroidism is "a condition caused by excessive production of iodinated thyroid hormones."[9] It is characterized by a variety of symptoms, and among the most common are weight loss and muscular weakness. When a person's thyroid activity is speeded up they are usually very thin.

Surprisingly, people with hyperthyroidism experience a number of other related problems, for example:

- Reduced circulating ghrelin levels[10] (a hormone to be discussed in greater detail later in this chapter),
- Increased insulin resistance,[11] (typically ghrelin and insulin resistance react inversely to one another),
- While experiencing abnormally low body weight, they at the same time experience an increased appetite.[12]

People being treated with medication for hyperthyroidism often experience weight gain, which is generally the result of decreased thyroid hormone concentrations, not because of their increased food intake.[13]

Second, an under active thyroid is a *hypothyroid*. Hypothyroidism is a condition of decreased thyroid activity.[14] It is characterized by a variety of symptoms; among the most common is a decrease in basal metabolic rate, fatigue and lethargy. When a person's thyroid activity is slowed down they are usually overweight. Estimates, in the year 2000 indicated that between ten and twelve million people in the U.S. had been diagnosed with hypothyroidism.[15]

There are several thyroid hormones that not only relate closely to hypothyroidism but that are used to confirm its medical diagnosis.[16] Key among these hormones is:

- Tri-iodothyronine (T_3),
- Thyroxine (T_4),
- Thyrotropin, also know as Thyroid Stimulating Hormone (TSH).[17]

T_3 & T_4 in proper balance and in the proper amount have beneficial effects on the body (e.g. enhanced cardiac function, the promotion of weight loss, reduced serum cholesterol).[18] However, excess T_3 or T_4 are "associated with unwanted effects on the heart, bone and skeletal muscle,"[19] and the level of T_3 has been shown to increase with overeating.[20] Some researchers disagree with the effects of T_3, T_4 and TSH on body weight, claiming that thyroid function has little or nothing to do with obesity and vice versa.[21] Based on the favorable results that many overweight people have seen when treated for a thyroid deficiency, it seems that this belief represents a minority view. There has been at least one research study that has gone so far as to suggest that a pharmacologic approach to balancing T_3 & T_4 is unsafe.[22] Modest increases in TSH have also been related to weight gain.[23]

Although it may be tricky to balance these hormones properly in a patient with hypothyroidism, if the proper balance can be achieved, they do have the potential to be helpful, either individually or in combination, as part of a weight loss program. A word of caution is in order here. On the negative side, Edmonds claimed that too much thyroid hormone for an extended period may permanently impair the ability to burn excess calories and weight may tend to increase.[24]

Testosterone

Testosterone is the principle male sex hormone, secreted primarily by the testes and it is responsible for:

- "The growth and development of the male reproductive structures,
- Increased skeletal and muscular growth,
- Enlargement of the larynx accompanied by voice changes,
- Growth and distribution of body hair,
- Increased male sexual drive."[25]

For purposes of the following discussion it is important to understand that the research literature frequently refers to:

- Total Testosterone (TT),
- Sex Hormone Binding Globulin (SHBG), which is a globulin, or class of proteins in the blood, that binds with and transports testosterone,
- Free Testosterone (FT).

Overweight men generally experience low levels of all three.

"Androgens are important determinants of body composition; there is no body compartment that is not directly or indirectly affected by androgens."[26] Growing evidence suggests androgens also regulate fat mass.[27] For example, studies show that total testosterone levels in men, are inversely related to body weight;[28] therefore, obese men have lower than normal total testosterone concentrations.[29] Testosterone supplementation of middle-aged men with low-normal testosterone levels and mid segment obesity has been reported to decrease visceral fat mass, improve insulin sensitivity and reduce plasma glucose levels and blood pressure.[30] Similar studies in older men have also shown that testosterone supplementation may decrease overall body fat.[31] As an additional benefit those men who do supplement a low testosterone level may also minimize progressive metabolic decomposition and cardiovascular disease often associated with obesity and the metabolic syndrome,[32] and while high doses of testosterone decrease overall body fat mass, the loss of body fat is more evenly distributed throughout the body.

As men age they experience a gradual decline in their testosterone levels along with a loss of muscle mass, an accumulation of mid body fat, impaired mobility and an increased risk of bone fractures.[33] Not just the aging process itself, but lifestyle and disease profiles contribute to a progressive decline in testosterone levels.[34] Additionally, hypogonadism (i.e. a condition resulting from abnormally decreased gonad function) has been related to low testosterone production. Hypogonadism can result in decreased lean body mass, loss of bone mineral density and increased body fat. "In relatively healthy men who have hypogonadism, testosterone replacement therapy has been shown to improve sexual function, mood, lean body mass and bone density."[35]

The evaluation of androgen levels in older men is made somewhat difficult by the "high prevalence of obesity and other confounding factors, such as chronic illness, lifestyle and medications, all of which can affect TT [total testosterone] levels."[36] However, caution needs to be exercised since "exclusive reliance on TT [total testosterone] alone in the diagnostic workup of androgen deficiency could result in misclassification and inappropriate treatment choices."[37]

At this point a couple of words of caution are in order:

- Metformin is an agent that potentiates the action of insulin and is widely used in the treatment of type 2 diabetes. "Metformin treatment combined with a hypocaloric diet lead [sic] to a decrease of FT in nondiabetic obese men and to a decreased TT in obese men with type 2 diabetes."[38]

- Testosterone supplementation increases growth hormone secretion and decreases leptin concentration in men.[39] The increase in growth hormone may or may not be problematic but a drop in leptin levels, as discussed later in this chapter, may signal the brain to encourage the body to consume food to overcome the depletion of energy stores, which for the already overweight man, is undesirable.

Estrogen / Progesterone

Estrogen and Progesterone are the two groups of female sex hormones that are produced primarily in the ovaries and are responsible for:

- "The development of the breasts,
- Distribution of fat evidenced in the hips, legs and breasts,
- Maturation of reproductive organs such as the uterus and vagina."[40]

Women going through menopause tend to gain weight, for various reasons.[41] One reason put forth by some researchers is that those who are on a program of estrogen replacement therapy (ERT) or a more complete hormone replacement therapy (HRT), usually consisting of estrogen plus additional hormones (e.g. progesterone) commonly complain of weight gain. This makes no sense, as a reason for weight gain, because if estrogen were to cause weight gain then menopausal women should lose weight, since their estrogen levels are dropping.

There are studies that agree with me, indicating that ERT/HRT, do not cause appreciable weight gain during midlife.[42] Several studies have shown that weight gain during midlife can be attributed to lifestyle changes associated with aging,[43] specifically decreased resting energy expenditure.[44] Moreover, reduced sex hormones at menopause may cause a decrease in resting energy expenditure.[45] While resting energy expenditure accounts for in excess of two thirds of the total daily energy expenditure, it decreases with age and physical inactivity.[46] Interestingly, further research has demonstrated that a lack of the appropriate amount of estrogen causes body fat to shift to the waist area. By adding ERT this shift is reduced.[47]

Additionally there are health risk factors, like the risk of cardiovascular disease and the risk of osteoporosis,[48] that respond favorably to HRT. Also women who maintain their pre-menopause body weight avoid the increased risk of breast cancer, which often accompanies increased body weight.[49] HRT seems to be able to counteract the negative affects of an unhealthy lifestyle.[50] That might be a lot of pie in the sky, but if you are struggling to lose weight why not consider HRT, if you need it and couple it with an improved lifestyle in order to give yourself twice the chance of success. In addition, it is important for women on ERT to include progesterone in their therapy if they are to receive the benefit of reducing the risk factors mentioned above.[51]

But wait, there may be a downside risk with ERT/HRT. "Overweight and obese women taking oral estrogen and those who combined estrogen plus progesterone are more insulin resistant than non-hormone users."[52]

Growth Hormone

"Growth Hormone (GH) is a protein that stimulates the growth of bones, muscles and other organs by promoting protein synthesis."[53] Growth hormone is a product of the pituitary. It has been highly studied and has been shown to be of great value in slowing the aging process. The question here is does growth hormone have a place in a weight loss program?

Human growth hormone (hGH) administered to growth hormone deficient, overweight adults has been shown to result in decreased body fat, increased lean body mass and weight loss.[54] However, hGH is comprised of a variety of bioactive components, which give it a broad range of physiological effects.[55] Studies have shown that hGH by itself may also have limited potential as a useful weight loss agent, because of several undesirable side effects, mainly on glucose intolerance, insulin resistance, edema and hypertension.[56]

There have been certain synthetic fragments of hGH that have been identified and show promise in the stimulation of weight loss. Although more study is needed, one of the studied fragments is a carboxy terminus of the hGH molecule known as AOD-9401. Research suggests that when given orally AOD-9401 may be useful in the treatment of obesity because of its ability to increase fat oxidation and the decomposition or the splitting up of fat, while decreasing the formation of further fat.[57]

The relationship between obesity and a GH deficiency is a chicken and egg routine. The question is does either one cause the other? The answer is not clear, but what is known is that there is often a deficiency of GH in the obese person, and several studies have suggested that the clearance of GH from the body occurs more frequently in obese people.[58] However, some suggest that GH clearance from the body is generally no more profound in the obese person than it is in those of normal weight, but exogenous (i.e. developed or produced outside the body) recombinant 22-kDa human growth hormone (rhGH) is cleared from the circulation at a higher rate in obese than in normal weight people.[59] Additionally, "rhGh treatment, if performed at adequate doses, appears to be effective in obese patients when associated with severely hypocaloric diets [diets consisting of restricted calories]."[60]

Obese individuals usually show low readings of Insulin-Like Growth Factor I (IGF-1). The good news is that when rhGH is given to these individuals in quantities sufficient to achieve proper levels of IGF-1, weight loss results and the weight loss is due entirely to a loss of body fat without a loss of muscle mass. Further there should be improvement in HDL cholesterol without detrimental side effects on fasting blood glucose, fasting insulin levels or measures of insulin sensitivity.[61] Finally, when GH and IGF-1 are added to a sensible program of diet and exercise, postmenopausal women have been shown to achieve a greater loss of weight and fat than their counterparts who engage in diet and exercise alone or diet and exercise combined with either GH or IGF-1 alone.[62] As these hormones relate to exercise, studies of GH and IGF-1 didn't appear to "improve aerobic fitness or promote greater gains in muscle strength in obese postmenopausal women than did diet and exercise alone."[63]

There are several substances that are known to stimulate the release of growth hormone from the pituitary gland; among them are amino acids, drugs, exercise[64] and secretagogues. Secretagogues are substances that stimulate the secreting organs. From personal experience I learned this. I was taking a high quality bio-identical growth hormone injection, which cost $1,000 per month. There were two things about this situation that I found disconcerting. First, of course was the high cost. Second, was the concern that sustained growth hormone supplementation might send a signal to my pituitary that as long as my body was being supplied, externally with the growth hormone that it needed, the pituitary's production of the hormone may no longer be needed, ultimately leaving my body completely dependent on the external supply. My solution has been to incorporate the use of secretagogues in an attempt to stimulate pituitary production of growth hormone, with the goal of eliminating the need for the growth hormone injections.

After initially incorporating the use of a couple of different secretagogues and eliminating my growth hormone injections the level of growth hormone in my blood stream did decline, but by experimenting with the secretagogues I was able to substantially increase my growth hormone level. The good news is that as of this writing my personal physician and anti-aging specialist feels strongly that a bit more refinement of the secretagogue usage should result in the desired level of growth hormone production from the pituitary, without any injections. My goal has been to preserve the "feedback mechanisms that modulate GH response in generation of...GH release, which more closely mimics natural secretion,"[65] and I am hopeful that I will achieve that goal. It should be noted that people have safely used growth hormone supplementation for years, but when they stop they usually return to their original baseline.

Ghrelin

The main hormone produced in the intestinal tract is grehlin. "Grehlin is the first circulating hormone demonstrated to stimulate food intake in man."[66] It is produced in the stomach, intestines and to a lesser extent in the pancreas. There is evidence that "grehlin plays a role in premeal hunger and meal initiation as well as long-term energy balance."[67] Ghrelin levels rise prior to a meal and fall after the meal, and interestingly they also rise after weight loss.[68] One study showed that as obese children lost weight, grehlin concentrations begin to rise, along with a related improvement in insulin sensitivity.[69] Here is where the body seems to be trying to play a nasty trick on us. After we have lost a few pounds ghrelin production increases, signaling the brain that we need to eat. Perhaps this is one of the reasons that weight loss is so difficult to maintain.

Ghrelin levels in the obese are substantially lower than they are in lean individuals.[70] It appears that "ghrelin is downregulated in human obesity...which may be a consequence of elevated insulin or leptin."[71]

While ghrelin is a contributor to the weight management process it also "plays a role in a variety of other body systems, including circulatory, digestion and cell proliferation."[72] Clinical applications of ghrelin have already been tested, although further study is needed. In the future ghrelin might become a useful tool for the treatment of a variety of conditions, including obesity.[73]

Leptin

For years fat tissue was regarded as simply passive fuel storage sites. However, with the discovery that adipose tissue secretes various hormones, with leptin being the most important, adipose tissue has been raised to the status of an endocrine gland.[74] Recent studies "provide further evidence of the key role of adipose tissue as a base from which neuronal signals regulating feeding and fuel metabolism are sent."[75] "Leptin is an adipocyte [fat cell] hormone that functions as the afferent signal in a negative feedback loop regulating body weight."[76] It reports nutritional information, including the size of the body's energy stores, to the brain.[77] Leptin is known to act on specific receptors in the hypothalamus and leptin levels correlate strongly with the degree of adiposity.[78] "Up to 10 percent of obese people have relatively low leptin levels."[79] The idea that obesity is largely the result of biological rather than psychological factors is certainly not a new concept and is supported by substantial data.[80]

Circulating concentrations of leptin appear to mirror fat cell stores, increasing with overfeeding and decreasing with starvation. During starvation leptin levels fall signaling the brain to encourage the body to consume food to overcome the depletion of energy stores. Conversely during weight gain leptin levels rise signaling the brain to encourage the body to reduce food consumption in order to reduce energy stores. This leads to the logical conclusion that this feedback system is a primary factor in regulating body weight in humans.[81]

"It is not surprising that in an underweight individual with anorexia nervosa, plasma leptin levels have been found to be consistently reduced,"[82] and during their recovery a progressive increase in leptin concentrations can be observed.[83] "In normal weight individuals with bulimia nervosa, circulating leptin has been reported to be either decreased our normal."[84]

Leptin concentrations in humans are positively correlated with fat mass and a lack of leptin is often accompanied by some rather extreme brain abnormalities including reduced brain weight, reduced brain volume, delayed maturation of neurons and glial cells and an increased susceptibility to neurodegeneration.[85] The administration of leptin "to obese humans only has a modest and variable effect on body weight."[86] The supplementation of leptin seems to work well when used on leptin deficient subjects but also tends to have little effect on diet-induced obesity.[87] "Leptin resistance may underlie the failure to regulate energy stores as seen in common forms of obesity."[88]

When it comes to how well leptin works to assist the overweight person in reducing their food consumption, a couple of potential problems exist:

- There might be impairment in the body's ability to deliver leptin to the brain[89] and one of the reasons might be elevated triglycerides, since it has been shown that triglycerides can impair the movement of leptin across the blood brain barrier.[90] This may account in part for the leptin resistance seen in obesity.[91] Study data has also indicated that, "it is difficult to explain human obesity on the basis of [central nervous system] CNS leptin resistance, in that leptin is released in the brain, and at a higher level in the obese."[92]

- The leptin receptor signaling system might be defective.[93] Although there are many possible factors that could override leptin induced satiety and cause weight gain, based on the available data, leptin functions as a satiety hormone, with greater degrees of body fat resulting in greater leptin induced satiety. Leptin therapy in the leptin deficient individual has been clearly associated with a reduction in caloric intake.[94]

Care must be exercised when evaluating leptin performance data in lean vs. overweight people, using the Body Mass Index (BMI), since using BMI produces erroneous results, whereas data based on percent body fat is much more accurate.[95] I would suggest that this is very likely true in evaluating other hormones, as well, since it is widely known that the BMI calculation is substantially flawed, while percent body fat provides a more reliable picture of body composition.

Leptin has several other body influencing connections that are closely associated with important body functions. For example:

- Insulin Resistance - A connection exists between leptin levels and insulin resistance. We hear a lot about how obesity leads to or at least contributes to diabetes. Studies have shown that a high leptin level, as typically seen in the overweight person, is directly related to insulin resistance.[96]

- Blood Pressure - Normal circulating leptin levels mediate both obesity and blood pressure.[97]

- Sex Hormones - Leptin levels may themselves be influenced by body weight and sex hormones.[98]

- Brain Size - There is an inverse relationship between the increased leptin levels seen in the obese and the size of the brain. High leptin levels appear to contribute either directly or indirectly to a reduced amount of gray matter in the brain.[99]

Adiponectin

Another important hormone secreted by fat tissue is adiponectin, which promotes fatty acid oxidation. This "adipose-specific protein, is negatively associated with adiposity, insulin sensitivity, diabetes,"[100] and "expression of Metabolic Syndrome and its individual traits in obese individuals."[101] Adiponectin "has been associated with the risk for a number of obesity-related diseases, such as diabetes, hypertension and coronary heart disease."[102]

Adiponectin is related to a gene known as the APM1 gene. This gene has been implicated in energy homeostasis in obesity and relates directly to the metabolic syndrome, specifically insulin resistance and obesity. Since the existence of a relationship between adiponectin and the APM1 gene is real, it is clear that "adiponectin does indeed play a role genetically in the development of obesity."[103]

Finally, adiponectin levels have been shown to be higher in women than in men.[104] Experts report that adiponectin may be an inherited factor in exceptional longevity.[105] It is interesting to think of the possibilities for men. If adiponectin levels could be elevated in men without pushing them into a metabolic syndrome related condition, it may be possible to improve their longevity, to match that of their female counterparts.

Cortisol

Cortisol is a hormone, produced by the adrenals, that is primarily a response to stress. It is often referred to as the stress hormone. It increases blood pressure, blood sugar levels and has immunosuppressive action. In humans stress-induced cortisol may play a role in obesity and it may be part of the explanation of stress-induced eating.[106] In tests where cortisol was given to healthy men for as little as four days, it led to increased energy expenditure and dramatically increased food intake.[107] In another laboratory setting women with high cortisol levels consumed more calories following a stressful situation than did those with low cortisol levels. In addition caloric intake was positively associated with negative mood feelings following the stressful situation.[108] In rodents it has been shown that adrenal steroids influence the selection of macronutrients by both: (1) increasing their appetite for carbohydrates and fat, and (2) regulating the timing of eating.[109] It appears that visceral fat has a somewhat high affinity for cortisol and abdominal obesity is associated with hormonal changes that often affect more visceral than subcutaneous fat tissue. In fact Bjorntorp & Rosmond speculated that, "elevated cortisol secretion is probably involved in abdominal obesity."[110]

Dehydroepiandrosterone (DHEA)

"DHEA and its sulfate DHEA-S are the most abundant circulating steroids in man and are the precursors for most steroid hormones."[111] DHEA is produced mainly in the adrenal glands, with a small amount coming from the brain and an additional small amount from the gonads in men. "Serum concentrations of DHEA and DHEA-S are age dependent; in man, they rapidly increase at puberty, reach their peak levels between 20 and 30 years of age, and then decrease gradually."[112] "DHEA administration in aged rats fed a high-fat diet significantly reduced their energy intake, body weight and body fat."[113] Since DHEA treatment is associated with a reduction in protein digestibility, the result is a reduction in fat and protein preservation, which has been suggested as the reason for DHEA's anti-obesity and anti-aging properties.[114]

"In a human study it was shown that 7-oxo-DHEA is a well tolerated and an effective weight loss aid."[115] When 7-oxo-DHEA was used in combination with exercise and a reduced caloric intake it was shown to be more effective in reducing body weight and body fat than exercise and a reduced caloric diet alone.[116]

Melatonin

"Melatonin is a hormone synthesized by the pineal gland."[117] "In mammals it influences hormone production and in many species it regulates seasonal changes such as reproductive patterns and fur color."[118] "In humans it is implicated in the regulation of sleep, mood, puberty and ovarian cycles."[119] A study of rats fed a high fat diet showed that not only was melatonin able to limit body weight gain but, "it also appears to prevent some of the side effects on lipid metabolism and on glucose homeostasis, such as decreased insulin sensitivity."[120] The obvious implications are that humans might receive the same weight loss benefit that the rats experienced.

Parathyroid Hormone (PTH)

Parathyroid Hormone is a hormone secreted from the parathyroid glands and is a regulator of blood calcium levels. It acts to increase blood calcium by increasing:

- The calcium that is released from the bones,
- Calcium re-absorption from the kidneys,
- The absorption of calcium in the intestines.[121]

There were a couple of small population studies, done in the mid nineties that suggested an inconclusive relationship between PTH and BMI.[122] One later and much larger study has shown a significant positive relationship between PTH and BMI. It revealed that both men and women who fell within the highest PTH quartile had an approximately 50 percent greater risk of being obese.[123]

Corticotropin-Releasing Hormone

Corticotropin-Releasing Hormone (CRH) is a hormone that during times of stress acts on the pituitary gland to stimulate it to produce corticosteroids.[124] Although CRH is primarily thought to involve the stress response, it has been known for years that it opposes energy storage and at the same time tends to foster energy expenditure. It has been demonstrated that "CRH can lower the body weight threshold that triggers food hoarding behavior in the male rat."[125] "The CRH system forms an important network of receptors and neurons capable of interactions with the effectors of food intake and energy expenditure,"[126] and when it is activated it is capable of strong appetite suppression and a thermogenic or heat producing action, which ultimately results in energy loss.[127]

This hormone is not to be confused with the stress hormone cortisol.

Prolactin

Prolactin is a hormone that is known for its milk stimulating effect of the mammary glands, in lactating women. It plays an essential role in the maintenance of immune system function in both men and women. The existence and importance of the relationship between prolactin and body weight is one that is not well recognized among clinicians. It is interesting to note that, especially in men, a clear association has been found between high prolactin levels and increased body mass and significant weight loss is possible by prolactin lowering therapy.[128]

Lesser Known Gut Hormones and Peptides

"The gastrointestinal tract (GIT) is the body's largest endocrine organ and produces around 30 different peptidic hormones, which act on several tissues, such as exocrine glands, gastrointestinal tract and CNS [central nervous system]."[129] The secretion of many gastrointestinal tract hormones and peptides[130] is influenced by the contents of the intestines. Intestinal hormones and peptides are intended to signal the central nervous system of current levels of nutrition in the body.[131]

Determining Your Hormone Levels

Having read this far, you now understand the impact that hormones could have on maintaining a reasonable body weight. Even if you have gained an undesirable amount of body weight, if you determine that your hormones are out of balance, you may be able to help yourself lose that weight by making the proper hormonal adjustments, along with the appropriate lifestyle changes. At this point the question is how do you determine your hormone levels and balance?

There is some hype surrounding hormone testing. Two recognized, reliable yet cost-effective methods for testing hormones are:

- Blood test,
- Saliva test.

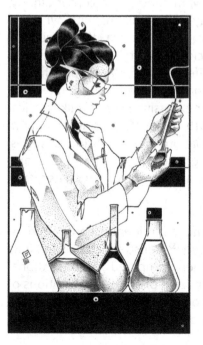

A blood test is the more complicated of the two. In order to get a blood test you will need a prescription from your doctor. Your doctor will usually suggest a lab that he/she works with and which is conveniently located in your area. You then go to the lab and submit to the blood test. The lab will forward the test results to your doctor and you must return to the doctor to get the results. During the office consultation you will have the benefit of your doctor's interpretation of the results.

A saliva test is much simpler to conduct but may prove less effective. You may contact a lab of your choice. Some health care providers might suggest a lab that they have experience with or you can Google, *saliva test labs*, to find one yourself. The lab will provide you with the necessary test kit, usually laboratory vials, and directions for the saliva test. You can prepare the samples at home and mail the test to the lab. Once the test is complete the lab will mail the results to you and they will guide you in the interpretation of the results.

Although this approach seems much simpler, there are a couple of problems. First, you can make serious errors during your interpretation of the results. Second, even if you interpret the results correctly, but your hormone levels are out of balance, you may not know what to do to correct them. In either case you will need a knowledgeable health care professional to help you interpret the results, recommend the proper adjustments, and provide you with any required prescriptions. So you may still need to go to your doctor's office for a consultation.

Synthetic Vs Bio-Identical Hormones

All hormones are not created equal. Although many doctors make little or no distinction between synthetic hormones and bio-identical or bio-available hormones, increasingly we are hearing more about their pros and cons. "Although known to be different with respect to molecular structure, receptor affinity, metabolism and other physiological traits most have been treated as if they were clinically identical."[132] Bio-identical, hormones are identical to those produced in the body, while bio-available are only available to the target tissues. "Synthetic hormones are not the same as their counterparts that are manufactured by the body, hence they are not recognized or metabolized as such."[133] Synthetic hormones, which are commonly referred to as hormone replacement therapy (HRT) should really be referred to as hormone substitution therapy, since they do not precisely match those produced in the body.[134]

A growing body of evidence brings the safety of synthetic hormones into question. There are numerous factors that affect the action, risks and benefits of various hormones. Among them are the "method of administration, absorption, bio-availability, metabolism, receptor affinity, receptor specificity and molecular structure."[135] One of today's big concerns with synthetic hormone replacement is that of blood clots. A good example is Provera, the frequently prescribed synthetic female hormone substitution therapy. A close look at Provera will reveal a host of possible serious side effects. The more common side effects include: "Acne, anaphylaxis (life-threatening allergic reaction), *blood clot in a vein, lungs, or brain*, breakthrough bleeding (between menstrual periods), breast tenderness or sudden or excessive flow of milk, cervical erosion or changes in secretions, depression, excessive growth of hair, fever, fluid retention, hair loss, headache, hives, insomnia, itching, lack of menstruation, menstrual flow changes, spotting, nausea, rash, skin discoloration, sleepiness, weight gain or loss, yellowed eyes and skin."[136] Ladies, if your doctor prescribes Provera and says there are no problems with its safety, you may want to ask a few questions.

One recent study revealed that in contrast to synthetic hormones a bio-identical progesterone cream was found to show no markers for inflammation or clotting.[137] Transdermal combinations of these bioidentical hormones are often advantageous when compared to conventional oral HRT. "In particular, the risk of blood clotting may be minimized for some combinations of hormones consisting of topical estrogen administration with progesterone rather than synthetic progestin."[138] Finally, "recombinant growth hormone (GH), has an identical structure to human growth hormone and is not associated with the risks attributable to human or animal derived products."[139]

Summary

We have all heard the statement that weight loss is simply the expending of more calories than we consume. While that principle still has truth today, there are a lot of people who find this concept frustrating. Many people continued to gain weight, even while they are reducing their caloric intake and doing more exercise. "This unfortunate process takes place largely due to the hormonal changes that occur with age."[140]

As mentioned, your body produces 125 different hormones that are transported in the bloodstream and used to regulate activities throughout your body. Not only are they critical for proper cellular functioning, many play a significant role in controlling body weight. Hormone levels need to be monitored and if found to be deficient may need to be stimulated or supplemented.

Hertoghe & Nabet began a section of their book by saying that "If nothing else gets you, middle-age spread will."[141] They later said that in addition to diet and exercise, you must address the hormone deficiencies that underlie almost all accumulation of excess weight. "Any diet that doesn't take hormones into account won't provide lasting results."[142] Special attention needs to be given to the sex steroids because they have been shown to "directly alter both food intake and body fat distribution."[143]

We saw that two of the more significant hormones in the process of body weight stabilization are ghrelin and leptin.

- Ghrelin is principally created in the intestinal track and it signals the brain that the body needs more energy, in effect telling the brain that it is time to eat.
- Leptin is primarily created in the fat cells and signals the brain that the body has plenty of stored energy, in the form of fat, therefore making eating unnecessary.

Interfering with the actions of these hormones may be impediments in their receptor systems.

This chapter has gone to great lengths to identify a variety of additional hormones and to make you aware of the role they can play in weight management. In order to determine the extent to which hormones could be affecting your weight you will need to locate a doctor that is knowledgeable in dealing with hormone issues, have your hormones tested, and make the necessary adjustments.

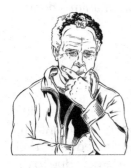

In this chapter you learned the subtle but important distinction between synthetic and bio-identical hormones. Armed with this information, I hope you will think twice before you allow anyone to convince you a synthetic hormone has no risks to your health. At this point I do need to offer one caveat. Be aware that the potential cost of some bio-identical hormones can be very high, but don't let their cost carry too much weight in your evaluation of the health pros and cons of synthetic vs bio-identical hormones.

Endnotes

1. "Hormone," *Dorland's Illustrated Medical Dictionary*, 30th ed: 862.
2. A.P. Coli, I.S. Farooqi, S. O'Rahilly, "The hormonal control of food intake," *Cell* 129 (2007) 251-262.
3. Ibid.
4. A.W. Norman, G. Litwack, *"Hormones"* 2nd ed, (San Diego, CA: Academic Press, 1997) 9.
5. M.A. Michalaki, A.G. Vagenakis, A.S. Leonardou, M.N. Argentou, I.G. Habeous, M.G. Makri, A.I. Psyrogiannis, F.E. Kalfarentzos, V.E. Kyriazopoulou, "Thyroid function in humans with morbid obesity," *Thyroid* 16 (2006) 73-78.
6. J. Marniemi, E. Kronholm, S. Aunola, T. Toikka, C.E. Mattlar, M. Koskenvuo, T. Ronnemaa, "Visceral fat and psychosocial stress in identical twins discordant for obesity," *J Int Med* 251 (2002) 35-43.
7. M.E. Hadley, J.E. Levine, "Endocrinology," 6th ed, (Upper Saddle River, NJ: Pearson Prentice Hall, 2007) 289.
8. "Hormone," *Dorland's Illustrated Medical Dictionary*, 30th ed: 862.
9. "Hyperthyroidism," *Dorland's Illustrated Medical Dictionary*, 30th ed: 889.
10. A.E. Altinova, F.B. Toruner, M. Akturk, S. Elbeg, I. Yetkin, N. Cakir, M. Arslan, "Reduced serum acylated grehlin levels in patients with hyperthyroidism," *Horm Res* 65 (2006) 295-299.
11. Ibid.
12. Ibid.
13. M. Abid, C.J. Billington, F.Q. Nuttall, "Thyroid function and energy intake during weight gain following treatment of hyperthyroidism," *J Am College Nutr* 18 (1999) 189-193.
14. "Hypothyroidism," *Dorland's Illustrated Medical Dictionary*, 30th ed: 900.
15. S. Danzi, I. Klein, "Recent considerations in the treatment of hypothyroidism," *Cur Opin Invest Drugs* 9 (2008) 357-362.
16. S. Danzi, I. Klein, "Recent considerations in the treatment of hypothyroidism," *Cur Opin Invest Drugs* 9 (2008) 357-362.
17. Ibid.
18. G. Brenta, S. Danzi, I. Klein, "Potential therapeutic applications of thyroid hormone analogs," *Nat Clin Prac Endocrin Metab* 3 (2007) 632-640.
19. Ibid.
20. E. Danforth, Jr., E.S. Horton, M. O"Connell, E.A.H. Sims, A. G. Burger, S.H. Ingbar, L. Braverman, A.G. Vagenakis, "Hormone metabolism during overnutrition," *J Clin Invest* 64 (1979) 1336-1347.

21. A. Strata, G. Ugolotti, C. Contini, G. Magnati, C. Pugnoli, F. Tirelli, U. Zuliani, "Thyroid and obesity: survey of some function tests in a large obese population," *Int'l J Obes* 2 (1978) 333-341.

22. E. Ortega, N. Pannacciulli, C. Bogardus, J. Krakoff, "Plasma concentrations of free triiodothyronine predict weight change in euthyroid persons," *Am J Clin Nutr* 85 (2007) 440-445.

23. C.S. Fox, M.J. Pencina, R.B. D'Agostino, J.M. Murabito, E.W. Seeley, E.N. Pearce, R.S. Vasan, "Relations of thyroid function to body weight: cross-sectional and longitudinal observations in a community-based sample," *Arch Intern Med* 168 (2008) 587-592.

24. M.W. Edmonds, "Fatigue, weight gain, and the thyroid (or is the thyroid why I am so tired and can't lose weight)," Thyrobulletin 19 (1998).

25. E.J. Applegate, "*The Anatomy & Physiology Learning System,*" 2nd ed, (Philadelphia, PA: Saunders, 2000) 218-219.

26. S. Bhasin, "Regulation of body composition by androgens," *J Endocrin* 26 (2003) 814-822.

27. Ibid.

28. N. Lima, H. Cavaliere, M. Knobel, A. Halpern, G. Medeiros-Neto, " Decreased androgen levels in massively obese men may be associated with impaired function of the gonadostat," *Int'l J of Obes* 24 (2000) 1433-1437.

29. Ibid.

30. S. Bhasin, "Regulation of body composition by androgens," *J Endocrin* 26 (2003) 814-822.

31. Ibid.

32. L. Niskanen, D.E. Laaksonen, K. Punnonen, P. Mustajoki, J. Kaukua, A. Rissanen, "Changes in sex hormone-binding globulin and testosterone during weight loss and weight maintenance in abdominally obese men with the metabolic syndrome," *Dia obes & metab* 6 (2004) 208-215.

33. A.M. Isidori, E. Giannetta, E.A. Greco, D. Gianfrilli, V. Bonifacio, A. Isidori, A. Lenzit, A. Fabbri, "Effects of testosterone on body composition, bone metabolism and serum lipid profile in middle-aged men: a meta-analysis," *Clin Endrocrin* 63 (2005) 280-293.

34. Ibid.

35. R.R. Kalyani, S. Gavini, A.S. Dobs, "Male hypogonadism is systemic disease," *Endrocrin Metab Clin N Am* 36 (2007) 333-348.

36. B.A. Mohr, S. Bhasin, V|C.L. Link, A.B. O'Donnell, J.B. McKinlay, "The effect of changes in adiposity on testosterone levels in older men: longitudinal results from the Massachusetts male aging study," *Euro J Endocrin* 155 (2006) 443-452.

37. Ibid.

38. M. Ozata, C. Oktenli, N. Bingo, I.C. Ozdemir, "The effects of metformin and diet on plasma testosterone and leptin levels in obese men," *Obes Res* 9 (2001) 662-667.

39. L. Adan, L. Bussieres, C. Trivin, J.C. Souberbielle, R. Brauner, "Effect of Short-term testosterone treatment on leptin concentrations in boys with pubertal delay," *Horm Res* 52 (1999) 109-112.

40. E.J. Applegate, "*The Anatomy & Physiology Learning System,*" 2nd ed, (Philadelphia, PA: Saunders, 2000) 219.

41. A.S. Ryan, B.J. Nicklas, D.M. Berman, "Hormone replacement therapy, insulin sensitivity and abdominal obesity in postmenopausal women," *Diabetes Care* 25 (2002) 127-133.

42. K.M. Davies, R.P. Heaney, R.R. Recker, M.J. Barger-Lux, J.M. Lappe, "Hormones, weight change and menopause," *In'l J Obes* 25 (2001) 874-879.

43. E.J. Anderson, H.B. Lavoie, C.C. Strauss, J.L. Hubbard, J.L. Sharpless, J.R. Hall, "Body composition and energy balance: lack of effect of short-term hormone replacement in postmenopausal women," *Metabolism* 50 (2001) 265-269.

44. Ibid.

45. D.S. Day, W.S. Gozansky, R.E. Van Pelt, R.S. Schwartz, W.M. Kohrt, "Sex hormone suppression reduces resting energy expenditure and B-Adrenergic support of resting energy expenditure," J Clin Endocrin Metab 90 (2005) 3312-3317.

46. E.J. Anderson, H.B. Lavoie, C.C. Strauss, J.L. Hubbard, J.L. Sharpless, J.R. Hall, "Body composition and energy balance: lack of effect of short-term hormone replacement in postmenopausal women," *Metabolism* 50 (2001) 265-269.

47. K.M. Davies, R.P. Heaney, R.R. Recker, M.J. Barger-Lux, J.M. Lappe, "Hormones, weight change and menopause," *Int'l J Obes* 25 (2001) 874-879.

48. E.J. Anderson, H.B. Lavoie, C.C. Strauss, J.L. Hubbard, J.L. Sharpless, J.R. Hall, "Body composition and energy balance: lack of effect of short-term hormone replacement in postmenopausal women," *Metabolism* 50 (2001) 265-269.

49. D. Han, J. Nie, M.R. Bonner, S.E. McCann, P. Muti, M. Trevisan, F.A. Ramirez-Marrero, D. Vito, J.L. Freudenheim, "Lifetime adult weight gain, central adiposity and the risk of pre and postmenopausal breast cancer in the western New York exposures and breast cancer study," *Int'l J Cancer* 119 (2006) 2931-2937.

50. C. Li, C. Borgfeldt, G. Samsioe, J. Lidfeldt, C. Nerbrand, "Background factors influencing somatic and psychological symptoms in middle-age women with different hormonal status: a population-based study of Swedish women," *Maturitas - Euro Men J* 52 (2005) 306-318.

51. M. L. Stefanick, "Estrogen, progestogens and cardiovascular risk," *J Reprod Med* 44 (1999) 221-226.

52. A.S. Ryan, B.J. Nicklas, D.M. Berman, "Hormone replacement therapy, insulin sensitivity and abdominal obesity in postmenopausal women," *Diabetes Care* 25 (2002) 127-133.

53. E.J. Applegate, "*The Anatomy & Physiology Learning System*," 2nd ed, (Philadelphia, PA: Saunders, 2000) 210.

54. M. Heffernan, R.J. Summers, A. Thorburn, E. Ogru, R. Gianello, W-J Jiang, F.M. Ng, "The affects of human GH and its lipolytic fragment (AOD9604) on lipid metabolism following chronic treatment of obese mice and B$_3$-AR knock-out mice," *Endocrinology* 142 (2001) 5182-5189.

55. M.A. Heffernan, A.W. Thornburn, B. Fam, R. Summers, B. Conway-Campbell, M.J. Waters, F.M. Ng, "Increase of fat oxidation and weight loss in obese mice caused by chronic treatment with human growth or a modified C-terminal fragment," *Int'l J Obes* 25 (2001) 1442-1449

56. M.A. Heffernan, W.J. Jiang, A.W. Thorburn, F.M. Ng, "Effects of oral administration of a synthetic fragment of human growth hormone on lipid metabolism," *Am J Physiol Endocrin Metab* 279 (2000) E501-E507

57. Ibid.

58. J.G. Langendonk, A.E. Meinders, J. Burggraaf, M. Frolich, C.A.M. Roelen, R.C. Schoemaker, A.F. Cohen, H. Pijl, "Influence of obesity and body fat distribution on growth hormone kinetics in humans," *Am J Physiol Endocrin Metab* 277 (1999) 824-829.

59. Ibid.

60. M. Tagliaferri, M. Scacchi, A.I. Pincelli, M.E. Berselli, P. Silvestri, A. Montesano, S. Ortolani, A. Dubini, F. Cavagnini, "Metabolic effects of biosynthetic growth hormone treatment in severely energy-restricted obese women," *Int'l J Obes* 22 (1998) 836-841.

61. S.G. Albert, A.D. Mooradian, "Low-dose recombinant human growth hormone as adjuvant therapy to lifestyle modifications in the management of obesity," *J Clin Endocrin Metab* 89 (2004) 695-701.

62. J.L. Thompson, G.E. Butterfield, U.K. Gylfadottir, J. Yesavage, R. Marcus, R.L. Hintz, A. Pearman, A.R. Hoffman, "Effects of human growth hormone, insulin-like growth factor I, and diet and

exercise on body composition of obese postmenopausal women," *J Clin Endocrin Metab* 83 (1998) 1477-1484.

63. Ibid.
64. J. Jamieson, L.E. Dorman, , V. Marriott, "Growth hormone: reversing human aging naturally," 7nd ed, (St. Louis, MO: Jamieson, 1997) 35.
65. Ibid., 36.
66. A.M. Wren, L.J. Seal, M.A. Cohen, A.E. Brynes, G.S. Frost, K.G. Murphy, W.S. Dhillo, M.A. Ghatel, S.R. Bloom, "Ghrelin enhances appetite and increases food intake in humans," *J Clin Endocrin Metab* 86 (2001) 5992-5995.
67. T. McLaughlin, F. Abbasi, C. Lamendola, R.S. Frayo, D.E. Cummings, "Plasma ghrelin concentrations are decreased in insulin-resistant obese adults relative to equally obese insulin-sensitive controls," *J Clin Endocrin Metab* 89 (2004) 1630-1635.
68. K.E. Foster-Schubert, A. McTierman, R.S. Frayo, R.S. Schwartz, K.B. Rajan, Y. Yasui, S.S. Tworoger, D.E. Cummings, "Human plasma ghrelin levels increase during a one-year exercise program," *J Clin Endocrin Metab* 90 (2005) 820-825.
69. K. Krohn, C. Boczan, B. Otto, W. Heldwein, R. Landgrat, C.P. Bauer, B. Koletzko, "Regulation of ghrelin is related to estimated insulin sensitivity in obese children," *Int'l J Obes* 30 (2006) 1482-1487.
70. P. Koutkia, S. Schurgin, J. Berry, J. Breu, B.S. Hang Lee, A. Klibanski, S. Grinspoon, "Reciprocal changes in endogenous ghrelin and growth hormone during fasting in healthy women," *Am J Psych Endocrin Metab* 289 (2005) E814-E822.
71. M. Tschop, C. Weyer, P.A. Tataranni, V. Devanarayan, E. Ravussin, M. L. Heiman, "Circulating grehlin levels are decreased in human obesity," *Diabetes* 50 (2001) 707-709.
72. H. Ueno, H. Yamaguchi, K. Kangawa, M. Nakazato, "Ghrelin: a gastric peptide that regulates food intake and energy homeostasis," *Regulatory Peptides* 126 (2005) 11-19.
73. Ibid.
74. T. Yamada, H. Katagiri, "Avenues of communication between the brain and tissues/organs involved in energy homeostasis," *Endocrin J* 54 (2007) 497-505.
75. Ibid.
76. J.M. Friedman, "The function of leptin in nutrition, weight and physiology," *Nutrition Reviews* 60 (2002) S1-S14.
77. Ibid.
78. N. Eikelis, G. Wisner, G. Lambert, M. Esler, "Brain leptin resistance in human obesity revisited," *Reg Pep* 139 (2007) 45-51.
79. A.P. Coli, I.S. Farooqi, S. O'Rahilly, "The hormonal control of food intake," *Cell* 129 (2007) 251-262.
80. G.C. Kennedy, "The role of depot fat in the hypothalamic control of food intake in the rat," *Proc R Soc* 140 (1953) 578-592.
81. A.F. Heini, C. Lara-Castro, K.A. Kirk, R.V. Considine, J.F. Caro, R.L. Weinsier, "Association of leptin and hunger-satiety ratings in obese women," *Int'l J Obes* 22 (1998) 1084-1087.
82. P. Monteleone, "Endocrine disturbances and psychiatric disorders," *Curr Opin Psych* 14 (2001) 605-610.
83. Ibid.
84. Ibid.
85. K. Sriram, S.A. Benkovic, D.B. Miller, J.P. O'Callaghan, " Obesity exacerbates chemically induced neurodegeneration," *Neuroscience* 115 (2002) 1335-1346.

86. A.P. Coli, I.S. Farooqi, S. O'Rahilly, "The hormonal control of food intake," *Cell* 129 (2007) 251-262.
87. Ibid.
88. Ibid.
89. S. Dagogo-Jack, "Human leptin regulation and promise in pharmacotherapy," *Current Drug Targets* 2 (2001) 181-195.
90. W.A. Banks, A.B. Coon, S.M. Robinson, A. Moinuddin, J.M. Shultz, R. Nakaoke, J.E. Morley, 'Triglycerides induce leptin resistance at the blood brain barrier," *Diabetes* 53 (2004) 1253-1260.
91. S.A. Farr, K.A. Yamada, D.A. Butterfield, H.M. Abdul, L. Xu, N.E. Miller, W.A. Banks, J.E. Morley, "Obesity and hypertriglyceridemia produce cognitive impairment," *Endocrin* 149 (2007) 2628-2636.
92. N. Eikelis, G. Wisner, G. Lambert, M. Esler, "Brain leptin resistance in human obesity revisited," *Reg Pep* 139 (2007) 45-51.
93. S. Dagogo-Jack, "Human leptin regulation and promise in pharmacotherapy," *Current Drug Targets* 2 (2001) 181-195.
94. S. Dagogo-Jack, "Human leptin regulation and promise in pharmacotherapy," *Current Drug Targets* 2 (2001) 181-195.
95. J.A. Marshall, G.K. Grunwald, W.T. Donahoo, S. Scarbro, S.M. Shetterly, "Percent body fat and lean muscle mass explain the gender difference in leptin: analysis and interpretation of leptin in Hispanic and non-Hispanic white adults," *Obesity Research* 8 (2000) 543-552.
96. Z. Maghbooli, A. Hossein-Nezhad, M. Rahmani, A.R. Shafaei, B. Larijani, "Relationship between leptin concentration and insulin resistance," *Horm Metab Res* 39 (2007) 903-907.
97. G. Livshits, I. Pantsulaia, L.M. Gerber, "Association of leptin levels with obesity and blood pressure: possible common genetic variation," *Int'l J Obes* 29 (2005) 85-92.
98. K.M. Sudi, S. Gallistl, M.H. Borkenstein, D. Payerl, R. Aigner, R. Moller, E. Tafeit, "Effects of weight loss on leptin, sex hormones, and measures of adiposity in obese children," *Endocrine* 14 (2001) 429-435.
99. N. Pannacciulli, D.S.N.T. Le, K. Chen, E.M. Reiman, J. Krakoff, "Relationships between plasma leptin concentrations and human brain structure: voxel-based morphometric study," *Neuroscience Letters* 412 (2007) 248-253.
100. I. Miljkovic-Gacic, X. Wang, C.M. Kammerer, C.H. Bunker, V.W. Wheeler, A.L. Patrick, L.H. Kuller, R.W. Evans, J.M. Zmuda, "Genetic determination of adiponectin and its relationship with body fat topography in multigenerational families of African heritage," *Metab Clin & Exper* 56 (2007) 234-238.
101. A.M. Xydakis, C.C. Case, P.H. Jones, R.C. Hoogeveen, M-Y Liu, E.O. Smith, K.W. Nelson, C.M. Ballantyne, "Adiponectin, inflammation, and the expression of the metabolic syndrome in obese individuals: the impact of rapid weight loss through caloric restriction," *J Clin Endocrin Metab* 89 (2004) 2697-2703.
102. I. Miljkovic-Gacic, X. Wang, C.M. Kammerer, C.H. Bunker, V.W. Wheeler, A.L. Patrick, L.H. Kuller, R.W. Evans, J.M. Zmuda, "Genetic determination of adiponectin and its relationship with body fat topography in multigenerational families of African heritage," *Metab Clin & Exper* 56 (2007) 234-238.
103. B.S. Sutton, S. Weinert, C.D. Langefeld, A.H. Williams, J.K. Campbell, M.F. Saad, S.H. Haffner, J.M. Norris, D.W. Bowden, " Genetic analysis of adiponectin and obesity in Hispanic families: the IRAS family study," *Human Genet* 117 (2005) 107-118.

104. I. Miljkovic-Gacic, X. Wang, C.M. Kammerer, C.H. Bunker, V.W. Wheeler, A.L. Patrick, L.H. Kuller, R.W. Evans, J.M. Zmuda, "Genetic determination of adiponectin and its relationship with body fat topography in multigenerational families of African heritage," *Metab Clin & Exper* 56 (2007) 234-238.

105. A.R. Shuldiner, J. Crandall, T.I. Pollin, K. Tanner, M. Rincon, R. Lipton, et al, "Adiponectin: an inherited survival factor in families with exceptional longevity," Abstract presented at the Annual American Society for Human Genetics Meeting, Salt Lake City, Utah, October 25-29, 2005.

106. E. Epel, R. Lapidus, B. McEwen, K. Brownell, "Stress may add bite to appetite and women: a laboratory study of stress-induced cortisol and eating behavior," *Psychoneuroendocrin* 26 (2001) 37-49.

107. P.A. Tataranni, D. Larson, S. Snitker, J. Young, J. Flatt, E. Ravussin, "Effects of glucocorticoid in energy metabolism and food intake in humans," *Am J Physio* 271 (1996) E317-E325.

108. E. Epel, R. Lapidus, B. McEwen, K. Brownell, "Stress may add bite to appetite in women: a laboratory study of stress-induced cortisol and eating behavior," *Psychoneuroendocrin* 26 (2001) 37-49.

109. D. Temple, S. Leibowitz, "Adrenal steroid receptors: interactions with brain neuropeptide systems in relation to nutrient intake and metabolism," *J Neuroendocrin* 6 (1994) 479-501.

110. P. Bjorntorp, R. Rosmond, "Obesity and cortisol," *Nutrition* 16 (2000) 924-936.

111. N. Orentreich, J.L. Brind, R.L. Rizer, J.H. Vogelman, "Age changes and sex differences in the serum dehydroepiandrosterone sulfate concentrations throughout adulthood," *J Clin Endocrin Metab* 59 (1984) 551-555.

112. T. Yamaji, H. Ibayashi, "Plasma dehydroepiandrosterone sulphate in normal and pathological conditions," *J Clin Endocrin* 29 (1969) 273-278.

113. F.P. de Heredia, D. Cerezo, S. Zamora, M. Garaulet, "Effect of dehydroepiandrosterone on protein and fat digestibility, body protein and muscular composition in high-fat-diet-fed old rats," *Brit J Nutr* 97 (2007) 464-470.

114. Ibid.

115. D.S. Kalman, C.M. Colker, M.A. Swain, G.C. Torina, Q. Shi, "A randomized double-blind placebo-controlled study of 3-acetyl-7-oxo-dehydroepiandrosterone in healthy overweight adults," *Curr Ther Res* 61 (2000) 435-442.

116. D.S. Kalman, C.M. Colker, M.A. Swain, G.C. Torina, Q. Shi, "A randomized double-blind placebo-controlled study of 3-acetyl-7-oxo-dehydroepiandrosterone in healthy overweight adults," *Curr Ther Res* 61 (2000) 435-442.

117. "Melatonin," *Dorland's Illustrated Medical Dictionary*, 30th ed: 1118.

118. Ibid.

119. Ibid.

120. B. Prunet-Marcassus, M. Desbazeille, A. Bros, k. Louche, P. Delagrange, P. Renard, L. Casteilla, L. Penicaud, "Melatonin reduces body weight gain in sprague dawley rats with diet induced obesity," *Endocrinology* 144 (2003) 5347-5352.

121. E.J. Applegate, *"The Anatomy and Physiology Learning System,"* 2nd ed, (Philadelphia, PA: Saunders, 2000) 213.

122. E. Kamycheva, J. Sundsfjord, R. Jorde, "Serum parathyroid hormone level is associated with body mass index: the 5th Tromso study," *Euro J Endocrin* 151 (2004) 167-172.

123. Ibid.

124. "Corticotropin," *Dorland's Illustrated Medical Dictionary*, 30th ed: 426.

125. D. Richard, Q. Huang, E. Timofeeva, "The corticotrophin-releasing hormone system in the regulation of energy balance in obesity," *Int'l J Obes & Relat Metab Disord* 24 (2004) S36-S39.
126. Ibid.
127. Ibid.
128. Y. Greenman, K. Tordjman, N. Stern, "Increased body weight associated with prolactin secreting pituitary adenomas: weight loss with normalization of prolactin levels," *Clin Endocrin* 48 (1998) 547-553.
129. H. Mendieta-Zeron, M. Lopez, C. Dieguez, "Gastrointensinal peptides controlling body weight homeostasis," *Gen & Comp Endocrin* 155 (2008) 481-495.
130. "Peptide," *Dorland's Illustrated Medical Dictionary*, 30th ed: 1396.
131. O.B. Chaudhri, V. Salem, K.G. Murphy, S.R. Bloom, "Gastrointestinal satiety signals," *Annu Rev Physiol* 70 (2008) 239-255.
132. D. Moskowitz, "A comprehensive review of the safety and efficacy of bio-identical hormones for the management of menopause and related health risks," *Alt Med Rev* 11 (2006) 208-223.
133. J. Jamieson, L.E. Dorman, , V. Marriott, "Growth hormone: reversing human aging naturally," 7nd ed, (St. Louis, MO: Jamieson, 1997) 95.
134. D. Moskowitz, "A comprehensive review of the safety and efficacy of bio-identical hormones for the management of menopause and related health risks," *Alt Med Rev* 11 (2006) 208-223.
135. Ibid.
136. Drugs.com, http://www.drugs.com/pdr/provera.html
137. D. Moskowitz, "A comprehensive review of the safety and efficacy of bioidentical hormones for the management of menopause and related health risks," *Alt Med Rev* 11 (2006) 208-223.
138. J.W. Schmidt, D. Wollner, J. Curcio, J. Riedlinger, L.S. Kim, "Hormone replacement therapy in menopausal women: past problems and future possibilities," *Gyn Endocrin* 22 (2006) 564-577.
139. R.G. Smith, M.O. Thorner, eds. *Human growth hormone: Research and clinical practice,* (Totowa, NJ Humana Press, 2000) 227.
140. J. Jamieson, L.E. Dorman, , V. Marriott, "Growth hormone: reversing human aging naturally," 7nd ed, (St. Louis, MO: Jamieson, 1997) 77.
141. T. Hertoghe, J. Nabet, *The hormone solution: Stay younger, longer with natural hormone and nutrition therapies*, (New York, NY: Harmony Books, 2002) 85.
142. Ibid.
143. H.R. Berthoud, C. Morrison, "The brain, appetite, and obesity," *Ann Rev Psych* 59 (2008) 55-92.

Part Three

How to Make a Difference

7   The Driving Force Within

Today, everywhere we look the glitzy Madison Avenue marketing schemes are suggesting that if we buy one product we will look younger, if we buy another we will feel better, or if we buy still another we will be more successful or socially acceptable. Often times the suggestion is so powerful that we end up doing exactly what they want us to do, and the worst part is that frequently we do something that we had no intention of doing. In reality this is simply the *law of stimulus-response*, where "individuals react or respond to stimuli in the environment or stimuli within themselves."[1]

How do these people know what we want even before we know ourselves? The answer is simple. Their success lies in having a clear understanding of exactly:

- What drives us or what turns us on,
- What can be done, if need be, to alter what drives us,
- How to tap into that drive.

They arrive at those answers by analysis of what moves us to action. Then they apply that knowledge to their advertising campaign.

Likewise, our weight loss efforts are driven by those same factors. This chapter is intended to help you better understand:

- Your motives for losing weight,
- What self-discipline it will take,
- How to effectively set reasonable weight loss goals,
- How to build and utilize an effective support system,
- How you might alter some of those drives, to better align them with your goals.

Motivation

Motivation is "any of the forces that activate behavior toward satisfying needs or achieving goals."[2] In plain words motivation is the arousal to action. Locke says there are four key concepts in motivation. They are:

- Needs - the requirements of the person,
- Values - that which the person considers beneficial or valuable,
- Goals and Intentions - the targets of action,
- Emotions - the form that the person uses to experience value appraisals.[3]

He goes on to say that, "motives, values and goals affect action in three ways. First, they affect what facts we choose to act on…Second, values and goals affect the intensity of the action…based on how important the value is held to be…Third, values and goals also affect the persistence of action, how prolonged it is."[4] In short if we keep Locke's four concepts in mind, as they relate to our goal of weight loss, and if we align our goals with our feelings about these concepts, the motivation we need to accomplish the goals should follow. The subject of motivation involves a variety of processes that provide behavior with both energy and direction, and the way people approach the desired outcome has a major impact on the energy they can muster to pursue their goals.[5]

Here are the two dominant theories of behavior change, both of which are applicable to weight loss:

- **The Theory of the Reasoned Action** (TRA) - proposed in the 1960's holds that behavior is generally determined by a conscious behavior intention, which turns out to be the strongest determinant of behavioral performance.[6]

- **The Theory of Planned Behavior** (TPB) - proposed in the 1980's, expands on the basic (TRA) by adding the requirement of perceived behavioral control. This change was intended to soften the behavior intention component of the (TRA), using the argument that behavior intention cannot be the major behavioral factor where the behavior is not entirely under the control of the individual.[7]

Even though the (TPB) makes intuitive sense, because health behaviors are greatly affected by perceptions of self-control, it suffers from some noteworthy inadequacies. It implies change can be accomplished by changing personal behavior, but doesn't offer solid suggestions as to how to change your mental state in order to accomplish the desired behavior change.[8] Having offered this negative aspect of behavior change theory, later in this chapter you will find several effective methods, among them good planning, that might be used to overcome this weakness.

Koo & Fishbach take a slightly different approach to motivation, but one that might seem logical to those of us that have a limited knowledge of psychology. They suggest two factors that tend to increase the motivation for individuals to work towards specific goals. The first is *goal commitment*, where people consider, (1) whether the goal is still worth pursuing, and (2) what they have accomplished to date, and the second is a *lack of goal progress*, where people consider what they have left to accomplish in order to attain the goal.[9] Interestingly, when people feel somewhat unsure about their level of commitment to the goal, evaluating performance data that shows progress-to-date can be motivating. Conversely when they are committed to the goal they automatically become more interested in goal progress, so evaluating performance data showing how far they have yet to go can be motivating.[10]

Here are some of the motivating factors that push many people toward exercise: "health, appearance, enjoyment, social interaction, stress relief, challenge, skill development, achievement, and personal satisfaction."[11] There are differences between what motivates men and women. In general terms, the motivations for exercise most often suggested by men are health and fitness and those suggested by women are social factors and release of tension.[12] If men are motivated enough to enter a weight loss program, they seem to forget health and fitness as motivational factors, rather they now become motivated by a desire to be more effective in the workplace.[13] Apparently going to the trouble of entering a weight loss program changes men's thinking.

On the other hand, weight loss or health-related goals may not be effective reasons for middle-aged women to begin exercising.[14] "Instead, healthcare providers and health promotion specialists might better facilitate long-term participation among healthy women if they emphasize physical activity as a means to enhance their quality of life."[15] Also age may alter the motivational factors among women, since it has been demonstrated that "dieting behavior among young girls is often a response to pressure from others to achieve thinness."[16] These same young women may be prone to diet if they are dissatisfied with their bodies or experience feelings of diminished self-worth.[17]

Frequently, the health care professional or personal trainer is faced with this question: How can I motivate my clients to lose weight? In my mind that question runs parallel to, how can I motivate my best friend to help me commit a robbery? Both questions are based on the assumption that one individual can control the motivation of another. While one individual can point out the benefits of changed behavior to another person, the true motivation for changing that behavior must come from within. Therefore, while I support the weight loss benefits you can achieve by altering your behavior, I cannot take responsibility for your motivation. To do so would put me in the position of an enabler and at the same time give you an easy excuse should you be unsuccessful.

When we talk about motivation we are really talking about self-efficacy, which is the ability to produce an effect, or to control the outcome of an event or series of events. "The evidence…is consistent in showing that efficacy beliefs contribute significantly to the level of motivation and performance."[18] Improvements in self-efficacy can support successful weight loss and among the tools that have been used to help individuals motivate themselves more effectively are: (1) improved goal setting, (2) verbal persuasion, (3) positive feedback, and (4) reinforcement of their success.[19] Self-efficacy results in better weight loss success if good role models are identified and appropriate environmental support is established.[20] External forces such as God or fate do not control eating behaviors, rather success comes from making the right decisions.[21]

One aspect of self-efficacy is the process of self-monitoring. An interesting study that followed the self-monitoring habits of low-income minority children showed that when one group of these children monitored their own behavior over a six-month period, they experienced significantly more weight loss than did another group who self-monitored less consistently.[22] The same study found that "parental self-monitoring was a significant predictor of child self-monitoring."[23] As a result if parents want their children to successfully lose weight they need to teach them self-monitoring, by setting that example.

Another interesting aspect of motivation comes into play when a physician gets involved in the obese person's struggle to lose weight. Some overweight individuals seek help from their personal physician; however, most people visit their doctors with health problems other than obesity. Women seek weight loss advice from their physicians more frequently than men do. This could be because they:

- Are more aware of their weight status than men are of theirs,
- Visit their physicians more frequently than men do,
- Generally undertake healthy lifestyle behaviors more often than men do,
- Are more willing to adopt changes to promote weight loss.[24]

When it comes to weight management conversations with their physicians most patients:

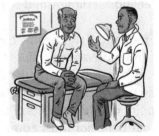

- Believe their doctor could help them lose weight although only a limited number have approached them,
- Want more help from their doctor than they are actually getting,
- Want dietary and exercise advice as well as help setting realistic weight loss goals.[25]

The bigger problem seems to be that physicians tend to drastically under report and under treat obesity. One study found that only 39 percent of obese adults received advice from their physician to lose weight,[26] while another reported that, "only 8.6% of all office visits had obesity reported, suggesting that office-based physicians seem to identify only one third of all of their obese patients."[27] There is a controversy regarding the benefits of obesity treatment for patients lacking some other obesity related disease (e.g. heart disease, diabetes, high blood pressure).

The reason is that there is supposedly little evidence supporting the long-term efficacy of weight reduction programs.[28] Perhaps the doctors that were the subject of the study need to look at the evidence cited throughout this book!

Apparently, if an obese patient goes to the doctor with a sore throat the physician treats the sore throat but does not proactively mention the subject of the patient's obesity, because he/she believes that either they or the patient are powerless to improve the situation. Wow, that's a little scary, since left unattended the obesity will surely lead to more serious problems. That seems to me like a wait until it's broke and then we will try and fix it approach, not to mention a complete dereliction of the doctor's ethical duty to the patient.

It is true that physicians have a limited time allotment during patient visits. It is equally true that many patients lack the motivation to lose weight. In the end people who receive "physician counseling about weight loss are 2 times more likely to report that they are currently trying to lose weight."[29] "In a national survey of 620 primary care physicians, over 40% agreed that obese patients could reach a normal weight if they were motivated, but that most patients would not be motivated enough to lose a significant amount of weight."[30]

Among physicians, low levels of attention to the problem of obesity may be based on two primary considerations: (1) the most effective use of their time, and (2) their ineffectiveness in treating obesity.[31] Experts have concluded that, "physicians provided insufficient guidance on weight management strategies, possibly because of inadequate counseling skills and confidence."[32] Others believe physician treatment of overweight patients is of limited effectiveness, because the patient's frequently set overly stringent weight loss goals.[33] How about this one! The real underlying reason for lack of physician interest in obesity is the, "physicians' lack of reimbursement for obesity treatment."[34]

Primary care physicians report that one of the key barriers to weight-loss counseling is their "self-perceived low competence in treating obesity."[35] Both the low physician competency coupled with the patient's inability to lose weight appears to be perceived by physicians as a blow to their egos, reflecting negatively on their personal success.[36] A low competence in treating obesity is not surprising. The typical medical school curriculum doesn't adequately prepare the physician to deal with the issue of obesity, since, "physicians receive virtually no training on nutrition or physical activity in medical school."[37]

How often do doctors say that if you want to lose weight you need to get some exercise and eat a low-fat diet? If doctors are pushed as to what they really mean by that statement, they usually have no further explanation. This criticism of limited physician competency is not intended to be an indictment of the western medical practitioner, but they simply are not trained in nutrition or exercise. For sound nutritional advice, a nutritionist should be consulted and if an effective exercise program is needed, a consultation with an exercise physiologist or personal trainer should prove beneficial.

Thuan & Avignon summed up the feelings of physicians they studied by citing these findings:

- Only 42 percent of physicians considered themselves well prepared to manage obesity,
- Only 51 percent found obesity management professionally rewarding,
- 66 percent believed that only a small percentage of patients could lose weight and maintain that loss,
- Only 34 percent believed that available drugs are effective,
- In general they do not consider collaboration with other health professionals (e.g. nutritionists, personal trainers) to be a priority.[38]

Call me old fashioned, but I don't care how professionally unrewarding the other 49 percent of the physicians cited in bullet two find obesity management, as long as they continued to charge for their health consultation services they owe it to their patients to delve into this obvious high risk health problem. In addition, this study fails to clarify why the physicians cited in bullet five don't feel it is a priority to collaborate with other health professionals. It strikes me as arrogant for them to blindly stumble forward when we have already seen and they know that: (1) they are not getting the desired weight loss results so many of their patients need, and (2) there are several other professional disciplines far more qualified to counsel in such areas as nutrition and exercise.

If a physician refers a patient to a complementary weight management program consultation, the patient is more likely to attend than if they were left to their own volition.[39] "Individuals often view doing things that their healthcare providers recommend to be healthy as something they are 'supposed to do' or 'should do.'"[40] However, when it comes to actually joining the weight management program, just the opposite is true. Physician referrals have a lower program enrollment rate than do personal referrals or self-referrals.[41] Among the explanations for these findings are:

- The obese are less motivated to lose weight when it's their physician's idea,
- Financial considerations may be more of an issue for physician referrals than for self-referrals,
- The patient may attend the consultation simply to appease the physician.[42]

Self-Discipline

This section is entitled *self-discipline* because I thought it would be more easily recognized, than the term self-regulation, which is used primarily in the psychological literature. "Regulation usually refers to controlling and making right some process that would otherwise run away or vary in undesirable ways."[43] Self-regulation or self-discipline obviously refers to personal activity that is self-controlled. Regulation can be simple; however in the context of self-discipline the complex human brain becomes involved, which can lead to either cognitive regulation or emotional regulation.[44] As we have already seen and as we will see later, both knowledge and feeling play important roles in the concepts discussed. If, as research has shown, the single most important factor affecting weight-loss is self-regulatory behavior,[45] then it should be of some comfort to realize the outcome is in your hands.

Good self-control goes hand-in-hand with good planning and poor self-control is closely related to impulsiveness.[46] One way of getting more self-control is by aggressively executing a well thought out plan. Good control for me results in my constantly asking two questions: (1) how can I get more control over the steps leading to the desired outcome, and (2) how can I simplify those steps to increase my probability of success? In the context of weight loss, the development of good self-control might be related to a greater awareness of the vulnerability to health risks and more sensible decisions about diet and exercise.[47]

Another method of gaining increased self-control is by acquiring more subject matter knowledge. Those who try to learn everything they can about a subject tend to procrastinate less and make more progress toward goal achievement, than those who shun the learning.[48] These individuals focus more on the search for information on self-improvement and less on self-validation,[49] which facilitates better planning and effective goal achievement. Think of how much progress you will make in your weight loss program if you begin reading about exercise, nutrition, etc. You don't have to become an expert on any of these subjects, but the more knowledge you have about how they apply to your particular situation, the better result you'll get. Here's another tightly knit circle: "the experience of mastering a task enhances self-efficacy… higher self-efficacy is assumed to facilitate mastery."[50] Increased mastery of one's cognitive skills tends to help the individual achieve higher levels of self-regulation.[51]

The strategy known as *mental contrasting* has an impact on self-discipline. The process of imagining a desired future outcome contrasts with the present reality. This process is "a self-regulation strategy that leads to goal commitment in line with a person's expectations of success."[52] Mental contrasting may be especially effective when one's expectations of success are high, because it helps provide the level of energy needed to accomplish the desired goal.

Exerting self-discipline can be difficult. Researchers often refer to the problem as ego depletion, a phenomenon of limited self-regulatory strength.[53] "The ability to exert self-control acts as a limited resource."[54] It takes energy to resist the persuasive efforts of others and as a result, during this self-discipline vs impulse tug-of-war, "people may lose their ability to resist after repeated exposure to persuasive appeals,"[55] (e.g. police interrogations, brainwashing, fraternity hazing). It has been shown that glucose, the body's major energy source, is depleted during active periods of self-discipline. As a result the ability to control thought and behavior is impaired until glucose levels are restored.[56] If the outside attempts to influence a person are weak, the person will be able to routinely dismiss them without a noticeable energy loss. Most individuals are aware of the drain that attempted outside influence places on their energy, so they tend to conserve it and use it as needed.[57]

Once energy depletion begins people tend to: (1) dig their heels in and feel stronger about their own point of view, and (2) seek information that confirms their own views.[58] Persuasive attempts are more successful against weakly held or newly formed attitudes than they are against established or firmly held attitudes.[59] Researchers have also found that:

- When an individual is presented with a goal and a temptation simultaneously, the value of the temptation relative to the goal increases, but when the goal and the temptation are presented apart from each other the value of the goal relative to the temptation increases.[60]

- When cognitive capacity is high, behavior is generally influenced by personal standards, and when cognitive capacity is low behavior is mostly influenced by automatic attitudes.[61]

- Decision-making and self-control are parallel psychological resources. "Making many decisions leaves the person in a depleted state and hence less likely to exert self-control effectively."[62]

The logical question is, what can be done to counteract ego depletion? A couple of answers seem quite simple. One is to sustain reasonable glucose levels in order to supply the body with the basic source of energy.[63] A second is to maintain a positive outlook, mood or emotional state.[64] But hold on, that may be easier said than done. In an ego depleted state it might be difficult to maintain a positive outlook. Study data suggests that the state of ego depletion: (1) retards people's ability to develop a positive attitude about themselves, (2) causes them to lose optimism regarding their own capability, (3) reduces their sense of control, and (4) causes them to be less optimistic about their future.[65] So which situation controls? The answer lies in your personal strength. If you have the ability to maintain an optimistic focus you will be less prone to ego depletion.

Another problem frequently encountered in a weight-loss program, is that of self-defeating behavior. Self-defeating behavior is any behavior where costs are greater than benefits. Self-defeating behavior leads to mistakes, personal detriment or suffering and is detrimental to goal achievement.[66] What causes self-defeating behavior? A fundamental human motivation is the need for social inclusion. People who are deprived of important social links can experience emotional harm, often leading to self-defeating behavior.[67] For example, exclusion from a desired group may lead to feelings of isolation.

Today, in Western society communicating with other people via email, phone and text messaging is commonplace, instead of communicating face-to-face. This type of communication leads to feelings of exclusion. To break this cycle, try pursuing your weight loss goals in a group setting or one-on-one with another individual, where skill mastery and support are available (e.g. support group, personal trainer, nutritionist). The resulting feelings of inclusion and support are sure to outweigh any inconvenience you might experience.

Here are a few considerations for self-discipline/self-regulation that should prove useful to you:

- Distress ensues when goal failure becomes a possibility. A person will normally engage in self-regulation in an attempt to make the necessary adjustments to achieve the goal.[68] Don't be alarmed or overwhelmed if you feel distress as a result of concluding you may fail to reach your goal. Realize the distress will not drive you into further self-regulation; it is strictly pushing you to come to grips with the idea that your goal is threatened.

- There are two important cognitive mechanisms that drive self-regulation: (1) self-efficacy appraisals, and (2) goal representations.[69] Self-efficacy appraisals occur when people reflect on their own ability to produce a desired result, and goal representations exist when people develop mental pictures of what they want to achieve in the future. Comparing your current weight loss performance against your perceived capability and allowing yourself to dream or fantasize about how good the outcome might be, are natural and healthy processes. These processes are to be encouraged and used as yardsticks against which you plan and measure your results.

- What it costs you to carry out your weight-loss program in time, money, energy, etc., compared to the benefit that you will receive from successful completion, is called a *cost-benefit analysis*. Costs occur at the time of performance, benefits occur sometime later. It is possible to gain the benefits that help us develop significant self-discipline, which in turn drives consistent performance over time.[70]

- A behavioral cue is a signal that triggers a specific behavioral response. Studies have shown that certain "cues may alter key-goal related processes that undermine self-regulatory objectives."[71] This is especially true for people who are attempting to control their eating behavior. Pleasurable food cues may influence eating behavior in a way that results in over eating.[72] For example the visual cue of seeing a plate full of cookies may spark the desire to eat some or all of them. The objective is to alter or remove the cue entirely. If the cookies were not in plain sight the temptation would not occur as easily. If they were not in the house at all, even if the thought of them was triggered, the act of eating them would be curtailed. This is not to imply that all cues are bad; some support desirable behavior as well.

Finally, the cornerstone of any weight control program is self-monitoring.[73] You must continually monitor and, where possible, measure your progress. You will be either making progress toward your weight loss goal, or you will be losing ground. It is unlikely you will hold a completely neutral position for a prolonged period. The only way to know where you are, at any given time, is to monitor yourself regularly. Monitoring may be as simple as checking your weight on a scale, measuring your waist with a tape measure, applying my Belt-Hole-Rule, using a percent body fat monitor or simply standing naked in front of a mirror and looking at yourself. I don't care how you do it but you must monitor your progress and react appropriately to the results.

Goal Setting

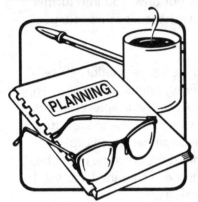

Setting goals, especially written goals, is a frequently overlooked factor in the pursuit of an objective, even though it can be of great benefit. "Setting goals is a standard management procedure and a common start to any project."[74] Goal setting is the process of clearly defining and targeting objectives to be accomplished, and it "operates primarily as a motivational mechanism to influence the degree of effort in striving toward a goal."[75] "Strategic goal setting refers to the intentions to attain a specific standard of proficiency usually within a specified amount of time."[76] When we set goals we specify what we want to happen and the steps necessary to make it happen. It is important to set an achievable goal, since, "people are more likely to select a particular goal if they expect that they can reach this goal."[77] Interestingly, goal setting is sometimes referred to as a discrepancy creating process, "it implies discontent with one's present condition and the desire to attain an object or outcome."[78]

People who are asked to achieve stringent criterion frequently performed better than people asked to merely do their best.[79] In studies where goal setting was related directly to exercise, the results demonstrated "that: (a) goal setting is an effective performance enhancement strategy, and (b) difficult and specific goals prompt higher levels of performance than objective 'do your best goals.'"[80] In addition, when good planning and organizational skills are coupled with sound goal setting, a valuable link is found to exist between the establishment of the goal and its achievement.[81]

Incentives may be used to enhance goal achievement. As might be expected, monetary incentives frequently improve performance, and the larger the incentive the greater the performance improvement, unless achievement of the goal is too difficult.[82] If monetary incentives enhance goal achievement, other favors, benefits or items that you value, could do the same. In attempting to reach your goal don't hesitate to include incentives, which you value, in your plan.

Two other important considerations in determining progress toward your goal are: (1) what information will you need, and (2) how will you get it. It is equally important to understand how you will interpret the feedback you get during the process of goal achievement, because until that becomes clear the feedback you get will be of little value.

Although health benefits are often given, by women, as reasons for establishing weight loss goals, in reality they often establish such goals in order to reshape their bodies and improve their appearance. Much of this drive to achieve the ideal body size and shape results from cultural beauty norms and the images women see in the media. As might be expected, with increasing age women often deemphasize these goals.[83.]

When researchers use the words goal orientation, they are referring "to the goals that are implicitly pursued by individuals while attempting to attain or achieve a certain level of performance."[84] Within the actual goal-setting framework are two goal orientation processes: (1) performance goal orientation, (an outcome-based behavior), and (2) learning goal orientation (an understanding or knowledge based behavior).[85] In the early stages of your weight loss program, goals that focus on learning or knowledge enhancement may prove helpful, but don't get stuck too long in that mode. If you are to reach your final objective your goals should quickly evolve into outcome-based behaviors.

Many goal-setting theories exist in the psychological literature. Five of the most applicable are outlined below. The one most relied upon in the weight loss research studies is the goal setting theory.

- **Goal Setting Theory** - was first described by Edwin Locke in the mid 1960's and later studied at great length, by the tandem of Locke and fellow researcher Gary Latham. The Goal Setting Theory is based on the two hallmark attributes of: (1) specificity, and (2) difficulty.[86] Goals that are specific and difficult lead to higher performance, when compared to easy goals or goals that require a person to just do their best,[87] "so long as the person is committed to the goal, has the requisite ability to attain it, and does not have conflicting goals."[88] Locke & Latham believe there are four mechanisms that have a substantial impact on goal performance. They are:
  - High goals lead to greater effort and/or persistence,
  - Goal pursuit focuses effort on goal-relevant actions rather than non-relevant actions,
  - Goal achievement depends on having the necessary knowledge and skill set,
  - Goals may motivate individuals to utilize their existing abilities more fully.[89]

  Most likely the enduring success of this theory is that it is rooted in real world common sense. It takes little imagination to figure out how the four mechanisms may be applied to a weight loss endeavor. This theory will be discussed in greater detail later in this chapter.

Here are four other theories that although of seemingly lesser value, should be understood because their consideration might lend additional strength and support to your goal-setting effort.

- **Social Cognitive Theory** - is based on the confidence that an individual has in his/her own ability to achieve the goal, in light of perceived barriers.[90] Study data greatly supports the notion that individual self-confidence in overcoming goal related barriers is a very positive factor in goal attainment. Furthermore, this theory dovetails very nicely with the goal setting theory.

- **Health Action Process Approach** - is a two-phased approach suggesting that during phase 1 goal intentions are developed, and during phase 2 specific plans are implemented that link goal intentions and goal achievement activity.[91] This theory is based to a large extent on an all-important planning component. More about planning will be discussed later in this chapter.

- **Self Determination Theory** - is a theory of human motivation that "emphasizes need fulfillment as a primary determinant of psychological well-being and successful goal pursuit."[92] The backbone of this theory is the presumption that people have three basic psychological needs: (1) to be competent, (2) to remain self-directed, and (3) to care for and relate to others.[93]

- **Fantasy Realization Theory** - is a recent (1990's) psychological exercise that differentiates between realities and fantasies. "Fantasies are thoughts and images of future events or behaviors that appear in the mind."[94] Attempting to realize one's fantasies could be a very slippery slope. The previously mentioned four theories should have positive, useful application in your weight loss program; the reason I mentioned this theory is so you understand there is little or no place for a fantasy-based goal in your weight loss program. If you are the type of personality that tends to fantasize freely, I hope before you finish reading this chapter you will realize fantasy goals are next to impossible to attain.

There are some subtle differences that exist between goal setting and other related factors that can easily be confused with actual goal setting.

- **Hope** - Hope was defined by Snyder, who was the originator of a theory he called the *hope theory*. Snyder said that hope is the "perceived capacity to: (1) develop workable goals, (2) find routes to those goals… and (3) become motivated to use those pathways."[95] It is interesting, and I must say confusing, that Snyder uses the word goal several times to define his hope theory. Others disagree with Snyder, as do I, that you can develop workable goals on the basis of hope.

  Hope is far different from a goal because it is more of a perception than a reality. Hope does not require a concrete path toward goal achievement or a thought process aligned with reality; in fact it is possible for individuals to have high hopes, yet never reach their goals.[96] It is this lack of a concrete path toward goal achievement that should suggest to you, it would be best not to base your weight loss effort on some kind of hope.

- **Implementation Intentions** - Implementation intentions "are plans that specify the when, where and how of goal striving in advance and have been shown to enhance rates of goal attainment compared to merely forming respective goal intentions."[97] By forming implementation intentions the individual becomes perceptually ready to move forward, without the need for conscious intent, once the opportunity presents itself.[98] Implementation intentions could be used as an initial stage of planning but they don't form a complete plan, because they lack key elements, such as, measurement and time restrictions. Once you are past the intention phase you still have to take action that will carry you the rest of the way to final achievement of the goal.

- **Goal Pursuit** - Researchers claim goal setting deals with the motivational factors for developing a goal, while goal pursuit involves all the decision processes and actions involved in achieving the goal.[99] Obviously goal setting, the topic of this section, is quite different than goal pursuit. Goal setting occurs on the front end and goal pursuit occurs on the back end of the process of accomplishing your goal.

- **Reaction to a Threat** - Goal setting deals with planning for goal attainment and involves realism and a degree of functional optimism, whereas the reaction to a threat may be more of a knee-jerk reaction dealing with defense optimism, posturing or manipulation.[100] When considering how people react to threats, one question that arises is whether or not a threat can be beneficial during goal setting. The answer may lie in how strongly the individual values achievement of the goal, rather than the discomfort associated with it. We might be inclined to believe that people always want to feel good; however, recent research "demonstrates that people want to feel unpleasant emotions, such as anger or fear, when these emotions promote the attainment of their long-term goals."[101]

- **Life Longings** - Life longings are "recurring, emotionally ambivalent representations of ideal (optimal or utopian) states of life."[102] People identify more closely with their goals than they do with their life longings because goals are "more closely linked to everyday actions, more strongly linked to the future, and more controllable."[103] There appear to be a number of aspects that differentiate goals and life longings. Goals are normally related to the individual's physical well being, and are viewed as concrete, highly attainable and strongly linked to action when they can be accomplished and are valuable.[104] Life longings closely parallel hope and dreams because they are difficult to translate into functional, useful action.

- **Goal Framing** - Goal framing is the act of defining the goal in terms of either a positive or negative state, [e.g. a positively framed weight loss goal might be - ("it would be good if I lost more than ten pounds in the next three months,") while a negatively framed goal might be - ("it would be bad if I didn't lose ten pounds in the next three months")]. Researchers studied this concept in an educational environment and their research "suggests that goals if they are construed as defining a state that one wants to avoid, can adversely affect performance."[105] So just how important is an optimistic mindset as opposed to a pessimistic one? So long as the goals are high-priority goals, "optimistic individuals would indeed increase goal engagement and would be more likely to attain their goal relative to individuals low in optimism."[106]

It is important to make the distinction between goal achievement and goal maintenance. As mentioned earlier goal achievement involves a discrepancy between where we are today and where we want to be; therefore goal achievement is about progressing forward from our current state, in order to reach the desired state. Goal maintenance is about preventing a current state from deteriorating. Since goal achievement and goal maintenance are quite different situations, it is easy to see that each may require a different strategy. Goal achievement is a process of adding to what has already been accomplished,[107] and involves nurturance and advancement.[108]

Goal maintenance, on the other hand, is the process of holding on to what we already have accomplished,[109] and involves security and safety.[110] It is interesting to note that while "vigilance characterizes a prevention focus, vigilance can be served either by conservative or risky tactics."[111] Once you become comfortable with making decisions that are sometimes conservative and other times risky, your planning will become much easier and will help you achieve better results. One outcome is that you will be able to initiate processes that help you make the least costly errors.

In order to set effective, achievable goals it "is generally agreed that a good goal is specific, measurable, achievable, realistic/relevant and timed (SMART)."[112][113] Using the (SMART) acronym, here are some examples of how you might apply each step:

- **Specific** - A goal to lose ten pounds will be far more effective than the more general goal to just lose weight.

- **Measurable** - If the ultimate goal is to improve your health by losing weight, it is much easier to measure weight loss than it is to measure improved health.

- **Achievable** - A weight loss of one pound per week is far more achievable that one pound per day.

- **Realistic / Relevant** - If you are 50 pounds overweight, it makes a lot more sense to set a goal to lose ten pounds than it does to set a goal to lose 50 pounds, then once that goal is accomplished set another goal to lose an additional ten pounds.

- **Time Restricted** - A goal to lose ten pounds in two months will have a much better chance of success then leaving the time frame open. The open time frame actually allows for never losing the ten pounds.

Some have attempted to refute the idea that realistic goals are much better than unrealistic goals, even though they avoided making that claim outright. For example one study said that, "our results augment the literature suggesting that unrealistic goals are not detrimental to weight loss."[114] First of all, their data only *suggests* that unrealistic goals are not detrimental. Second, none of the previous data cited, implies that unrealistic goals are detrimental to success, just that they are not as effective as realistic goals. These researchers went on to say that: "the evidence does not convincingly support the prevalent clinical practice of counseling people to adopt modest weight loss goals,"[115] however, their study does not convincingly support the opposing idea either. Apparently they haven't seen any of the studies cited below! The numerous research studies cited make the claim that realistic weight loss goals are important, rather than modest weight loss goals. If it were realistic to establish much bolder weight loss objectives then a modest weight loss goal would not be realistic.

The selection of a proper goal is of great importance. Generally, when considering weight loss goals we either consciously or unconsciously engage in the following considerations:

- **Perceived Health Risk** - Our possible susceptibility to disease and the severity of its manifestation.
- **Outcome Expectancies** - What it will cost and what the resulting benefits will be.
- **Social Influence** - What other important people in our lives think of us.
- **Self-Efficacy** - Our perceived ability to carry out the intended behavior.[116]

Once the goal is clearly in focus, the size of the goal becomes important because of its relationship to the number and frequency of possible incremental successes. Research has shown that goal setters "who experienced repeated successes set higher personal goals than did those with only a single success."[117] "Multiple, specific goals act as stepping stones to the greater goal people are striving toward."[118] One reason why you have a greater chance of success by setting small bite-sized goals is that there is a great sense of accomplishment that comes with achieving each goal. By setting five different ten pound weight loss goals you will experience the joy of achieving five successes rather than setting one, 50 pound weight loss goal and having to wait until you reach that single goal to feel the joy of success.

Individuals who indicate that only large weight loss goals are acceptable to them, lose significantly less weight when compared to people with less stringent goals.[119] "Effort should be made during weight-loss treatment to minimize the relative importance of reaching an unrealistic personal goal."[120] Study results found "participants who have modest goals were more likely to achieve them…those who reached their weight loss goals also did better in the long term than those who did not."[121]

As one might expect, the setting of smaller bite-size goals automatically results in more frequent goal-setting. In weight management programs, frequent goal setting has been found to be more successful than less frequent goal setting.[122] "Theoretically, frequency of goal setting may indicate the level of commitment to diet and physical activity behavior change."[123] I like to think of frequent goal setting in a weight loss context as goal readjustment, since we are really redefining the steps along the path to greater goal accomplishment.

The good news is that even if you never achieve the 50 pound goal, in the example above, with 10, 20, 30 pounds of weight loss you will have achieved several small successes and more importantly you will have gained the health benefits associated with even modest weight loss. Researchers constantly talk about the fact that "significant health benefits are associated with modest weight losses that fall short of healthy and aesthetic ideals."[124]

People who are about to tackle a self-change program should understand the difficulty of the task they are undertaking. The two pillars of effective goal pursuit are: (1) the selected goal has to be personally meaningful, and (2) there has to be a specific, detailed action plan, describing how the goal will be achieved.[125] Once the goal is formulated it provides a roadmap for getting from point A to point B, and offers valuable guidance if you get off track. "When one's expectations are out of line with what can be achieved, self-confidence may become overconfidence, leading from hope to false hope."[126] "False hope is based on a mistaken belief that change is easily attainable and likely to produce exaggerated benefits."[127] It is important to realize that study data lends credence to the idea that, "people possess quite accurate knowledge of their chances of success."[128] Perhaps this is the reason that such things as New Year's resolutions are often successful. "Contrary to widespread public opinion, a considerable proportion of New Year's resolvers do in fact succeed, at least in the short run...the success rate of resolutions is approximately ten times higher than the success rate of adults desiring to change their behavior but not making a resolution."[129]

Let's take a look at actual processes for setting viable goals so you can get out of the gate on the right foot. First, do an exceptionally good job of planning, and (2) effectively manage the process of implementation.[130] Put another way, "plans are the designs we construct to guide our attempts to reach a goal in a given environment."[131] Planning typically defines the (who, what, where, when and how) to perform the behavior. "Planning enhances information processing in terms of increased accessibility, recall, detection, and discrimination of critical cues."[132] Individuals who take the time to develop a plan, are much more likely to engage in the desired behavior, than they would be if they hadn't prepared the plan.[133] Note that a good plan: (1) reduces procrastination, (which affects 95 percent of the population), by increasing energy levels,[134] (2) reduces the vulnerability to being distracted by time pressure,[135] and (3) is tightly linked to the well-being of the individual.[136]

The planning process has been divided into the following two subcategories:

- Action Planning - involves selecting behaviors that will help attain the desired goal,[137] and it works best when intentions are high.[138]

- Coping Planning - anticipates the range of difficulties or barriers that might inhibit a person from acting upon his/her intentions and implements appropriate plans to deal with those situations.[139]

Action planning and coping planning have a positive effect on health behaviors.[140] For those of you who have attempted a weight-loss program in the past, I am certain that you understand the difficulty of restructuring your already hectic schedule to incorporate time-consuming exercise activities. Macdonald & Palfai emphasize the importance of good planning related to an exercise program by saying that "possessing strong regulatory skills may be necessary for maintaining exercise behavior over time."[141] They also maintain that people who are good at planning: (1) naturally experience less setbacks when faced with minor goal failures, and (2) are better able to utilize those planning skills to move smoothly from exercise goal setting to exercise goal achievement.[142] Even if you aren't currently very good at planning, by utilizing the knowledge that you have already acquired in this chapter and the tools and techniques developed later in this book, your skills will improve enough to substantially benefit your weight loss program.

Research demonstrates that a number of individual psychological characteristics can have a big impact on goal setting. Those that you possess will be of benefit. Here they are:

- **Optimism** - has been shown to be a functional asset once the individual has determined the goal;[143] however, "people have a tendency to err from realism in an optimistic direction when making predictions about future events."[144] You need to keep your optimism under control and be realistic while you are setting a goal then allow your optimism to grow while you are in pursuit of the goal. Even though there may be a tendency to be overly optimistic, people can demonstrate optimism without increasing their vulnerability to failure.[145]

- **Mood** - is a psychological state of mind that will have a favorable impact on task performance, in pursuit of a goal, if it is positive or upbeat. Your "mood state can bias judgments of performance or progress toward the goal."[146]

- **Perfectionism** - has been debated by some as an asset and by others a detriment in athletic performance; however, when it comes to achieving performance goals, perfectionism predicts training performance and competitive performance.[147] Since training is an integral part of any weight loss program, it appears that a little bit of perfectionism should serve program participants well.

- **Personal Power** - refers to those individuals who have power over their personal situations. The ability to act boldly "facilitates goal pursuit by increasing the readiness to act in a goal consistent manner, and by increasing persistence, flexibility, and ability to seize good opportunities."[148] Powerful acting individuals are better at adjusting their performance to the demands of the task at hand, pursuing the opportunities offered and ignoring lesser activities.[149]

The physical mechanisms and considerations for establishing a goal, or multiple goals, can take a variety of forms. They can be simple or complex. I prefer simple! There is a very interesting bit of research that deals directly with the pursuit of body weight control and proposes a very straightforward and simple goal setting approach. The bottom line goal, or schema, as they prefer to call it can be uncovered by asking a series of probing questions, with each question delving into the reasons behind the answer to the prior question. "The result is a structured network comprised of sequences of reasons (i.e. subordinate goals) explaining why one holds a particular body weight goal."[150]

This technique is nothing more than the *Five Why* root-cause analysis technique popularized years ago by the Toyota Motor Corporation. Toyota uses this successive question asking method to explore the cause-and-effect relationship underlying the problem to be solved. It should be noted that there is nothing sacred about asking the why question specifically five times, it may be asked more or less times depending on the situation.

Here's an example of how it might work in a weight-loss program:

Q1	Why do you want to achieve X body weight?
A1	I want improved health.
Q2	Why do you want improved health?
A2	I want to live a longer, happier life.
Q3	Why do you want to live a longer happier life?
A3	To do normal activities and live a normal lifespan.
Q4	Why normal activities and a normal lifespan?
A4	To participate in my kid's activities.
Q5	Why participate in your kid's activities?
A5	To be the best possible parent that I can be.

The series of questions and answers provides a solid framework and gives you a better understanding of why you want to achieve your desired body weight. The real value is in the answer to the last question, because that is the real reason for the overall weight loss goal. Once you have drilled down the list, establishing logical, incremental (mini) goals becomes much simpler. In this example the real reason for wanting to lose weight is not to look better, not to satisfy your doctor, not to get health insurance, but it is specifically to be the best possible parent. Formulating your goals around this understanding makes properly focusing on the necessary tasks easier.

If you're working in a group setting "the aim of the why question is to enable different stakeholders to authentically express themselves so that they can discover deep commonalities and appreciate differences."[151] Through this process stakeholders can more easily commit to goals they deem valuable. "It also enables them to question their own goals, reframe them, and discover new ones."[152]

A big component of goal setting is determining how difficult the goal should be. Researchers disagree as to how goal difficulty impacts goal achievement. Some suggest that if a goal is set too high, the possibility of not reaching it can threaten the individual and can also lead to feelings of helplessness.[153] If individuals have a high degree of control over the tasks required to meet the goal at least they will maintain their level of motivation.[154] However, as logic dictates, goal achievement is only possible if the person striving for the goal has the requisite skills or capability.[155] So don't set any goal for yourself or let anyone else set a goal for you until it is clear that you have the necessary skills to accomplish it.

Another critical aspect of goal setting is whether we set our own goals or someone else sets them for us. If we set our own goals and consistently fail to meet them, the perceived discrepancy is generally seen to be maladaptive; whereas, when someone else sets our goals, especially when the standards are high, we may experience feelings of depression, anger and fear of negative evaluation.[156] The bottom line here is that the needs of the individual attempting to achieve the goal, are of paramount importance.[157] [158] In addition, we may experience psychological distress if we set low goals but feel that others have overly high expectations for us.[159] Even though others may have input into your goals, I strongly suggest that you set them yourself, since you must ultimately own them.

This book is intended for use in one of two different settings. First, it is complete and detailed enough to be used by individuals attempting to lose weight working alone. Second, it is common for fitness centers, churches, etc. to form groups to help individuals accomplish their weight loss objectives and it will prove valuable in that setting, as well. If goals are established in a group setting they usually fall into two categories: (1) goals that are set by individuals, for their own benefit, but which might be subject to peer review (e.g. each member of the group sets a weight-loss goal, which will be posted for review by group members), and (2) goals that are set by the group, for the benefit of the group, to be pursued by the group. We will concern ourselves with only those goals that fall in the first group.

Group participation can have a positive affect on the achievement of individual goals. If individual goals are established in a group setting and it happens that there are group goals as well, and if the individual goals and group goals are compatible with one another, higher overall group performance will result.[160] Group participants will benefit most from group participation by doing whatever they can to ensure that when group goals are established, those goals are not in opposition to their own individual goals.

Group participation in goal setting increases group identification, and the desire to identify with a successful group motivates the individual to perform better individually.[161] This is basically teambuilding, "which can be viewed as a method to promote an increased sense of unity and cohesiveness and enable the team to function together."[162] In addition, it has been shown that when goals are established in a group, moderately difficult goals are more easily achieved if they were preceded by an easy goal.[163] The reason seems to be that participant buy-in increases as incremental successes are achieved.

One of the important aspects of goal achievement is the ability to juggle multiple tasks. (e.g. in a weight-loss program we need to juggle the tasks of exercise and diet simultaneously). Two problems exist: (1) you must first determine the order in which the tasks will be performed (they may also be performed at the same time), and (2) you must periodically switch between tasks. Frequently, when the demands of difficult, multiple goals are placed on individuals, and they believe those demands exceed their capabilities, the result is one goal is sacrificed to ensure that the other is reached.[164] Here's where good planning helps. Once the plan is set in place and the order of task performance is established, switching between tasks becomes more fluid[165] and people who set performance goals switch tasks less frequently.[166]

Another interesting thing happens when individuals establish personal goals in a group setting, and here the study data supports what our logic and experience already tell us. The threat of having to share personal performance data with peers increases one's performance.[167] Does peer evaluation affect different people in different ways? Parker answered that question by stating that people who are: (1) sensitive to evaluation, (2) have high self esteem concerns, (3) have strong social identities, or (4) have strong personal identities, all demonstrate the highest performance.[168] Quite simply "competition acts as an incentive to enhance performance."[169]

What are the potential pitfalls to goal setting? Latham and Locke answered that question in great detail. Here are the ten potential pitfalls they found to both individual and group goal setting:

- People lacking the knowledge and skill to achieve a difficult goal perform better when they simply attempt to do their best,
- If there is a conflict between a group goal and an individual goal, the individual goal will have a detrimental effect on group performance,
- Goal setting may be viewed as a threat rather than a challenge,
- A chilling effect may exist if failure to attain a goal results in punishment,

- Past successes frequently lead to the setting of higher subsequent goals even if that is unreasonable,
- Performance is frequently overstated when money is tied to goal attainment,
- When the goal outcome is tied to individual identity, risky or irrational actions may be employed to achieve the goal,
- Non-goal performance measures often get ignored,
- Goals can increase personal stress,
- If individuals or groups are assigned progressively higher goals as a result of past successes, in effect they are being punished for those past successes.[170]

Individuals or groups entering the goal setting process are well advised to study these ten potential pitfalls closely before beginning. Avoiding the inclusion of any of these weaknesses in your performance goals will prove to be of substantial benefit.

Apart from the establishment, implementation and pursuit of goals, the goal setting process itself has other inherent benefits. Goal setting works through a motivational mechanism to positively affect performance by enhancing an individual's self-perception of efficacy.[171] "Irrespective of which goal is chosen, or how attractive it is, the decision process by which the selection occurs has in and of itself, motivational benefits that help to sustain pursuit, enact the decision, and eventually realize the chosen goal."[172]

What about weight loss maintenance, once the desired goal has been reached? "It has been suggested that the failure to reach a self-determined weight may discourage the person's belief in his/her ability to control his weight, which will result in the abandonment of weight maintenance behaviors."[173] Self-control of weight maintenance is of vital importance. When creating a weight maintenance program special attention needs to be given to employing methods or strategies that: (1) help you optimize your ability to regulate and control your weight yourself, and (2) enhance your belief and understanding that you can control your own weight.[174] One such strategy may be regular self-weighing. It has been found that frequent self-weighing is a simple technique that can be used to maintain long-term weight loss results.[175] Increases in the frequency of self-weighing, and increases in physical activity, coupled with increased dietary restraint and decreased depression have been shown to improve weight loss and maintenance.[176]

Once goals are established and goal pursuit begins, it is vitally important to have the proper feedback, in a timely manner, in order to monitor progress and make any needed adjustments to the plan. However, "for feedback to be most effective it must be associated with behavioral consequences."[177] Feedback contributes to the goal setting process by adding a much needed evaluation dimension. Donaldson & Normand stated that "feedback in combination with goal setting can effectively increase the productivity of adults across a variety of settings."[178] Previously, in this section, I mentioned the importance of small, bite sized, incremental, measurable goals. As they relate to feedback, "multiple, specific goals act as stepping stones to the greater goal people are striving toward, and feedback acts as encouragement along the way."[179] Normand examined the real value of feedback and determined that, "self-monitoring, goal setting, and feedback can be used to increase the daily activity level of healthy adults at a level that might prevent weight gain typically observed as individuals age."[180]

"Feedback on goal attainment also influences goal performance by allowing individuals to gauge the relationship between their current performance and their goal."[181] There are several different feedback methods and the effect of the feedback is dependent on the value that individuals place on it or the amount of pain or gain that they will receive from it. Where an individual is working alone to achieve a goal the simplest and most useful feedback method is to keep statistics, data or other performance records. Where an individual is working in a group the publication of achievement results may have a bigger impact. Loewy & Bailey found that "delivering feedback verbally may…produce different results than when feedback is delivered through public posting."[182] They didn't make it clear under which circumstances each might prove to be the better method, although as discussed earlier a public posting is simply another method of sharing individual performance data among group participants, which often puts pressure on them to increase their performance.

One important question is whether or not unfavorable feedback results could have negative consequences with respect to performance. Researchers have found that "repeated failure led to adverse changes in mood/motivation."[183] This is not a surprising outcome, but should your mood or motivation decline in response to negative feedback? Frequently, if feedback is increasingly negative, individuals adjust their goals downward and the size of the goal adjustment tends to be in proportion to the amount of bad news; therefore, it is important to maintain a small gap between performance and the goal.[184] The converse holds true for positive feedback.

Finally, to avoid psychological distress you must keep your personal expectations in line with reality, so that you do not consistently fail to meet your own standards.[185] However, participants in one weight loss program, who had unrealistically high expectations but experienced only minimal psychological distress, actually lost more weight than their lower expectation counterparts.[186] What should you do if you discover that one or more of your goals are unrealistic? Change them! "People who are better able to disengage from unattainable goals and reengage with alternative goals…may experience better physical health."[187]

Building a Support System

"Historically, people banded together to improve their chances for survival by pooling their social and economic resources; however, contemporary groups are more likely to organize around a theme or problem."[188] Whenever a sports team relies on the support of its fans, we refer to that support as the teams' home-field advantage. In everyday life we frequently get support and counsel from family, friends or others that have an interest in our success, in effect using them as a classic form of social support. Because of the security we normally find within the family, we often subconsciously view non-family social support as an extension of the family. Even though there is some conflicting research data as to the effectiveness of social support, the good news is that much of that data "suggests beneficial effects of the inclusion of social support in interventions aimed at long-term health behavior change."[189]

This section analyzes psychological research data, in the area of social support, and uses that data to build a framework for its application in a weight loss program. Many times in our life's endeavors, when the going gets tough, we enlist the help of others and seemingly gain strength from their encouragement. On one hand we may seek the help of professionals (e.g. physicians, nutritionists, personal trainers), and on the other we may turn to social support. This is not meant to imply that we must make an either or decision, in reality both work nicely together. In fact, social support "is not a substitute for professional services, but rather, it serves a different purpose for members, and the findings suggest that it may lead to more confident and appropriate use of existing services, as well as challenging them."[190]

As you will see social support, also referred to as group support, can be a useful tool if constructed and used properly. In the research literature these groups are referred to as *support groups*, *self-help groups*, *mutual help groups* or *mutual aid groups*. Regardless of what they're called these groups all share several common characteristics. They:

- Are an informal, non-professional association of people with common interests,
- Are voluntary and confidential,
- Pool resources,
- Gather, share and evaluate information,
- Share individual experiences (including successes and failures),
- Provide sympathetic understanding and support,
- Offer group members a sense of belonging.

The difference between support groups and self-help groups is very subtle. Support groups tend to focus most of their energy on offering emotional support for group members, whereas self-help groups act more proactively to find and implement problem solutions. Since the group itself determines its function and direction these subtleties become relatively unimportant. I will use the terminology *support group* from this point forward, unless cited research does otherwise.

There are some common features that if operated effectively can help a support group succeed and thrive. Among these features are:

- A clear understanding of the group's purpose,
- A convenient meeting time,
- A comfortable environment,

- A skilled facilitator,
- A good grasp of resources and services available in the area,
- An ability to assist members to gain access to resources and services,
- An ability to identify and attract speakers for group education,
- A balanced program of support, education and socialization,
- Effective printed handouts distributed at the meetings,[191]
- Involvement of the participants in the design, trial and evaluation of interventions.[192]

Usually the strongest and most supportive group is the family. "Weight-loss interventions targeting food intake and/or physical activity might be most effective if they…involve family members appropriately."[193] We have all learned from experience, the benefit of having solid family support in most of life's experiences, so it should come as no surprise that dependable family support in the choice and preparation of the food we eat and encouragement in our exercise program can certainly have a positive effect on outcomes. This is especially true when dealing with adolescent obesity, where it has been shown that "the most effective treatments include substantial parental involvement."[194] Childhood obesity benefits tremendously from quasi-family groups consisting of parents and medical professionals.[195] Actually, parental involvement is extremely important in childhood obesity, since the children don't have the knowledge, experience or resources to bring about the needed changes themselves. When parents assume the necessary role of the primary change agent in their child's weight loss effort good things can happen, like: (1) the child loses weight, (2) the child maintains the weight loss better, (3) the process is more cost effective, and (4) typical dieting side effects are avoided.[196]

Family support incorporates four separate and distinct types of support:

- Emotional support (e.g. caring and empathy),
- Instrumental support (e.g. providing tangible assistance or materials),
- Informational support (e.g. providing information to solve problems),
- Appraisal support (e.g. providing information to aid in self-evaluation).[197]

By effectively tapping into one or more of these types of support the individual can make progress that may not be made alone. For example, it has been shown that overweight and obese mothers who improved their dietary habits also saw a resulting improvement in the dietary habits of their young children.[198]

Care must be taken when using family members as a major part of the support system. Occasionally there is a great deal of disparity between family members' body weight. Households that were studied in Brazil, China and Russia showed that many of them simultaneously had both overweight and underweight family members and weight loss programs needed to deal with one situation, would not prove helpful at the other extreme.[199] The implications are: (1) in your attempt to lose weight you may find it difficult for thin family members to understand and properly support your effort, and (2) if other family members are also overweight they may not want you to break from the pack, therefore you may get opposition rather than support. While family support can be very powerful, pick your supporting cast carefully.

Much like the family, ethnic identity can play a critical role in one's support system. "Strong ties to one's ethnic group, both in behavioral practices and in affect, have a health-protective element."[200] In addition to ethnic identity active church members may benefit from church based support groups. Researchers successfully combined the two in a cardiovascular health promotion study with sixteen Baltimore African American church based support groups. While the study was aimed at improving the cardiovascular health of female participants, the improvements obtained were the result of improved nutrition and exercise, and weight loss was one of the risk factor improvements.

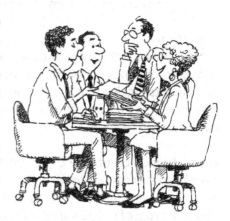

The favorable results appeared to come from two important factors: (1) the participants were in an environment that was comfortable for them and supportive of them, and (2) they had confidence in the leadership of their groups, which was evidenced by the fact that once the leadership changed to lay leaders, group attendance tapered off substantially.[201] It seems logical that similar results might be obtained in other support group settings, for example groups organized in health clubs or nutrition centers.

Support groups operate in any of a number of ways.

- **Location** - Frequently support group members come together, at a designated physical location, to discuss group concerns.

- **Leadership** - Usually, a leader is appointed: (1) who assists the group in planning its direction, (2) guides the discussion, and (3) marshals the necessary resources. This method of operation has been used for years as an effective weight loss and health improvement tool.

- **Identity** - There are two identities to consider: (1) personal identity, and (2) social identity. Individuals benefit most when their personal identity blends smoothly with the group's identity, since "both personal and social identities are important and influential."[202]

- **Peer Pressure** - Peer pressure plays an important role in the functioning of a support group. For example, peer pressure among young girls may be tremendous. Young girl's perceptions of what their friends think about them can easily predict their individual actions, and those who perceive their friends as an important source of influence, frequently are very concerned about such things as body image and dieting.[203] Peer pressure can prove to be beneficial if the pressure comes from the group, in the form of group support for individuals, and works as a catalyst to support them in accomplishing their goals.[204]

The effectiveness of the group may depend on how distressed the participants are. Experts experimented with cancer patients and demonstrated that while distressed participants in the support group may benefit from the presence of non-distressed participants the non-distressed participants received little or no benefit from their participation. The reality is that the group might have been more effective if it consisted entirely of either distressed or non-distressed participants.[205]

With a broad acceptance of the Internet, online support groups have become popular. They have been successfully used to offer support and information to people with eating disorders.[206] When surveyed, facilitators of an online cancer survivor support group were highly optimistic about the role of online support groups in providing care for those that need it, and they cited patient anonymity, easy participation and limited social commitment to the group, among the positive attributes of this approach. The downside of this approach was that group members appeared to feel little or no commitment to the group, by not joining many of the online group sessions, coming online late or drifting in and out at will.[207] Another weight-loss study found that those who took the most advantage of the online program lost the most weight; however, that study did not answer the question of whether it was the online program or the participants own off line work that led to the weight-loss.[208]

Phone-based coaching coupled with monthly in-person support group sessions appears to be another good approach for helping disabled, obese adults reduce their body weight and increase their physical activity. It was determined that this technique worked because it: (1) sustained interventions over a period of time, (2) minimized transportation difficulties, and (3) provided the needed assistance at times convenient for the individuals.[209]

In addition, those with the most optimism have the most social support. One of the ways to increase both optimism and social support is to join a support group, "where new, more optimistic interpretations about the future weight loss and healthy dietary habits would take place."[210] On the flip side pessimistic behavior has been shown to result in both less support from family and friends and lower quality support.[211] Most likely this is because pessimistic people are less likeable. So, if you want to benefit as much as possible from a support group, maintain a positive attitude.

At some point the structure of the support group becomes important. Above I mentioned several support group characteristics that cause people to join them. Psychologists tell us that from that list of characteristics people mainly join support groups to avoid feeling alone, and to gather information. It has been shown that people: (1) who are younger, (2) from a higher socioeconomic status, (3) lacking other social support, (4) having a positive attitude, (5) perceiving a higher degree of group control, and (6) having the ability to get to group meetings the easiest, all tend to join support groups more freely.[212]

In order to satisfy participant needs effective group leadership is needed. Group participants judge the quality of the group leader by: (1) whether or not they allow people the opportunity to talk, (2) their personality, (3) their empathy and understanding, and (4) their qualifications.[213] Interestingly, the most preferred group leaders are not professionals but rather people who have the same problem or have overcome the problem the participants are struggling with.[214]

Even with all the good that can come from participation in a support group, some argue that there are inherent weaknesses. Among the weaknesses cited are:

- A lack of formal procedures, which may include:
  o Screening of new members,
  o Follow up with participants,
- Inadequate record-keeping,
- A lack of formal leadership training,
- A fairly high attrition rate,
- Limited accountability.

While these arguments may have a kernel of truth, I think that the research data cited has proven that the positive aspects certainly outweigh the negatives. I am sure that your main concern is with losing the undesirable body weight in a healthy manner and thereafter maintaining your desired weight. Since I am personally all about results, I believe that any reasonable tools employed in that effort are justified. Studies have shown: (1) not only can a support group coupled with a low calorie diet help individuals lose weight, but (2) the combination of both can help with weight maintenance for years to come.[215] Therefore, if you can benefit from participation in a support group, to hell with all the background noise about why it might not be optimal.

Summary

At this point, you should be fairly comfortable with what is driving you to go forward with a weight loss program and how to effectively tap into that force. As discussed in the beginning of this chapter, motivation is driven by personal: (1) needs, (2) values, (3) goals and intentions, and (4) emotions. Having a good understanding of what these four concepts mean to you should prove useful in your weight loss program.

While psychological theories attempt to explain how motivation works, they generally fall short because they fail to offer concrete actions that can be taken to increase motivation. Interestingly, among the factors that have a big impact on motivation, are:

- Goal commitment: (1) determining whether the goal is still worth pursuing, and (2) evaluating what has been accomplished to date,
- Progress made towards that goal (either good progress or a lack of desirable progress),
- The amount of control you have over the outcome, since the more control you feel you have the greater the level of motivation and performance,
- Improved goal setting,
- Positive feedback and support.

Here are some additional points to keep in mind.

- Men and women are motivated differently. If you and your spouse or a significant other, are attempting to lose weight together, don't try to reach a common consensus as to what the motivating factor is. For one of you it may be improved health and for the other it may be improved appearance.

- Don't fall into the trap of trying to find someone else to motivate you. The driving force must come from within. If you're looking to a doctor, nutritionist, personal trainer, family member, friend or someone else to motivate you, you will be very disappointed with your progress.

- If you do not have sufficient control over your life, look for ways to change things. If you are caught in the vicious circle of work and family obligations, with no time left for you to take care of yourself, you must make adjustments to your schedule that will provide you the time you need. You have to get to the point where you feel that you have the power to control your own destiny.

- If you need professional help seek it, but don't attempt to dump your responsibility on the professional. You need to be in control of and responsible for your own actions. You are responsible for your own personal successes and failures.

Hand-in-hand with motivation is the principle of self-discipline. If self-discipline seems like a problem for you here are some considerations that should help you improve that situation:

- One of the best ways to bolster self-discipline is through good planning. A detailed plan based upon reasonable goals helps clarify the methods to be employed in order to get from point A to point B. Once the plan of attack is clearly defined, the stress of moving from the planning phase to the action phase is minimized substantially and weak self-discipline tends to abate.

- Increasing your subject matter knowledge is a great way to increase self-discipline and motivation. If, for example, you find it difficult to begin a much needed exercise program, by learning more about exercise benefits and techniques, the mystery will disappear. You will procrastinate less about getting involved in an exercise program, your self-confidence will soar knowing that you possess the understanding needed to go forward and you will make more progress toward achievement of your goal.

- Through the process of mentally comparing the desired future outcome to your present condition, you will experience a greater sense of: (1) goal commitment, (2) self-confidence, (3) self-discipline, and (4) goal directed energy.

The down side of struggling to maintain self-discipline is that it depletes your energy. The ability to maintain a positive outlook is a major factor in sustaining self-discipline. Although at times it may be difficult to maintain a positive outlook, that situation should be the exception rather than the rule. It is important to your weight loss effort and overall health as well, to maintain a positive outlook. If you are naturally inclined to be a negative person, consider engaging the help of a psychologist or joining a support group, or both.

As mentioned earlier, one of humanity's most fundamental motivations is the need for social inclusion and people lacking strong social ties often act out their distress through self-defeating behavior. To minimize self-defeating behavior, participation in a group activity (especially a weight loss support group) is a good way of breaking that cycle.

In any weight loss program setting and pursuing powerful goals will prove to be invaluable. What are powerful goals? Earlier in this chapter we described SMART goals as *written* goals that are: (1) Specific, (2) Measurable, (3) Achievable, (4) Realistic/Relevant, and (5) Time Restricted. If your goals are not written they may be no more than thoughts, hopes, or dreams and if they don't include the five step SMART goal criteria, your chance of success is limited. Be sure to keep your optimism under control and be realistic during goal setting. Too much optimism tends to be tantamount to fantasy.

Understand that while both *process goals* and *outcome goals* are acceptable; process goals focus on the methods used to achieve the desired results while outcome goals focus on the results themselves. Use both whenever they are appropriate for you. Both may be needed and can be beneficial as long as they follow the SMART criteria. Remember too that your weight loss program is a personal, individual thing; therefore, even though you may take advice from others, as to the character or composition of your goals, they ultimately need to be your goals. Don't let somebody else set your goals! In addition, the goal setting process itself has inherent benefits. For example, it can have a positive impact on performance, by enhancing your perception of self-control, which helps in the pursuit of the chosen goal. Ultimately, a goal will serve as a roadmap or GPS system that will guide you on the journey to your destination.

Active training in lifestyle modification, which includes social support, will help you achieve a far better result than sitting on your butt and doing nothing.[216]

Here is something to look out for. Psychologists believe that the theories of substitution and compensation play an important role as to where we turn for support. The *Theory of Social Network Substitution* is defined as "the extent to which…individuals can derive support from alternative social ties," while the *Theory of Compensation* "refers to the extent to which these alternative social ties enhance well-being."[217] Research shows that low-income mothers, (the majority of whom were unmarried), with a weak social network, may be likely to substitute their children (ages one-sixteen years old) for their missing network and rely on these kids for support. The problem is that the children as well as the mother are under a great deal of stress from their daily struggles and the children's inability to deal effectively with this role puts added pressure on them. In fact, the mother not only doesn't get the support she needs but both the mother and the children suffer negative health consequences.[218] So, mothers beware of this possible situation and look elsewhere for your support.

When thinking about where to get support, consider:

- Family - Look for strong ties with adult family members. Family members generally have the greatest interest in your well being, so if they are competent to serve as a sounding board and are interested in supporting you they should be your best option.

- Organized Support Groups - The quality of the support you get from an organized support group, because it is structured around people with common interests and frequently involves professionals, should be a good way of helping you achieve success. Use care in selecting a support group and don't be reluctant to leave one group and to join a different group if that seems right for you.

- Friends - Although friends frequently have an interest in your benefit, they may be hard pressed to understand the size of the task you face and may not be able to offer any expertise that you can rely on. In addition, if personal situations arise that you consider sensitive, friends may not respect your privacy to the extent that your family or an organized support group will.

Remember, this whole endeavor is about you! Since you are the person who will benefit by losing the unwanted weight, you must take full responsibility for planning for your success and then effectively executing your plan. "Motivated, free-living individuals, given appropriate support, can make and sustain major dietary changes,"[219] and the necessary exercise changes, attitude changes, etc.

Endnotes

1. M.E. Gredler, "Hiding in plain sight: the stages of mastery/self-regulation in Vygotsky's cultural-historical theory," *Ed Psych* 44 (2009) 1-19.

2. "Motivation," *Dorland's Illustrated Medical Dictionary*, 30th ed: 1175.

3. E.A. Locke, "Motivation, cognition, and action: an analysis of studies of task goals and knowledge," *Applied Psych* 49 (2000) 408-429.

4. Ibid.

5. G. Oettingen, "Mental contrasting and goal commitment: the mediating role of energization," *Person Soc Psycho Bull* 35 (2009) 608-622.

6. P.A. Hall, G.T. Fong, L.J. Epp, L.J. Elias, "Executive function moderates the intention-behavior link for physical activity and dietary behavior," *Psych & Health* 23 (2008) 309-326.

7. Ibid.

8. F.F. Sniehotta, "Towards a theory of intentional behavior change: plans, planning, and self-regulation," *Brit J Health Psych* 14 (2009) 261-273.

9. M. Koo, A. Fishbach," Dynamics of self-regulation: how (un)accomplished goal actions affect motivation," *J Person & Soc Psych* 94 (2008) 183-195.

10. Ibid.

11. N.E. Sherwood, R.W. Jeffery, "The behavioral determinants of exercise: implications for physical activity interventions," *Ann Rev Nutr* 20 (2000) 21-44.

12. Ibid.

13. M.S. Sabinsky, U. Toft, A. Raben, L. Holm, "Overweight men's motivations and perceived barriers towards weight loss," *Euro J Clin Nutr* 61 (2007) 526-531.

14. M.L. Segar, J.S. Eccles, C.R. Richardson, "Type of physical activity goal influences participation in helping midlife women," *Womens Health Issues* 18 (2008) 281-291.

15. Ibid.

16. K.G. Strong, G.F. Huon, "Controlled motivation and the persistence of weight loss dieting," *Euro Eat Disord Rev* 7 (1999) 136-146.

17. Ibid.

18. A. Bandura, E.A. Locke, "Negative self-efficacy and goal effects revisited," *J Applied Psych* 88 (2003) 87-99.

19. M.T. Warzinski, S.M. Sereika, M.A. Styn, E. Music, L.E. Burke, "Changes in self-efficacy and dietary adherence: the impact on weight loss in the PREFER study," *J Behav Med* 31 (2008) 81-92.

20. M. Reickshe, J. Mills, H. Henry, "Qualitative study of spirituality in a weight-loss program: contribution to self-efficacy and locus of control," *J Nutr Ed Behav* 36 (2004) 13-19.

21. Ibid.

22. J.N. Germann, D.S. Kirschenbaum, B.H. Rich, "Child and parental self-monitoring as determinants of success in the treatment of morbid obesity in low-income minority children," *J Ped Psych* 32 (2006) 111-121.

23. Ibid.

24. J.Y. Ko, D.R. Brown, D.A. Guluska, J. Zhang, H.M. Blanck, B.E. Ainsworth, "Weight loss advice U.S. obese adults receive from healthcare professionals," *Prev Med* 47 (2008) 587-592.

25. M.B. Potter, J.D. Vu, M. Croughan-Minihane, "Weight management: what patients want from their primary care physicians," *J Family Prac* 50 (2001) 513-518.

26. J.Y. Ko, D.R. Brown, D.A. Guluska, J. Zhang, H.M. Blanck, B.E. Ainsworth, "Weight loss advice U.S. obese adults receive from healthcare professionals," *Prev Med* 47 (2008) 587-592.

27. R.S. Stafford, J.H. Farhat, B. Misra, D.A. Schoenfeld, "National patterns of physician activities related to obesity management," *Arch Fam Med* 9 (2000) 631-638.

28. Ibid.

29. C.A. Befort, K.A. Greiner, S. Hall, K.M. Pulvers, N.L. Nollen, A. Charbonneau, H. Kaur, J.S. Ahluwalia, "Weight-related perceptions among patients and physicians: how well do physicians judge patients' motivation to lose weight," *J Gen Int Med* 21 (2006) 1086-1090.

30. Ibid.

31. R.R. Leverence, R.L. Williams, A. Sussman, B.F. Crabtree, "Obesity counseling and guidelines in primary care: a qualitative study," *Am J Prev Med* 32 (2007) 334-339.

32. J. Huang, H. Yu, E. Marin, S. Brock, D. Carden, T. Davis, "Physicians' weight loss counseling in two public hospital primary care clinics," *Acad Med* 79 (2004) 156-161.

33. A. Bocquier, P. Verger, A. Basdevant, G. Andreotti, J. Baretge, P. Villani, A. Paraponaris, "Overweight and obesity: knowledge, attitudes, and practices of general practitioners in France," *Obes Res* 13 (2005) 787-795.

34. J.Y. Ko, D.R. Brown, D.A. Guluska, J. Zhang, H.M. Blanck, B.E. Ainsworth, "Weight loss advice U.S. obese adults receive from healthcare professionals," *Prev Med* 47 (2008) 587-592.

35. C.A. Befort, K.A. Greiner, S. Hall, K.M. Pulvers, N.L. Nollen, A. Charbonneau, H. Kaur, J.S. Ahluwalia, "Weight-related perceptions among patients and physicians: how well do physicians judge patients' motivation to lose weight," *J Gen Int Med* 21 (2006) 1086-1090.

36. M. Jay, A. Kalet, T. Ark, M. McMacken, J.J. Messito, R. Richter, S. Schlair, S. Cherman, S. Zabar, C. Gillespie, "Physicians' attitudes about obesity and their associations with competency and specialty: a cross-sectional study," *BMC Health Services Res* 9 (2009) 1-11.

37. S.G. Aldana, "*The Culprit & the Cure*," (Mapleton, UT: *Maple Mountain Press,* 2005) vi.

38. J.F. Thuan, A. Avignon, "Obesity management: attitudes and practices of French general practitioners in a region of France," *Intl J Obes* 29 (2005) 1100-1106.

39. M. Binks, P. Mahlen, "Referral sources to a weight management program," *J Gen Int Med* 17 (2002) 596-603.

40. M.L. Segar, J.S. Eccles, S.C. Peck, C.R. Richardson, "Midlife women's physical activity goals: sociocultural influences and effects and behavioral regulation," *Sex Roles* 57 (2007) 837-849.

41. M. Binks, P. Mahlen, "Referral sources to a weight management program," *J Gen Int Med* 17 (2002) 596-603.

42. Ibid.

43. M.D. Lewis, R.M. Todd, "The self-regulating brain: cortical-subcortical feedback and the development of intelligent action," *Cognitive Develop* 22 (2007) 406-430.

44. Ibid.

45. E.S. Anderson, R.A. Winett, J.R. Wojcik, "Self-regulation, self-efficacy, outcome expectations, and social support: social cognitive theory and nutrition behavior," *Ann Behav Med* 34 (2007) 304-312.

46. T.A. Wills, C.R. Isasi, D. Mendoza, M.G. Ainette, "Self-control constructs related to measures of dietary intake and physical activity and adolescents," *J Adolesc Health* 41 (2007) 551-558.

47. Ibid.

48.   A.J. Howell, D.C. Watson, "Procrastination: associations with achievement goal orientation and learning strategies," *Person Indivual Differ* 43 (2007) 167-178.

49.   O. Janssen, J. Prins, "Goal orientations and the seeking of different types of feedback information," *J Occupation Org Psych* 80 (2007) 235-249.

50.   U. Scholz, F.F. Sniehotta, B. Schuz, A. Oeberst, "Dynamics in self-regulation: plan execution self-efficacy and mastery of action plans," *J Applied Soc Psych* 37 (2007) 2706-2725.

51.   M.E. Gredler, "Hiding in plain sight: the stages of mastery/self-regulation in Vygotsky's cultural-historical theory," *Ed Psych* 44 (2009) 1-19.

52.   G. Oettingen, "Mental contrasting and goal commitment: the mediating role of energization," *Person Soc Psych Bull* 35 (2009) 608-622.

53.   C. Martijn, H.J.E.M. Alberts, H. Merckelbach, R. Havermans, A. Huijts, N.K. DeVries, "Overcoming ego depletion: the influence of exemplar priming of self-control performance," *Euro J Soc Psych* 37 (2007) 231-238.

54.   E. Burkley, "The role of self-control in resistance to persuasion," *Person Soc Psych Bull* 34 (2008) 419-431.

55.   Ibid.

56.   M.T. Gailliot, R.F. Baumeister, C.N. DeWall, J.K. Maner, E.A. Plant, D.M. Tice, L.E. Brewer, B.J. Schmeichel, "Self-control relies on glucose as a limited energy source: willpower is more than a metaphor," *J Person & Soc Psych* 92 (2007) 325-336.

57.   M. Muraven, D. Shmueli, E. Burkley, "Conserving self-control strength," *J Person Soc Psych* 91 (2006) 524-537.

58.   P. Fischer, T. Greitemeyer, D. Frey, "Self-regulation and selective exposure: the impact of depleted self-regulation resources on confirmatory information processing," *J Person Soc Psych* 94 (2008) 382-395.

59.   E. Burkley, "The role of self-control in resistance to persuasion," *Person Soc Psych Bull* 34 (2008) 419-431.

60.   A. Fishbach, Y. Zhang, "Together or apart: when goals and temptations complement versus compete," *J Person Soc Psych* 94 (2008) 547-559.

61.   W. Hofmann, W. Rauch, B. Gawronski, "And deplete us not into temptation: automatic attitudes, dietary restraint, and self-regulatory resources as determinants of eating behavior," *J Exper Soc Psych* 43 (2007) 497-504.

62.   K. D. Vohs, B.J. Schmeichel, N.M. Nelson, R.F. Baumeister, J.M. Twenge, D.M. Tice, "Making choices and their subsequent self-control: a limited-resource account of decision-making, self-regulation, and active initiative," *J Person Soc Psych* 94 (2008) 883-898.

63.   M.T. Gailliot, R.F. Baumeister, C.N. DeWall, J.K. Maner, E.A. Plant, D.M. Tice, L.E. Brewer, B.J. Schmeichel, "Self-control relies on glucose as a limited energy source: willpower is more than a metaphor," *J Person & Soc Psych* 92 (2007) 325-336.

64.   D.M. Tice, R.F. Baumeister, D. Shmueli, M. Muraven, "Restoring the self: positive affect helps improve self-regulation following ego depletion," *J Exper Soc Psych* 43 (2007) 379-384.

65.   P. Fischer, T. Greitemeyer, D. Frey, "Ego depletion and positive illusions: does the construction of positivity require regulatory resources?" *Person Soc Psych Bull* 33 (2007) 1306-1321.

66.   E. Briones, C. Tabernero, A. Arenas, "Effects of disposition and self-regulation on self-defeating behavior," *J Soc Psych* 147 (2007) 657-679.

67.   Ibid.

68. D. DeRidder, R. Kuijer, C. Ouwehand, "Does confrontation with potential goal failure promote self-regulation? Examining the role of distress in the pursuit of weight goals," *Psych Health* 22 (2007) 677-698.

69. W.D. Scott, E. Dearing, W.R. Reynolds, J.E. Lindsay, G.L. Baird, S. Hamill, "Cognitive self-regulation and depression: examining academic self-efficacy and goal characteristics in youth of a Northern Plains tribe," *J Research Adol* 18 (2008) 379-394.

70. P.A. Hall, G.T. Fong, L.J. Epp, L.J. Elias, "Executive function moderates the intention-behavior link for physical activity and dietary behavior," *Psych Health* 23 (2008) 309-326.

71. T.P. Palfai, A. Macdonald, "Effects of temptations on the affective salience of weight control goals," *Behav Res Ther* 45 (2007) 449-458.

72. E.K. Papies, W. Stroebe, H. Aarts, "The allure of forbidden food: on the role of attention in self-regulation," *J Exper Soc Psych* 44 (2008) 1283-1292.

73. D. Kirschenbaum, J.N. Germann, B.H. Rich, "Treatment of morbid obesity in low-income adolescents: effects of parental self-monitoring," *Obes Res* 13 (2005) 1527-1529.

74. D.J. Schulman-Green, A.D. Naik, E.H. Bradley, R. McCorkle, S.T. Bogardus, "Goal setting as a shared decision making strategy among clinicians and their older patients," *Patient Ed & Counseling* 63 (2006) 145-151.

75. L. Evans, L. Hardy, "Injury rehabilitation: a goal-setting intervention study," *Res Quart Exer & Sport* 73 (2002) 310-319.

76. A. Kitsantas, "The role of self-regulation strategies and self-efficacy perceptions in successful weight loss maintenance," *Psych & Health* 15 (2000) 811-820.

77. R.M. Puca, "Action phases and goal setting: being optimistic after decision making without getting into trouble," *Motivation & Emotion* 28 (2004) 121-145.

78. E.A. Locke, G.P. Latham, "New directions in goal-setting theory," *Current Directions Phych Science* 15 (2006) 265-268.

79. S.G. Harkins, P.H. White, C.H. Utman, "The role of the internal and external sources of evaluation in motivating task performance," *Person & Soc Psych Bulletin* 26 (2000) 100-117.

80. D.S. Downs, R.N. Singer, "Goal setting and implementation intentions: preliminary support for increasing exercise behavior," *J Human Movement Studies* 45 (2003) 419-432.

81. Ibid.

82. D. O'Hora, K.A. Maglieri, "Goal statements and goal-directed behavior: a relational frame account of goal setting in organizations," *J Org Behav Mgmt* 26 (2006) 131-170.

83. M.L. Segar, J.S. Eccles, S.C. Peck, C.R. Richardson, "Midlife women's physical activity goals: sociocultural influences and effects and behavioral regulation," *Sex Roles* 57 (2007) 837-849.

84. B.T. Breland, J.J. Donovan, "The role of state goal orientation in the goal establishment process," *Human Performance* 18 (2005) 23-53.

85. Ibid.

86. L. Scobbie, S. Wyke, D. Dixon, "Identifying and applying psychological theory to setting and achieving rehabilitation goals," *Clin Rehab* 23 (2009) 321-333.

87. A.D. Stajkovic, E.A. Locke, E.S. Blair, "A first examination of the relationship between primed subconscious goals, assigned conscious goals, and task performance," *J Applied Psych* 91 (2006) 1172-1180.

88. E.A. Locke, G.P. Latham, "New directions in goal-setting theory," *Current Directions Phycho Science* 15 (2006) 265-268.

89. Ibid.

90.   L. Scobbie, S. Wyke, D. Dixon, "Identifying and applying psychological theory to setting and achieving rehabilitation goals," *Clin Rehab* 23 (2009) 321-333.

91.   Ibid.

92.   R.S. Lutz, P. Karoly, M.A. Okun, "The why and the how of goal pursuit: self determination, goal process cognition, and participation in physical exercise," *Pshcho Sports & Exer* 9 (2008) 559-575.

93.   Ibid.

94.   G. Oettingen, H-J Pak, K. Schnetter, "Self-regulation of goal setting: turning free fantasies about the future into binding goals," *J Pers & Soc Psych* 80 (2001) 736-753.

95.   C.R. Snyder, " Teaching: the lessons of hope," *J Soc & Clin Psych* 24 (2005) 72-84.

96.   D.B. Feldman, K.L. Rand, K. Kahle-Wrobleski, "Hope and goal attainment: testing a basic prediction of hope theory," *J Soc & Clin Psych* 28 (2009) 479-497.

97.   T.L. Webb, P. Sheeran, " How do implementation intentions promote goal attainment? A test of component processes," *J Exper Soc Psych* 43 (2007) 295-302.

98.   Ibid.

99.   R.P. Bagozzi, E.A. Edwards, "Goal setting and goal pursuit in the regulation of body weight," *Psych & Health* 13 (1998) 593-621.

100. R. Schwarzer, "Optimism, goals, and threats: how to conceptualize self-regulatory processes in the adoption and maintenance of health behaviors," *Psych & Health* 13 (1998) 759-766.

101. M. Tamir, "What do people want to feel and why? Pleasure and utility in emotion regulation," *Cur Dir Psych Science* 18 (2009) 101-105.

102. S. Mayser, S. Scheibe, M. Riediger, "An empirical differentiation of goals and life longings," *Euro Psych* 13 (2008) 126-140.

103. Ibid.

104. Ibid.

105. C.J.R. Roney, D.R. Lehman, "Self-regulation in goal striving: individual differences and situational moderators of the goal framing/performance link," *J Applied Soc Psych* 38 (2008) 2691-2709.

106. A.L. Geers, J.A. Wellman, G.D. Lassiter, "Dispositional optimism and engagement: the moderating influence of goal prioritization," *J Person Soc Psych* 96 (2009) 913-932.

107. J.C. Brodscholl, H. Kober, E.T. Higgins, "Strategies of self-regulation and goal attainment versus goal maintenance," *Euro J Soc Psych* 37 (2007) 628-648.

108. A.A. Scholer, S.J. Stroessner, E.T. Higgins, "Responding to negativity: how a risky tactic can serve a vigilant strategy," *J Exper Soc Psych* 44 (2008) 767-774.

109. J.C. Brodscholl, H. Kober, E.T. Higgins, "Strategies of self-regulation and goal attainment versus goal maintenance," *Euro J Soc Psych* 37 (2007) 628-648.

110. A.A. Scholer, S.J. Stroessner, E.T. Higgins, "Responding to negativity: how a risky tactic can serve a vigilant strategy," *J Exper Soc Psych* 44 (2008) 767-774.

111. Ibid.

112. T.J.H. Bovend'Eerdt, R.E. Botell, D.T. Wade, "Writing SMART rehabilitation goals and achieving goal attainment scaling: a practical guide," *Clin Rehab* 23 (2009) 352-361.

113. G.P. Latham, "A five-step approach to behavior change," *Org Dynamics* 32 (2003) 309-318.

114. J.A. Linde, R.W. Jeffery, R.L. Levy, N.P. Pronk, R.G. Boyle, "Weight loss goals and treatment outcomes among overweight men and women enrolled in a weight-loss trial," *Int'l J Obes* 29 (2005) 1002-1005.

115. J.A. Linde, R.W. Jeffery, R.L. Levy, N.P. Pronk, R.G. Boyle, "Weight loss goals and treatment outcomes among overweight men and women enrolled in a weight-loss trial," *Int'l J Obes* 29 (2005) 1002-1005.
116. S. Maes, P. Karoly, "Self-regulation assessment and intervention in physical health and illness: a review," *Int'l Assn Applied Psych* 54 (2005) 267-299.
117. C.J. Spieker, V.B. Hinsz, "Repeated success and failure influences on self-efficacy and personal goals," *Soc Behav & Person* 32 (2004) 191-198.
118. R.L. West, D.K. Bagwell, A. Dark-Freudeman, "Memory and goal setting: the response of older and younger adults to positive and objective feedback," *Psych & Aging* 20 (2005) 195-201.
119. P.J. Teixeira, S.B. Going, L.B. Houtkooper, E.C. Cussler, C.J. Martin, L.L. Metcalfe, N.R. Finkenthal, R.M. Blew, L.B. Sardinha, T.G. Lohman, "Weight loss readiness in middle-aged women: psychosocial predictors of success for behavioral weight reduction," *J Behav Med* 25 (2002) 499-523.
120. P.M. O'Neil, C.F. Smith, G.D. Foster, D.A. Anderson, "The perceived relative worth of reaching and maintaining goal weight," *Int'l J Obes* 24 (2000) 1069-1076.
121. R.W. Jeffery, R.R. Wing, R.R. Mayer, "Are smaller weight losses or more achievable weight loss goals better in the long term for obese patients" *J Consult Clin Psych* 66 (1998) 641-645.
122. F. Nothwehr, J. Yang, "Goal setting frequency and the use of behavioral strategies related to diet and physical activity," *Health Ed Res* 22 (2007) 532-538.
123. Ibid.
124. A.J. Zametkin, C.K. Zoon, H.W. Klein, S. Munson, "Psychiatric aspects of child and adolescent obesity: a review of the past 10 years," *J Am Acad Child Adol Psych* 43 (2004) 134-150.
125. M. Downie, R. Koestner, E. Horberg, S. Haga, "Exploring the relation of independent and interdependent self-construals to why and how people pursue personal goals," *J Soc Psych* 146 (2006) 517-531.
126. J. Polivy, "The false hope syndrome: unrealistic expectations of self change." *Int'l J Obes* 25 (2001) S80-S84.
127. Ibid.
128. Y. Benyamini, O. Raz, "'I can tell you if I'll really lose all that weight': dispositional and situated optimism as predictors of weight loss following a group intervention," *J Applied Soc Psych* 37 (2007) 844-861.
129. J.C. Norcross, M.S. Mrykalo, M.D. Blagys, "Auld Lang Syne: success predictors, change processes and self-reported outcomes of New Year's resolvers and nonresolvers," *J Clin Psych* 58 (2002) 397-405.
130. T. Reuter, J.P. Ziegelmann, A.U. Wiedemann, S. Lippke, "Dietary planning as a mediator of the intention-behavior relation: an experimental-causal-chain design," *Applied Psych* 57 (2008) 194-207.
131. A.K. MacLeod, E. Coates, J. Hetherton, "Increasing well-being through teaching goal-setting and planning skills: results of a brief intervention," *J Happiness Stud* 9 (2008) 185-196.
132. T. Reuter, J.P. Ziegelmann, A.U. Wiedemann, S. Lippke, "Dietary planning as a mediator of the intention-behavior relation: an experimental-causal-chain design," *Applied Psych* 57 (2008) 194-207.
133. Ibid.
134. P. Gropel, P. Steel, "A mega-trial investigation of goal setting, interest enhancement, and energy on procrastination," *Person Individual Differ* 45 (2008) 406-411.

135. O.J. Strickland, M. Galimba, "Managing time: the effects of personal goal setting and resource allocation strategy and task performance," *J Psych* 135 (2001) 357-367.

136. A.K. MacLeod, E. Coates, J. Hetherton, "Increasing well-being through teaching goal-setting and planning skills: results of a brief intervention," *J Happiness Stud* 9 (2008) 185-196.

137. F.F. Sniehotta, "Towards a theory of intentional behavior change: plans, planning, and self-regulation," *Brit J Health Psych* 14 (2009) 261-273.

138. U. Scholz, B. Schuz, J.P. Ziegelmann, S. Lippke, R. Schwarzer, "Beyond behavioral intentions: planning mediates between intentions and physical activity," *Brit J Health Psych* 13 (2008) 479-494.

139. U. Scholz, B. Schuz, J.P. Ziegelmann, S. Lippke, R. Schwarzer, "Beyond behavioral intentions: planning mediates between intentions and physical activity," *Brit J Health Psych* 13 (2008) 479-494.

140. F.F. Sniehotta, "Towards a theory of intentional behavior change: plans, planning, and self-regulation," *Brit J Health Psych* 14 (2009) 261-273.

141. A. Macdonald, T. Palfai, "Predictors of exercise behavior among university student women: utility of a goal-systems/self-regulation theory framework," *Person Individual Differ* 44 (2008) 921-931.

142. Ibid.

143. R.M. Puca, "Action phases and goal setting: being optimistic after decision making without getting into trouble," *Motivation & Emotion* 28 (2004) 121-145.

144. F.W. Wicker, J.E. Turner, J.H. Reed, E.J. McCann, S.L. Do, "Motivation when optimism declines: data on temporal dynamics," *J Psych* 138 (2004) 421-432.

145. R.M. Puca, "Action phases and goal setting: being optimistic after decision making without getting into trouble," *Motivation & Emotion* 28 (2004) 121-145.

146. M.A. Davis, S.L. Kirby, M/B. Curtis, "The influence of affect on goal choice and task performance," *J Applied Soc Psych* 37 (2007) 14-42.

147. J. Stoeber, M.A. Uphill, S. Hotham, "Predicting race performance in triathlon: the role of perfectionism, achievement goals, and personal goal setting," *J Sport & Exer Psych* 31 (2009) 211-245.

148. A. Guinote, "Power and goal pursuit," *Person Soc Psych Bulletin* 33 (2007) 1076-1087.

149. Ibid.

150. R.P. Bagozzi, E.A. Edwards, "Goal setting and goal pursuit in the regulation of body weight," *Psych & Health* 13 (1998) 593-621.

151. V.J. Friedman, H. Rothman, B. Withers, "The power of why: engaging the goal paradox in program evaluation," *Amer J Eval* 27 (2006) 201-218.

152. Ibid.

153. J. Bueno, R.S. Weinberg, J. Fernandez-Castro, L. Capdevila, "Emotional and motivational mechanisms mediating the influence of goal setting on endurance athletes' performance," *Psych Sports & Exer* 9 (2008) 786-799.

154. Ibid.

155. V.J. Fortunato, K.J. Williams, "The moderating effects of dispositional activity on performance and task attitudes in the goal-setting context," *J Applied Soc Psych* 32 (2002) 2321-2353.

156. N.W. van Yperen, M. Hagadoorn, "Living up to high standards and psychological distress," *Euro J Person* 22 (2008) 337-346.

157. K. Thedford, "Setting goals and empowering lifestyle modification," *J Amer Diet Assoc* 104 (2004) 559.

158. E.D. Playford, L. Dawson, V. Limbert, M. Smith, C.D. Ward, R. Wells, "Goal-setting in rehabilitation: report of a workshop to explore professionals' perceptions of goal setting," *Clin Rehab* 14 (2000) 491-496.

159. N.W. van Yperen, M. Hagadoorn, "Living up to high standards and psychological distress," *Euro J Person* 22 (2008) 337-346.

160. G.H. Seijts, G.P. Latham, "The effects of goal setting and group size on performance in a social dilemma," *Canada J Behav Science* 32 (2000) 104-116.

161. J. Wegge, S.A. Haslam, "Improving work motivation and performance in brainstorming groups: the effects of three group goal-setting strategies" *Euro J Work & Org Psych* 14 (2005) 400-430.

162. J. Senecal, T.M. Loughead, G.A. Bloom, "A season-long team-building intervention: examining the effect of team goal setting on cohesion," *J Sport & Exer Psych* 30 (2008) 186-199.

163. S.A. Haslam, J. Wegge, T. Postmes, "Are we on a learning curve or a treadmill? The benefits of participative group goal setting become apparent as tasks become increasingly challenging over time," *Euro J Soc Psych* 39 (2009) 430-446.

164. A.M. Schmidt, C.M. Dolis, "Something's got to give: the effects of dual-goal difficulty, goal progress, and expectancies on resource allocation," *J Applied Psych* 94 (2009) 678-691.

165. N. Chevalier, A. Blaye, "Setting goals to switch between tasks: effect of cue transparency on children's cognitive flexibility," *Dev Psych* 45 (2009) 782-797.

166. O.J. Strickland, M. Galimba, "Managing time: the effects of personal goal setting and resource allocation strategy and task performance," *J Psych* 135 (2001) 357-367.

167. R.J. Parker, "The effects of evaluative context on performance: the roles of self-and social-evaluations," *Soc Behav & Person* 29 (2001) 807-822.

168. Ibid.

169. V.B. Hinsz, "The influences of social aspects of competition in goal-setting situations," *Current Psych* 24 (2005) 258-273.

170. G.P. Latham, E.A. Locke, "Enhancing the benefits and overcoming the pitfalls of goal setting," *Org Dynamics* 35 (2006) 332-340.

171. L. Evans, L. Hardy, "Injury rehabilitation: a qualitative follow-up study," *Res Quart Exer & Sport* 73 (2002) 320-329.

172. U.M. Dholakia, R.P. Bagozzi, "Mustering motivation to enact decisions: how decision process characteristics influence goal realization," *J Behav Decision Making* 15 (2002) 167-188.

173. K. Elfhag, S. Rossner, "Who succeeds in maintaining weight loss? A conceptual review of factors associated with weight loss maintenance and weight regain," *Obes Rev* 6 (2005) 67-85.

174. A. Kitsantas, "The role of self-regulation strategies and self-efficacy perceptions in successful weight loss and maintenance," *Psych & Health* 15 (2000) 811-820.

175. J. Gokee-LaRose, A.A. Gorin, R.R. Wing, "Behavioral self-regulation for weight loss in young adults: a randomized controlled trial," *Int'l J Behav Nutri Phy Activity* 6 (2009) 1-9.

176. R.R. Wing, J.L. Fava, S. Phelan, J. McCaffery, G. Papandonatos, A.A. Gorin, D.F. Tate, "Maintaining large weight losses: the role of behavioral and psychological factors," *J Consult Clin Psych* 76 (2008) 1015-1021.

177. S. Loewy, J. Bailey, "The effects of graphic feedback, goal setting, and manager praise on customer service behaviors," *J Org Behav Mgmt* 27 (2007) 15-26.

178. J.M. Donaldson, M.P. Normand, "Using goal setting, self-monitoring, and feedback to increase calorie expenditure in obese adults," *Behav Intervent* 24 (2009) 73-83.

179. R.L. West, D.K. Bagwell, A. Dark-Freudman, "Memory and goal setting: the response of older and younger adults to positive and objective feedback," *Psych & Aging* 20 (2005) 195-201.

180. M.P. Normand, "Increasing physical activity through self-monitoring, goal setting, and feedback," *Behav Intervent* 23 (2008) 227-236.

181. D. O'Hora, K.A. Maglieri, "Goal statements and goal-directed behavior: a relational frame account of goal setting in organizations," *J Org Behav Mgmt* 26 (2006) 131-170.

182. S. Loewy, J. Bailey, "The effects of graphic feedback, goal setting, and manager praise on customer service behaviors," *J Org Behav Mgmt* 27 (2007) 15-26.

183. L. Venables, S.H. Fairclough, "The influence of performance feedback on goal-setting and mental effort regulation," *Moti Emot* 33 (2009) 63-74.

184. R. Ilies, T.A. Judge, "Goal regulation across time: the effects of feedback and affect," *J Applied Psych* 90 (2005) 453-497.

185. N.W. van Yperen, M. Hagedoorn, "Living up to high standards and psychological distress," *Euro J Person* 22 (2008) 337-346.

186. Y. Benyamini, O. Raz, "I can tell you if I'll really lose all that weight: dispositional and situated optimism as predictors of weight loss following a group intervention," *J Applied Soc Psych* 37 (2007) 844-861.

187. C. Wrosch, G.E. Miller, M.F. Scheier, S.B. dePontet, "Giving up on unattainable goals: benefits for health," *Person Soc Psych Bull* 33 (2007) 251-265.

188. Encyclopedia of Mental Disorders, http://www.minddisorders.com/Py-Z/Self-help-groups.html.

189. M.W. Verheijden, J.C. Bakx, C. van Weel, M.A. Koelen, W.A. van Staveren, "Role of social support in lifestyle-focused weight management interventions," *Euro J Clin Nutri* 59 (2005) S179-S186.

190. C. Munn-Giddings, A. McVicar, "Self-help groups as mutual support: what do carers value?" *Health Soc Care in Community* 15 (2006) 26-34.

191. Traumatic Brain Injury (TBI) Support Groups, Brain Injury Resource Center, http://www.headinjury.com/nw_tbi_support_group_intro.html.

192. S.L. Thomas, J. Hyde, A. Karunaratne, R. Kausman, P.A. Komesaroff, "They all work...when you stick to them: a qualitative investigation of dieting, weight loss, and physical exercise, in obese individuals," *Nutr J* 7 (2008) 1-7.

193. N. McLean, S. Griffin, K. Toney, W. Hardeman, "Family involvement in weight control, weight maintenance and weight-loss interventions: a systematic review of randomized trials," *Intl J Obes* 27 (2003) 987-1005.

194. A.J. Zametkin, C.K. Zoon, H.W. Klein, S. Munson, "Psychiatric aspects of child and adolescent obesity: a review of the past 10 years," *J Am Acad Child Adol Psych* 43 (2004) 134-150.

195. C. Weigel, K. Kokocinski, P. Legerer, J. Dotsch, W. Rascher, I. Knerr, "Childhood obesity: concept, feasibility, and interim results of a local group-based, long-term treatment program," *J Nutr Ed Behav* 40 (2008) 369-373.

196. M. Golan, A. Weizman, A. Apter, M. Fainaru, "Parents as the exclusive agents of change in the treatment of childhood obesity," *Am J Clin Nutr* 67 (1998) 1130-1135.

197. J. Paisley, H. Beanlands, J. Goldman, S. Evers, J. Chappell, "Dietary change: what are the responses and roles of significant others?" *J Nutr Ed Behav* 40 (2008) 80-88.

198. D.M. Klohe-Lehman, J. Freeland-Graves, K.K. Clarke, G. Cai, S. Voruganti, T.J. Milani, H.J. Nuss, J.M. Proffitt, T.M. Bohman, "Low-income, overweight and obese mothers as agents of change to improve food choices, fat habits, and physical activity in their 1-to-3 year old children," *J Am College Nutr* 26 (2007) 196-208.

199. C.M. Doak, L.S. Adair, C. Monteiro, B.M. Popkin, "Overweight and underweight coexist within households in Brazil, China and Russia," *J Nutr* 130 (2000) 2965-2971.

200. J.M. Siegel, M.S. Hyg, A.K. Yancey, W.J. McCarthy," Overweight and depressive symptoms among African-American women," *Prev Med* 31 (2000) 232-240.

201. L.R. Yanek, D.M. Becker, T.F. Moy, J. Gittelsohn, D.M. Koffman, "Project Joy: faith based cardiovascular health promotion for African American women," *Pub Health Rep* 116 (2001) 68-81.

202. W.B. Swann, Jr., A. Gomez, D.C. Seyle, J.F. Morales, C. Huici, "Identity fusion: the interplay of personal and social identities in extreme group behavior," *J Person & Soc Psych* 96 (2009) 995-1011.

203. D.M. Hutchinson, R.M. Rapee, "Do friends share similar body image and eating problems? The role of social networks and peer influences in early adolescence," *Behav Res Ther* 45 (2007) 1557-1577.

204. E. Kumakech, E. Cantor-Graae, S. Maling, F. Bajunirwe, "Peer-group support intervention improves the psychosocial well-being of AIDS orphans: cluster randomized trial," *Soc Science & Med* 68 (2009) 1038-1043.

205. C.L. Carmack-Taylor, J. Kulik, H. Badr, M. Smith, K. Basen-Engquist, F. Penedo, E.R. Gritz, "A social comparison theory analysis of group composition and efficacy of cancer support group programs," *Soc Science & Med* 65 (2007) 262-273.

206. A.M. Darcy, B. Dooley, "A clinical profile of participants in an online support group," *Euro Eat Disord Rev* 15 (2007) 185-195.

207. J.E. Owen, E. O'Carroll-Bantum, M. Golant, "Benefits and challenges experienced by professional facilitators of online support groups for cancer survivors," *Psych-Oncology* 18 (2009) 144-155.

208. K.H. Webber, D.F. Tate, J.M. Bowling, "A randomized comparison of two motivationally enhanced internet behavioral weight loss programs," *Behav Res Ther* 46 (2008) 1090-1095.

209. J.H. Rimmer, A. Rouworth, E. Wang, P.S. Heckerling, B.S. Gerber, "A randomized controlled trial to increase physical activity and reduce obesity in a predominantly African-American group of women with mobility disabilities and severe obesity," *Prev Med* 48 (200) 473-479.

210. H. Kelloniemi, E. Ek, J. Laitinen, "Optimism, dietary habits, body mass index and smoking among Finnish adults," *Appetite* 45 (2005) 169-176.

211. J. Ciarrochi, P.C.L. Heaven, "Learned social hopelessness: the role of explanatory style in predicting social support during adolescence," *J Child Psych & Psychiatry* 49 (2008) 1279-1286.

212. B. Voerman, A. Visser, M. Fischer, B. Garssen, G. van Andel, J. Bensing, "Determinants of participation in social support groups for prostate cancer patients," *Psycho-Oncology* 16 (2007) 1092-1099.

213. P.N. Butow, L.T. Kirsten, J.M. Ussher, G.V. Wain, M. Sandoval, K.M. Hobbs, K. Hodgkinson, A. Stenlake, "What is the ideal support group? Views of Australian people with cancer and their carers," *Psych-Oncology* 16 (2007) 1039-1045.

214. Ibid.

215. H. Lantz, M. Peltonen, L. Agren, J.S. Torgerson, "A dietary and behavioural programme for the treatment of obesity: a 4-year clinical trial and a long-term posttreatment follow-up," *J Int Med* 254 (2003) 272-279.

216. T.L. Pettman, G.M.H. Mosan, K. Owen, K. Warren, A.M. Coates, J.D. Buckley, P.R.C. Howe, "Self-management for obesity and cardio-metabolic fitness: description and evaluation of the lifestyle modification program of a randomized controlled trial," *Intl J Behav Nutri & Phy Act* 5 (2008) 1-15.

217. K.D. Mickelson, J.L. Demmings, "The impact of support network substitution on low-income women's health: are minor children beneficial substitutes?" *Soc Science & Med* 68 (2009) 80-88.

218. Ibid.

219. E. Lanza, A. Schatzkin, C. Daston, D. Corle, L. Freedman, R. Ballard-Barbash, B. Caan, P. Lance, J. Marshall, F. Iber, M. Shike, J. Weissfeld, M. Slattery, E. Paskett, D. Mateski, P. Albert, the PPT Study Group, "Implementation of a 4-y, high fiber, high fruit-and-vegetable, lo-fat dietary intervention: results of dietary changes in the polyp prevention trial," *Am J Clin Nutr* 74 (2001) 387-401.

8   Lesser-Known Weight Loss Considerations

There are some groups of overweight individuals that don't draw much attention among researchers. The reason is because: (1) research funding isn't readily available for research projects that don't demonstrate the potential for a large financial return, or (2) the group is small and has special characteristics that pull it away from the larger group of overweight people. I did not want to ignore these groups, which I have labeled *Special Needs Groups*.

Special Needs Groups

For the vast majority of people beginning weight loss it can be as simple as: (1) obtaining your physicians clearance, (2) planning your approach, and (3) embarking on your weight loss journey. However, some people fall into groups with special needs that require an approach to weight loss with more careful thought and monitoring. Those with special needs frequently require the intervention and oversight of skilled professionals, primarily because of the possibility of serious negative consequences that could result from limited knowledge of their special condition. Much of the discussion that focuses on those with special needs involves recommended diet and exercise limitations. This is a great place to keep in mind the old Clint Eastwood movie line, "A man's got to know his limitations."

There are numerous special needs that could be identified. For purposes of this book the four major categories of: (1) the chronically ill, (2) children, (3) the elderly, and (4) pregnant women are the groups that will be considered. This is because these groups include the majority of people with special needs, and because of the very limited research data available for other people with special needs. In each of the four special needs groups I will begin by explaining some of the significant differences between the group and the general population.

The Chronically Ill

Chronic means "persisting over a long period of time."[1]

Differences From the General Population

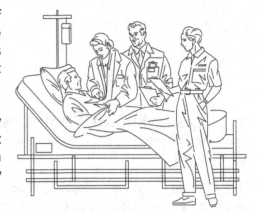

- The chronically ill are usually under the care of a physician, so it is of vital importance that the physician is the focal point of any weight loss attempt, in order not to disrupt the treatment already being provided.

- The body of the chronically ill person is already under stress as a result of its attempt to defeat the illness; therefore, the added stress of a weight-loss program needs to be carefully evaluated.

- During a chronic illness individuals may be too weak to engage in a weight-loss program that they might otherwise be able to actively participate in.

The battle against cancer is one of those situations. If you have undergone recent cancer surgery, radiation or chemotherapy your system is in a weakened state. An exercise program is likely to be more than your body is prepared to handle and dietary changes, unless supervised closely by an experienced nutritionist, could be downright dangerous. If you have completed cancer treatment and are currently diagnosed in remission you may have moved back into the general population where your doctor's approval for a weight-loss program usually means that less supervision is needed. One example is that of endometrial cancer. One study claims that the majority of endometrial cancer survivors are obese and that a weight loss intervention program is not only acceptable but also desirable.[2]

During the discussion of chronic conditions, another one that surfaces frequently is type 2 diabetes. It has been shown that "nutrition therapy and physical activity can assist persons with diabetes to achieve metabolic goals,"[3] with the primary metabolic goal being an improved blood glucose level. To me this means blood glucose improvement to the point of eliminating the diabetes altogether. Aside from obtaining physician approval prior to beginning a weight-loss regime, none of the studies cited here or in the chapter on exercise put undue restriction on people with type 2 diabetes. One scientist looked at type 2 diabetes primarily from a psychological standpoint and suggested that the most successful approach to treatment might be what she called the *Disability Limitation*. She attempted to stabilize the patient's weight wherever it was, and just prevent further weight gain, with the goal of not complicating the patient's existing psychological difficulties.[4] This study is troubling for a number of reasons: (1)

it doesn't make very clear the depth of the psychological problems that the participants may have had, (2) it gives very limited credence to the role of diet, (3) exercise is only mentioned in passing, and (4) it ignores a preponderance of the evidence demonstrating the value of weight loss for the type 2 diabetic.

Apart from limited study data to the contrary it is widely accepted that diabetics and those at risk for diabetes can benefit substantially from exercise and dietary improvement.[5][6] One research group didn't restrict their physical activity research to just diabetics, but when talking about chronically ill patients in general made the broader claim that, exercise "is especially important for adults with chronic illnesses because it may delay progression of some chronic illnesses and manage symptoms of others."[7]

Here is a great example of a chronic condition where exercise is a problem. Weight loss interventions that might work well for the general public, might not be appropriate for Parkinson's disease patients, because of a loss of physical function.[8] Let me say it one more time, if you have a chronic illness or are a weight-loss specialist about to begin working with someone who has a chronic illness, *do not proceed without physician involvement and clearance.*

Children

Differences From the General Population

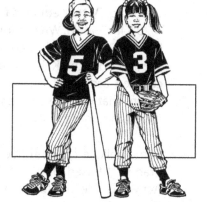

- The child's body is growing and developing at a hyper rate; therefore, extra caution must be used in the creation of any strenuous exercise or nutrition-limiting regime that competes for valuable growth resources.

- The optimum exercise capacity of children has not been clearly defined.[9]

- Since children cannot make health-related decisions, parental involvement is a necessity.

- Children cannot make the adjustments necessary for weight loss by themselves. Success requires a weight management plan that revolves around a healthy lifestyle for the whole family.[10]

- The linchpin of successful childhood weight reduction programs is strong parental intervention.[11]

Before delving into what might be done to help obese children lose weight, let me address the childhood obesity risk factors for those readers that are concerned about a child who might be headed toward obesity. Since there are numerous risk factors, the obvious approach is to mitigate or eliminate as many as possible, by addressing the easiest factors to correct first and progressing to the more difficult ones. So what is it that might lead a child into obesity?

- Sedentary Activities - In 2005 the Kaiser Family Foundation produced a massive report called "Generation M: media in the lives of 8-18 year-olds." They said that kids in that age group spent nearly 6.5 hours per day using recreational media, (note this does not include time spent in school and homework time outside school).[12] The percentage breakdown looks like this:

  o Screen Media - 45 percent,
  o Audio Media - 22 percent,
  o Print Media - 11 percent,
  o Computers - 11 percent,
  o Video Games - 9 percent.[13]

I realize the percentages only add up to 98 percent but that's how the Kaiser data was presented.

From the data you can see that if these kids spend 45 percent of their media time watching TV that equates to (45 percent x 6.5 hrs/day = 2.9 hrs/day x 7 days/week = 20.5 hrs/week). What might that number be today? Nielsen Company research in late 2009 claimed that children today, ages two-eleven (this age group is slightly skewed from the Kaiser study) are actually watching TV 28 hrs/week and younger children are watching as much as 32 hrs/week.[14] By connecting the dots this means that our kids are becoming increasingly sedentary, which coincides with an increasing obesity rate.[15]

Some believe children need "60 min of moderate to vigorous daily exercise in all grades."[16] Based upon US Department of Health and Human Services Physical Activity Guidelines for Americans, Bennett & Sothern went further by making it clear that moderate exercise alone was not sufficient and that at least three days a week children's physical activities need to include bouts of vigorous exercise.[17] Parents, if this kind of activity is not part of your plan or your local school districts plan for your kids, consider the following:

  o Attempt to get it included in your kids' school plan,
  o Limit the kids' total recreational media time to one-two hrs/day,[18]
  o Get them involved in organized sports outside of school,
  o Sign them up at a local park district fitness center,

- o Make them walk to school,[19]
- o Have them ride a bike to school.

"Interventions to increase exercise should lay the foundations for a healthy lifestyle that can be maintained throughout adulthood."[20]

- High Calorie Diet - The combination of a high calorie diet and a sedentary lifestyle have consistently been associated with an overweight population,[21] and today's *Super Size Me* mentality is not working in favor of our children. Not only are they eating more total calories than they need, they are eating a lot of calories with no nutritional value. Here's what you can do to help your kids eat better:

  - o Set an example by encouraging the Rule of Thirds at home,
  - o Limit the amount of junk food that you allow into your home, because it will be eaten,
  - o Increase your control over what they eat. In 1946 the US Congress enacted the National School Lunch Program and from its inception it has served a dual purpose: (1) to provide meals for hungry school kids, and (2) provide a place for farmers to get rid of their surplus crops.[22] Since it is overseen by the US Department of Agriculture (USDA) I bet you can guess which purpose takes priority. School lunches have been criticized for frequently exceeding maximum allowable fat recommendations for school children.[23] The most effective way to deal with this problem is to pack your kids school lunch and limit the amount of money they take to school, so you can better control what they're eating.

- Parental Obesity - "Research indicates that obesity aggregates within families."[24] The two major reasons are: (1) overweight parents pass on a genetic predisposition to their children, and (2) children learn eating and exercise habits from their parents, the combination of which can easily lead to a childhood weight problem.

- Inadequate Parental Involvement - "Parents are a critical part of treatment interventions involving youths, especially younger children under the age of 12, because of their influence on the home environment."[25] While dietary improvement, increased exercise, behavioral change and more parental involvement are all important factors in helping children lose weight,[26] "behavioral interventions for childhood obesity that target both the child and parent have demonstrated the greatest success in improving weight status."[27] As a matter of fact, parental involvement is so important that it has been stated that parental-only intervention could even be effective.[28] The biggest problem is that, "a lack of childhood role models for exercise and an adult pattern of sedentary lifestyles appear to be significant factors contributing to obesity."[29]

- <u>Dysfunctional Family Environment</u> - Appropriate family behavior might be one of the most helpful things for overweight kids.[30] The importance of the family on the actions of a child cannot be overstated. Children not only learn important lessons from their parents but they also learn from other family members. For example, they generally determine the level of their physical activity by watching what their siblings do.[31] Higher levels of family nurturance also relate to lower caloric intake.[32]

- <u>Prescription Drugs</u> - Some antipsychotic and anti-epileptic drugs have been associated with excess weight gain.[33] Obviously without prior doctor approval it would be a mistake to take your child off such medications, just because they may promote excess weight gain; however, be aware that they can contribute to a weight problem.

- <u>Socio-Economic Status</u> - Children from poor families in developed countries and affluent families in countries undergoing economic transition frequently are at a greater risk for childhood obesity.[34] Since socioeconomic related obesity is more prevalent among women than among men,[35] it is logical to believe that obesity will more readily trickle-down from the mother to her children, especially in low-income single parent homes. A typical low-income household spends about the same on food as their higher income counterparts; however their food choices tend to be higher calorie and lower nutrition.[36] Poor food choices are the result of limited knowledge, which can only be overcome when low-income women are trained in inexpensive, healthful eating and the diet-disease relationship.[37]

- <u>Medical Condition</u> - Although it is rare, some children suffer from a medical condition that promotes weight gain, for example hypothyroidism, hypercortisolism, a growth hormone deficiency, hypothalamic damage, etc.[38]

- <u>Lack of Adequate Breast Feeding</u> - Some data suggests breast-fed children tended to be less obese than formula fed children because they consume less total energy, less protein and fewer micronutrients. It has been speculated that this may be the result of a finer tuned ability to regulate their food intake.[39] Some later data restricts that claim by suggesting the effects may be somewhat diminished 20 years later.[40]

  I realize that there is not much you can do for a child in terms of breast-feeding if they are passed the infant nursing stage, but this information should be of value if you are now or will soon be nursing an infant. To benefit an infant the most, the recommended length of time for nursing them is at least six months.[41]

Pharmacotherapy or bariatric surgery should only "be considered if a formal program of intensive lifestyle modification has failed to limit weight gain or to mollify comorbidities in obese children."[42] Comorbidities are diseases or other pathologic process that occur simultaneous with another.[43] This should only be considered after extensive consultation with psychological and pediatric healthcare providers. The hurdles for bariatric surgery in children are much higher than for adults. Here they are:

- The Child has attained: (1) Tanner 4 or 5 pubertal development, and (2) they are at or near their final adult height,
- The Child has a BMI greater than 50, or a BMI greater than 40 and severe comorbidities,
- The Child has participated in a formal program of intensive lifestyle modification, without favorable results and severe obesity and comorbidities persist,
- Psychological evaluation confirms the stability of the family,
- Qualified and experienced surgical help is available.[44]

Like every other aspect of a child's life, the study data bears out that a weight loss effort requires a good parental example, a supportive family relationship, love, understanding and encouragement.

The Elderly

Differences From the General Population

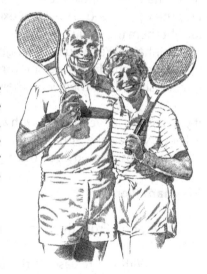

- In the elderly the body is in a more accelerated rate of decline than at any other time in life. For example cardiac output, VO_{2max}, muscle mass, metabolic rate, are all declining. "As the aging process continues, the frequency of contact between the elderly and their physicians increases substantially,"[45] which places the physician in a particularly strong counseling role.

- Injuries occur more easily and are more difficult to overcome.

Most of the research on weight loss in the elderly focuses on effective exercise routines. The elderly should only be limited by what they are capable of doing; therefore, it is important that they set exercise goals that meet their needs.[46] The health benefits of exercise for the elderly is well established; however, they seldom use it for health improvement and weight loss.[47] Muscle mass loss during weight loss is a danger for all of us but especially so for the elderly, since they tend to lose muscle mass with the passage of time anyway. It has been suggested that progressive resistance training when coupled with a proper diet reduces muscle mass loss during weight-loss and increases muscle strength in frail, obese older adults.[48] Exercise also improves physical function[49] and ameliorates frailty in these same adults.[50] Even though I don't usually think of walking as exercise, for the general population, it may be all that many older adults can do. If that is the case, one way for them to get the health benefits of increased exercise is to drive less and walk more, since lower rates of auto use have been associated with a lower BMI.[51]

There are often exercise barriers for the elderly, which may include: (1) illnesses, (2) misinformed belief systems, (3) lack of a peer group, (4) no access to exercise equipment, (5) financial constraints, (6) a sense of disempowerment, and (7) fear of injury.[52] Perceived barriers to exercise are so ingrained in the elderly that a long-term exercise program may be a challenge, however since they hold their physician's opinion in high regard these barriers can frequently be overcome with the physician's encouragement.[53]

Elderly women may be more disproportionately affected by various exercise barriers than are their male counterparts. For example, postmenopausal women typically experience weight gain as their estrogen levels decline, while at the same time they become more sedentary. Insufficient exercise is an important and modifiable cause of postmenopausal associated weight gain.[54] A group of African-American women were studied, with interesting results. This group has the highest incidence of overweight in the United States, at 48 percent. The result was their perceived barriers to exercise were almost endless, (e.g. inclement weather, no one taught them the value of exercise, never exercised before, never played sports, they might mess up their hair).[55] Yes, you read it right they might mess up their hair! Apparently they don't mind the world around them seeing them as overweight or maybe even obese, but God forbid that anyone should see them with their hair messed up.

If you wish to move forward with a weight loss program that includes exercise and you find that it keeps you awake at night thinking of excuses why you can't do it, go back and reread the chapter on psychology. You must get beyond these problems if you are to be successful.

Pregnant Women

Differences From the General Population

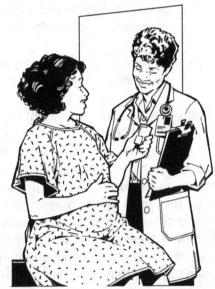

- "With the release of the hormone relaxin, joints become looser, increasing the risk for injury during exercise."[56]

- Body temperature regulation can be substantially altered and difficult to maintain and it has been suggested that severe overheating may damage the central nervous system of the fetus.[57]

- Nutritional requirements are increased and since dieting often tends to work against nutritional support, dieting during pregnancy is not recommended. In addition harsh dieting during pregnancy may produce a phenomenon known as *Accelerated Starvation in Pregnancy*, which results in an increase in the level of ketones in the mother's blood, raising the possibility of harm to the fetus.[58]

Here weight loss and health considerations fall into three pregnancy categories:

- Pre-Pregnancy - One good reason for losing weight if you are trying to get pregnant is that weight loss is one of the best ways of increasing fertility in infertile, overweight or obese women.[59] The health of the mother, including her weight status, prior to a pregnancy certainly has an impact on both her health during the pregnancy and the ultimate health of her baby.

  Women with a normal BMI before pregnancy have been shown to be more likely to maintain their recommended weight during pregnancy, (that's a good thing).[60] However a high pre-pregnancy BMI is a risk factor for high weight gain and a high BMI during pregnancy, (that's a bad thing). [61] Others have gone further when they demonstrated that a high pre-pregnancy BMI and gestational hyperglycemia are risk factors for adverse pregnancy outcomes.[62] Mothers that experience a BMI increase between their first and second pregnancy are at higher risk of negative pregnancy outcomes.[63]

- Pregnancy - Gaining some weight during pregnancy is a normal occurrence, but an important factor to be concerned about is that pregnancy is considered a risk factor for the development of obesity.[64] If you are concerned about your weight during pregnancy, four important questions frequently arise: (1) whether obesity jeopardizes the health of the developing baby, (2) whether obesity complicates the delivery, (3) is it safe to diet, and (4) is it safe to exercise? One study answered the first two by explaining that obesity may drive adverse pregnancy outcomes by affecting either the mother (e.g. maternal morbidity) or the infant (e.g. infant development), or both.[65] However, on the other side of the weight loss argument, the main reason that doctors are concerned about excess weight loss during pregnancy is that it has been associated with an increased risk of preterm birth and preterm birth is a leading cause of infant mortality.[66] One key to enhancing the probability of a normal pregnancy, delivery, and baby is to maintain a proper body weight during pregnancy. The second two questions will be answered below.

  Caveat - Be careful with this whole weight loss idea during pregnancy. One important question is, "could extraordinary attention to diet, exercise, and weight-management create stress and feelings of hopelessness in overweight pregnant women, leading them to increase their intake of high-calorie or high-fat foods, or to reduce their motivation to exercise?"[67] The important thing to be avoided during pregnancy is the development of an obsession with weight loss that actually produces the opposite result. The wiser approach might be to suspend your weight-loss program until after the baby is born.

Over the years a lot of questions have been raised about whether pregnant women should diet or exercise during pregnancy. Let's address these two issues now.

o   Dieting - Generally dieting for weight loss during pregnancy is discouraged because of the mothers' increased nutritional requirements.[68] Thin women are especially at an increased risk of under nutrition during pregnancy.[69]

o   Exercising - Unless otherwise directed by a physician, exercise during pregnancy is generally considered to be of value; however, pregnancy is an accurate predictor of an impending decrease in the amount and intensity of normal exercise.[70] Pregnancy increases both physical and psychological stress on the mother's body, through such changes as: (1) unwanted weight gain, (2) altered posture, (3) additional dietary requirements, and (4) cardiovascular and gastrointestinal dysfunction.[71] "Despite these demands, exercise during pregnancy and postpartum is a beneficial and a recommended activity for alleviating negative physical and psychological symptoms."[72] The US Department of Health and Human Services reiterates that sentiment by stating that, "physical activity during pregnancy benefits a woman's overall health."[73]

Does exercise affect the fetus? Research suggests that in the absence of medical complications more than 30 minutes per day, of moderate exercise, performed most days of the week does not: (1) have a negative effect on the developing fetus, (2) shorten the pregnancy prematurely, (3) result in a low birth weight baby, and (4) produce obstetrical complications.[74]

Although there are a few highly trained female athletes that have continued running programs late into their third trimester, this is certainly the exception rather than the rule. Unless there are contraindications, doctors usually recommend that fit, well-trained, athletic pregnant women may continue their exercise routine, well into their pregnancy, although they highly favor modifying the routine to eliminate high impact activities (e.g. running). On the other hand women attempting to begin an exercise routine should start easily by selecting an exercise intensity, duration and frequency that does not result in pain, shortness of breath or excess fatigue, and they should progress at a rate that avoids significant discomfort.[75]

What exercises are best? What exercises should be avoided? Here is what the American Pregnancy Association suggests.

Recommended Exercise Protocol

- o   Kegel Exercises - exercises that contract and relax the muscles of the pelvic floor intended to improve the ability to hold urine,
- o   Swimming,
- o   Walking,
- o   Running and Jogging - only: (1) if you were a runner prior to getting pregnant, and (2) with the approval of your physician, but they may still prove to be too high impact,
- o   Bicycling,
- o   Stair Climbing Machines,
- o   Yoga,
- o   Aerobics - especially water aerobics,
- o   Dance,[76]
- o   Extend warm-up and cool-down periods,
- o   Eat a light snack before exercising,
- o   Drink plenty of water during exercising.[77]

Exercises to Avoid - (These include anything that is high impact, has a risk of falling or requires exceptional balance or extreme range of motion):[78]

- o   Skiing,
- o   Water Skiing,
- o   Horseback Riding,[79]
- o   Strenuous exercises in hot or humid conditions,
- o   Exercises performed in the supine position (i.e. on your back) after the first trimester,[80]
- o   Exercises that require straining or holding your breath during exertion.[81] While exercising the benchmark for appropriate intensity is your own personal impression of how you feel, often referred to as your *Rate of Perceived Exertion*.[82]

Under certain pregnancy related situations your doctor is very likely to forbid you from exercising. The March of Dimes produced a quick reference fact sheet of such conditions:

- o   Heart disease that compromises blood flow,
- o   Preterm labor,
- o   Incompetent cervix,

- o   Restrictive lung disease,
- o   Multiple gestation,
- o   Persistent vaginal bleeding,
- o   Pregnancy related high blood pressure.[83]

- <u>Postpartum</u> - This is a time when women are trying to get back to normal and they have the added burden of being a 24-hour caregiver for a new baby.[84] The authorities tell us that many mothers need to change their health behaviors during the first four months after delivery, by losing weight and improving nutrition and exercise regimes,[85] because it has been shown that 15 to 20 percent of postpartum mothers retain in excess of 11 pounds of body weight 6-18 months after delivery.[86] Although I am not sure whether or not the cultural differences between the Middle East and the West might skew study data produced in one area and applied to the other, an interesting study from Iran found, "weight gain during pregnancy was the most important determinant of weight retention at three years postpartum."[87]

Here is where knowledge seems to pay off. It has been demonstrated that women with more nutritional knowledge were able to maintain lower postpartum weight retention than their less knowledgeable counterparts.[88]

Here's some great news for women who have recently given birth. Breast-feeding mothers have significantly larger reductions in hip circumference and are closer to their pregnancy weight within one month of delivery.[89] A whole host of additional benefits accrue to mothers who are breast-feeding. Breast-feeding:

- o   Promotes faster shrinking of the uterus,
- o   Reduces postpartum bleeding,
- o   Decreases risk of breast and ovarian cancer,
- o   Delay's resumption of the menstrual cycle,
- o   Improves bone density,
- o   Decreases risk of hip fracture,
- o   Improves glucose profile in gestational diabetics.[90]

Here are some suggestions that may help you with postpartum weight loss:

- o   If it is not already too late, take steps to achieve a normal BMI prior to or during pregnancy,
- o   Involve any or all of the following to assist you; physician, nurse, dietitian, nutritionist, psychologist, or personal trainer,
- o   Join a support group,
- o   Consider a longer period of breast-feeding,
- o   Investigate ways of increasing your activity level.[91]

Be careful of a one-size-fits-all approach to postpartum weight management, because it has been shown that postpartum women participating in a weight management program, customized especially for them, have the greatest success.[92]

The Relationship Between Sleep and Weight Loss

Human beings evolved in a world that alternated between periods of daylight and darkness. That meant they went to bed at sundown and got up at dawn. Consequently our food seeking behavior coupled with the vigilance to avoid predators became paired with the daylight hours. Similarly, satiety and sleep became paired with the darkness.[93] Not until recently did we have lights to illuminate the darkness, nighttime entertainment like TV and the Internet to keep us awake into the wee morning hours and night shift work, all of which serve to disrupt the normal human circadian rhythm.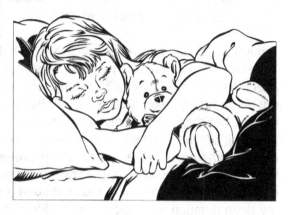

Why do we need to sleep in the first place? There are a number of theories as to why sleep is necessary, several of which have little or no connection with a weight loss effort. The one that appears to be the most generally accepted in the health community, the easiest to understand and the most logical is called the Repair and Restoration Theory. It holds that the sleep cycle provides the body with an opportunity to do a number of things:

- Repair the damage that we have done during the day - During the sleep cycle we normally stop smoking cigarettes, drinking alcohol, eating food that has been sprayed with chemical fertilizers and pesticides, taking prescription drugs, and setting in traffic breathing auto exhaust fumes. During the day all of these activities have caused untold damage to the body. At this point the body gets a sort of mini vacation while it attempts to clean up the mess. This is the time when muscles damaged by severe exercise are repaired and rebuilt,[94] the immune system is strengthened[95] (to better wage the war against infection),[96] and muscle tone and skin appearance are rejuvenated.[97]

- Restore the body back to a state of homeostasis - The body's goal during the time of damage repair is to return to a state of normalcy, and the sleep state is when that happens. As discussed in chapter 1, our bodies always try to achieve health stabilization, and while the body's daily challenges are postponed during sleep it works on neutralizing health threats.

- • <u>Conduct a general housecleaning</u> - In conjunction with damage repair, as we sleep the body engages in an extensive cleanup. The generally overworked liver, lungs, kidneys, digestive system and lymphatic system attempt to play catch-up as they remove dead cells and pathogens from the system. If you have been ill or exposed to an exceptionally high amount of pollution the cleanup task becomes even more difficult, which means that more than normal sleep may be required or else the cleanup process may be incomplete. This is exactly the reason your doctor recommends more rest during a time of illness.

Today it is estimated that between 50 and 70 million Americans suffer chronic sleep deprivation. This sleep deprivation has a negative impact on the daily functioning of the body and adversely affects health and longevity.[98] The long-term effects of sleep deprivation and/or sleep disorders, not only is poorly recognized as a public health problem, but is now being linked a wide range of adverse health consequences which include an increased risk of: (1) hypertension, (2) diabetes, (3) <u>obesity</u>, (4) heart attack, and (5) stroke.[99] How much sleep should we get? It is hard to make a generalization because normal sleep patterns change with such things as age, exercise level and general health status. For example we all know that a year-old baby normally sleeps considerably more than a 30-year-old adult. I personally know that my activity level impacts my sleep duration (e.g. when I am working, playing or getting a lot of exercise on a beautiful summer day, I sleep considerably more than I do when I am cooped up in the house watching sports on a cold winter day).

Here's how one Mayo Clinic researcher answers the question of, "how many hours of sleep are enough for good health?" Appropriate sleep duration depends on a variety of factors, especially age:

- • Infants sleep at least 16 hours a day,
- • Preschoolers need at least 11 hours of sleep a night,
- • School age children need at least ten hours of sleep a night,
- • Teenagers need about nine hours of sleep a night,[100]
- • Adults are good with seven to eight hours of sleep a night.[101] [102]

That same researcher found that adults who sleep considerably more or less than seven hours per night have a higher mortality rate than adults who sleep about seven hours a night.[103] Based on this data it seems logical to shoot for seven to eight hours of good quality sleep per night.

The growing sleep debt in America may be contributing to increased obesity and diabetes by leading to an increased food intake.[104] Prior to this study, it was demonstrated that adults who only sleep on average five hours per night have a higher BMI and in addition women have a higher incidence of diabetes.[105] Adolescent studies show that longer duration sleep is associated with an increased risk of being overweight but this only holds true among males, not among females.[106] Older female adolescence may hold weight gain at bay by replacing recreational Internet time with sleep and by avoiding alcohol consumption.[107] Later work not only supported this thinking but took it further by claiming that chronic partial sleep loss may increase the risk of obesity and diabetes via multiple pathways; among them are: (1) altered glucose metabolism, (2) increased appetite, (3) decreased energy expenditure,[108] (4) impaired carbohydrate metabolism, (5) altered endocrine function, and (6) decreased insulin sensitivity.[109] Wow, that seems like a lot of potential negative consequences for being sleep deprived!

Here is where the research gets a little dicey. Three primary questions persist:

- Does a chronic lack of sleep cause obesity?
- Does obesity cause a diminished sleep pattern?
- Does no cause and effect relationship exist between an abnormally short or long sleep duration and obesity, or do they simply coexist?

From existing evidence, neither short nor long sleep duration can be associated with obesity in adults, however in children and adolescents short sleep patterns are consistently associated with a higher BMI.[110] Parents, here is important information for you. Studies of preschool children concluded that a short sleep duration is definitely associated with obesity in preschool children and get this, short sleep duration is significantly related to sleeping with caregivers, that means you the parent.[111] So if you want to do your kids a favor, and probably yourself at the same time, make them sleep in their own beds.

As you might expect, other study data disagrees with the idea that adult sleep deprivation unfavorably affects weight status. Horne maintains that there is no study data proving that a diminished sleep pattern in either adults or children causes any more than about a one kilogram (i.e. two pounds) per year weight gain.[112] That's just great but guess what? In twenty years at that rate of gain, you will be forty pounds overweight and that is not good. Worse yet, couple that with an increasingly sedentary lifestyle and perhaps a more calorie rich diet and you could find yourself eighty or a hundred pounds overweight, and that's deadly. This whole short sleep duration versus weight gain concept is completely supported by research showing that short sleep duration is associated with lowered physical activity levels and poor nutrition, which we already know promote weight gain and obesity.[113]

If you wanted to know what your personal sleep requirements are; how might you find out? Here's what I recommend. If you had an occasion to be off work for a week or so and didn't have to get up with an alarm clock, go to bed between 10 PM and 11 PM and sleep until you wake up. A vacation might allow you the opportunity to conduct this test, but be aware you may experience a somewhat abnormal or erratic sleep pattern because of later than normal evening meals, late night hours, excess drinking or simply the typical vacation excitement of getting going in the morning.

I understand that this simple little test may be somewhat difficult to orchestrate in today's hectic environment, but give it a try and see if it tells you something of value. Although I wouldn't claim that this is a scientifically precise analytical technique it should give you a decent benchmark. If you did this test and figured out that your body would really like to sleep seven and a half-eight hours a night, but under normal circumstances you are only sleeping five-six hours, then you might work toward improving the situation. I know in my case I have for years had the luxury of working a job that allows me to sleep until I wake up. My normal bedtime is 11 PM and I consistently sleep between seven and a half and eight and a half hours a night, depending on the day's level of physical activity and exercise.

There are other things that might make you sleep longer than normal, for example people who are depressed often sleep much longer than they normally would and various pharmaceuticals have the same effect.

Here are some suggestions that you might try if you aren't sleeping as soundly as you think you should and are serious about developing a more effective sleep pattern.

- Make sure your room is dark,
- Make sure your room is quiet,
- Wear loose comfortable clothing (or none at all),
- Moderate the temperature,
- If you suffer from allergies continuously run a HEPA filter in your room,
- Don't let children or pets sleep with you,
- Don't eat heavily after the normal dinner hour,
- Don't work too late into the evening,
- Don't watch TV or movies that get you agitated or excited close to bedtime,
- Don't drink alcohol or coffee in the evening.

Study data certainly has not proven short duration sleep patterns actually cause obesity, but what they have concluded is, "that short duration of sleep might represent a risk marker rather than a causative risk factor for obesity."[114] Inadequate sleep has the possibility of influencing body weight by making it difficult to maintain a healthy lifestyle and study data does suggest that sleep deprivation could play in pivotal role in obesity in select individuals.[115] There are no claims that a sizable weight loss might be accomplished by sleeping an extra hour a night; however, based on the research data cited it does seem logical that due consideration should be given to sleep deprivation as one more possible body weight contributor.

Caveat - The subjects in the remainder of this chapter are not mainstream weight loss topics, primarily because: (1) there is limited research data, if any, to support them, and (2) the amount of improvement from using any one or a combination of these techniques pales in comparison to diet and exercise. This doesn't automatically mean that they are of no value. All of them have been used for years by a variety of natural healers and/or other health devotees.

The obvious question is that if they are any good why isn't there research data to support that fact? They lack research support because those entities spending money on research don't see a potential return on such an investment. Today healthcare research costs massive amounts of money. That money comes principally from the large pharmaceutical companies with a much smaller portion coming from the government [e.g. the Food and Drug Administration (FDA), the National Institute of Health (NIH), the Center for Disease Control (CDC)]. Pharmaceutical's interest is to conduct research that will lead to patented products, where they control the distribution, sale and price for the life of the patent. On the other hand the government's interest is supposedly to benefit us citizens. Some have suggested that a strong symbiotic relationship has developed between the pharmaceutical companies and the government, perhaps resulting in an arrangement where we the people have been forgotten, and where all research expenditures are spent to facilitate research leading to patentable products. I will let you judge that one for yourself.

I offer the following topics with the hope they may not only broaden your understanding of the various facets of weight loss, but more importantly they may help you in your effort to lose weight as well. In addition to what I offer, I suggest that you do your own research on any subject of interest to you, especially utilizing the Internet, where you will find a lot of thought provoking discussion on all of these topics. Don't ignore the Internet because some of what you read may be inaccurate. I suggest you look for recurring themes and use your common sense in determining whether the material you have found can benefit you.

Acupuncture

The Chinese created acupuncture 5000 years ago and have been using it successfully, in a wide variety of applications, ever since. Among these applications are Chinese acupuncture clinics that specialize in weight loss. Minimal Chinese research is available for two reasons: (1) apparently the Chinese haven't felt much of a need to prove acupuncture's effectiveness to the rest of the world, and (2) most of the research that has been done in China has not been translated into English. In recent years a modest amount of acupuncture research has been conducted in the United States and as a result it has gained expanded acceptance here. Most of us either have made use of acupuncture or know of others who have, with one of its highest profile successes having been in smoking cessation programs.

One recent Chinese study concluded that acupuncture definitely was effective in treating obesity,[116] and an Australian study suggested that acupuncture can be an effective weight loss tool if used in conjunction with diet and exercise, and its benefits were shown to extend beyond the results that can be obtained by diet and exercise alone.[117]

Acupuncture hasn't typically been claimed, by western health care practitioners, to be a contributing factor in weight loss, rather it is an adjunctive therapy that is used to treat some obesity related risk factors. Knowing that appetite, stress and depression are all risk factors for obesity, some researchers have used acupuncture to control them in the treatment of obesity.[118] When it comes to treating Major Depressive Disorder, one study found that "acupuncture therapy is safe and effective in treating MDD."[119] Finally, a study of the available research that has been done previously on acupuncture treatment for insomnia, concluded that most of the studies reviewed were of poor quality, leading to no clear conclusion, although they did offer promise for this application of acupuncture.[120]

Massage Therapy

Massage therapy is the technique of pressing, rubbing and manipulating the muscles and soft tissue of the body,[121] for the express purpose of promoting health and well-being.[122] Various types of well-being can be achieved but one with a big possibility of affecting weight loss is improvement in the symptoms of depression. After receiving massage therapy, aggressive adolescents become less anxious, and their immune systems are enhanced.[123] Additional study data has revealed massage therapy provides a psychologically soothing and sedating effect.[124] We know that improving either of these situations could positively impact obesity treatment.

Sauna / Steam Room

The sauna and the steam room both consist of a small, enclosed room with a source of high heat. The temperature and humidity levels are quite different for each. The sauna can be either wet or dry while the steam room is always 100 percent humidity. Sauna temperatures are much higher than those of the steam room, primarily because the body can tolerate higher heat in the dryer environment. As the humidity is increased in the sauna, the temperature is decreased and if the humidity were to reach 100 percent it would be a steam room. The object of both the sauna and steam room are similar, to relax, sweat out toxins, lower blood pressure and lose weight. However, since sweating is the primary weight-loss vehicle, the problem is that a drop in weight is merely a loss of water, which end's up only temporary because any weight loss is quickly regained by drinking water.

Like several of the other techniques mentioned in this chapter the sauna and steam room, can be effective weight-loss tools when coupled with appropriate lifestyle changes, but may not be of much value as a stand-alone technique. In addition, safety needs to be considered. For those individuals who are used to using a sauna (e.g. many Scandinavians), safety concerns are usually minimal. "For most healthy people...sauna bathing is well tolerated and safe;"[125] however, heart patients and pregnant women need to consult their physician before beginning sauna use. It should be noted that alcohol consumption during sauna bathing must be avoided.

Given the limited value of sauna and steam room use for weight loss, independent of other foundational weight-loss practices, I am reluctant to suggest them as weight-loss tools. In addition, if you decide to use either of them you will need to do further research to determine the appropriate duration and frequency for your particular needs.

Mind Machines

Today there is an emerging field of alternative health care that is based upon the use of specialized technical equipment called *Mind Machines*. These devices are intended to produce a deep state of relaxation or focused concentration in the user, by altering brain wave frequency from a higher level to a lower level, with a resulting state of consciousness that is frequently compared to that obtained from meditation or prayer. Although there are a multitude of different types of mind machines available today, by far the most popular and highly recognizable is the light/sound machine, (a.k.a. an Auditory Visual Stimulation Device), which consists primarily of a pair of headphones and strobe light goggles.

As you recall from the chapter on the psychological aspects of weight loss, some of the cofactors that can exist with obesity are stress, tension, anxiety and depression. Coexisting with obesity is extremely high levels of what has been referred to as arousability, meaning that the obese person is much more sensitive to external stimulation, often experiencing it as highly stressful.[126] The secret then is to find a way to minimize the stress and anxiety. By using mind machine technology to stimulate the normal reward system the obese individual may be able to mitigate destructive reward system behaviors like overeating or becoming sedentary.[127] In the future, I can envision this type of technology developing into popular tools, used for a variety of health treatments, including obesity.

Summary

The process of weight loss is not the same for all of us. Many people find themselves faced with special conditions that make it more difficult to vigorously pursue a weight-loss program. The chronically ill, children, the elderly and pregnant women often find that the two most important components of weight loss, diet and exercise, cannot be fully utilized because of their special condition. These groups frequently find themselves too weak or frail to exercise and they are often too run down or nutritionally depleted to diet. In addition a doctor may, for health reasons, restrict chronically ill people or pregnant women from dieting or exercising no matter how overweight they are. When it comes to all of these special conditions, there is no one-size-fits-all program. Special needs people must have a weight-loss regime created specifically for their individual circumstances.

Another important consideration is the amount of sleep we regularly get. As with the special needs person our individual sleep requirements vary with age, exercise level and general health status. Although it has not been demonstrated conclusively that sleep deprivation causes obesity it has been shown to be a risk factor. The best approach is to determine what your normal sleep pattern should be and then work towards achieving it regularly. From a general health standpoint I am often surprised when I hear a person say that all they require is five or five and a half hours sleep a night! In fact I have a friend that claims that if she sleeps more than five and a half hours a night she wakes up with a headache. My response is nonsense, that is classic insomnia. I don't believe for one minute that anybody can run full speed for 18 or 19 hours a day and sleep five or six without suffering major health consequences as a result.

As noted earlier acupuncture, massage therapy, sauna/steam room and mind machines all claim some limited value in weight reduction, even though supporting evidence is sparse. If you find any of these techniques appealing you may want to investigate them further and experiment with them to determine if they can help you.

The take away message from this chapter is that if you have a special need, you need special help! You must work closely with your doctor and I recommend that you consider engaging the services of an experienced nutritionist and/or exercise professional.

Endnotes

1. "Chronic," *Dorland's Illustrated Medical Dictionary*, 30th ed: 363.
2. V.E. von Gruenigen, K.S. Courneya, H.E. Gibbons, M.B. Kavanagh, S.E. Waggoner, E. Lerner, "Feasibility and effectiveness of a lifestyle intervention program in obese and endometrial cancer patients: a randomized trial," *Gyn Oncol* 109 (2008) 19-26.
3. M.J. Franz, "Lifestyle modifications for diabetes management," *Endocrin Metab Clin N Am* 26 (1997) 499-510.
4. M. Clark, "Is weight loss a realistic goal of treatment in type 2 diabetes? The implications of restraint theory," *Patient Ed Counsel* 53 (2004) 277-283.
5. T.P.J. Solomon, S.N. Sistrun, R.K. Krishnan, L.F. Del Aguila, C.M. Marchetti, S.M. O'Carroll, V.B. O'Leary, J.P. Kirwan, "Exercise and diet enhance fat oxidation and reduce insulin resistance in older obese adults," *J App Physiol* 104 (2008) 1313-1319.
6. E.P. Weiss, S.B. Racette, D.T. Villareal, L. Fontana, K. Steger-May, K.B. Schechtman, S. Klein, J. O'Holloszy, "Improvements in glucose tolerance and insulin action induced by increasing energy expenditure or decreasing energy intake: a randomized controlled trial," *Am J Clin Nutr* 84 (2006) 1033-1042.
7. V.S. Conn, A.R. Hafdahl, S.A. Brown, L.M. Brown, "Meta-analysis of patient education interventions to increase physical activity among chronically ill adults," *Patient Ed Counsel* 70 (2008) 157-172.
8. P.J. Tuite, R.E. Maxwell, S. Ikramuddin, C.M. Kotzd, C.J. Billingtond, M.A. Laseski, S.D. Thielen, "Weight and body mass index in Parkinson's disease patients after deep brain stimulation surgery," *Park Rel Disord* 11 (2005) 247-252.

9. *"Ace personal trainer manual-American Council on Exercise,"* 3rd ed (San Diego, CA: *American Council on Exercise*, 2003) 365.

10. A.F. Browne, T. Inge, "How young for bariatric surgery in children?" *Seminars Ped Surgery* 18 (2009) 176-185.

11. M. Yackobovitch-Gavan, N. Nagelberg, M. Phillip, L. Ashkenazi-Hoffnung, E. Hershkovitz, S. Shalitin, "The influence of diet and/or exercise and parental compliance on health-related quality of life in obese children," *Nutr Res* 29 (2009) 397-404.

12. D.F. Roberts, U.G. Foehr, V. Rideout, *"Generation M: media in the lives of 8-18 year olds,"* (A Kaiser Family Foundation Study 2005) 57. This study can be found online at http://www.kff.org/entmedia/entmedia030905pkg.cfm

13. Ibid.

14. The Nielsen Company, nielsenwire, *"TV viewing among kids at an eight-year high,"* http://blog.nielsen.com/nielsenwire/media_entertainment/tv-viewing-among-kids-at-an-eight-year-high/

15. L.H. McArthur, D. Holbert, M. Pena, "Prevalence of overweight among adolescents from six Latin American cities: a multivariable analysis," *Nutr Res* 23 (2003) 1391-1402.

16. G.P. August, S. Caprio, I. Fennoy, M. Freemark, F.R. Kaufman, R.H. Lustig, J.H. Silverstein, P.W. Speiser, D.M. Styne, V.M. Montori, "Prevention and treatment of pediatric obesity: an Endocrine Society clinical practice guideline based on expert opinion," *J Clin Endocrinol Metab* 93 (2008) 4576-4599.

17. B. Bennett, M.S. Sothern, "Diet, exercise, behavior: the promise and limits of lifestyle change," *Seminars Ped Surgery* 18 (2009) 152-158.

18. American Academy of Pediatrics, *"Children, adolescents, and television,"* http://www.pediatrics.org/cgi/content/full/107/2/423

19. R. Pabayo, L. Gauvin, T.A. Barnett, B. Nikiema, L. Seguin, "Sustained active transportation is associated with a favorable body mass index trajectory across the early school years: findings from the Québec Longitudinal Study of child development birth cohort," *Prev Med* (2009) 1-6.

20. A. McCall, R. Raj, "Exercise for prevention of obesity and diabetes in children and adolescents," *Clin Sports Med* 28 (2009) 393-421.

21. L.H. McArthur, D. Holbert, M. Pena, "Prevalence of overweight among adolescents from six Latin American cities: a multivariable analysis," *Nutr Res* 23 (2003) 1391-1402.

22. A. Demas, "Low-fat school lunch programs: achieving acceptance," *Am J Cardiol* 82 (1998) 80T-82T.

23. H.M. Hendy, K.E. Williams, T.S. Camise, "Kids choice school lunch program increases children's fruit and vegetable acceptance," *Appetite* 45 (2005) 250-263.

24. C.A. Limbers, E.A. Turner, J.W. Varni, "Promoting healthy lifestyles: behavior modification and motivational interviewing in the treatment of childhood obesity," *J Clin Lipidology* 2 (2008) 169-178.

25. B. Bennett, M.S. Sothern, "Diet, exercise, behavior: the promise and limits of lifestyle change," *Seminars Ped Surgery* 18 (2009) 152-158.

26. J.A. Snethen, M.E. Broome, S.E. Cashin, "Effective weight loss for overweight children: a meta-analysis of intervention studies," *J Ped Nursing* 21 (2006) 45-56.

27. C.A. Limbers, E.A. Turner, J.W. Varni, "Promoting healthy lifestyles: behavior modification and motivational interviewing in the treatment of childhood obesity," *J Clin Lipidology* 2 (2008) 169-178.

28. D.M. Janicke, B.J. Sallinen, M.G. Perri, L.D. Lutes, J.H. Silverstein, M.G. Huerta, L.A. Guion, "Sensible treatment of obesity in rural youth (STORY): design and methods," *Contemp Clin Trials* 29 (2008) 270-280.

29. M.T. Railey, "Patterns of obesity and African-American women," *J Nat Med Assoc* 92 (2000) 481-484.

30. K.M. Young, J.J. Northern, K.M. Lister, J.A. Drummond, W.H. O'Brien, "A meta-analysis of family-behavioral weight-loss treatments for children," *Clin Psych Rev* 27 (2007) 240-249.

31. P.W. Franks, E. Ravussin, R.L. Hanson, I.T. Harper, D.B. Allison, W.C. Knowler, P.A. Tataranni, A.D. Salbe, "Habitual physical activity in children: the role of genes and the environment," *J Clin Nutr* 82 (2005) 901-908.

32. H. Kitzman-Ulrich, R. Hampson, D.K. Wilson, K. Presnell, A. Brown, M. O'Boyle, "An adolescent weight loss program integrating family variables reduces energy intake," *J Am Diet Assoc* 109 (2009) 491-496.

33. L.A. Baur, J. O'Connor, "Special considerations in childhood and adolescent obesity," *Clin Derm* 22 (2004) 338-344.

34. Ibid.

35. K. Ball, D. Crawford, "Socio-economic status and weight change in adults: a review," *Soc Sci Med* 60 (2005) 1987-2010.

36. H. Stewart, N. Blisard, "The thrifty food plan and low-income households in the United States: what food groups are being neglected," *Food Policy* 31 (2006) 469-482.

37. K.W. Dammann, C. Smith, "Factors affecting low-income women's food choices and the perceived impact of dietary intake and socioeconomic status on their health and weight," *J Nutr Ed Behav* 41 (200(0 242-253.

38. L.A. Baur, J. O'Connor, "Special considerations in childhood and adolescent obesity," *Clin Derm* 22 (2004) 338-344.

39. N.F. Butte, "The role of breastfeeding in obesity," *Ped Clin N Am* 48 (2001) 189-198.

40. E. Kvaavik, G.S. Tell, K.I. Klepp, "Surveys of Norwegian youth indicated that breast feeding reduced subsequent risk of obesity," *J Clin Epidemiol* 58 (2005) 849-855.

41. G.P. August, S. Caprio, I. Fennoy, M. Freemark, F.R. Kaufman, R.H. Lustig, J.H. Silverstein, P.W. Speiser, D.M. Styne, V.M. Montori, "Prevention and treatment of pediatric obesity: an Endocrine Society clinical practice guideline based on expert opinion," *J Clin Endocrinol Metab* 93 (2008) 4576-4599.

42. G.P. August, S. Caprio, I. Fennoy, M. Freemark, F.R. Kaufman, R.H. Lustig, J.H. Silverstein, P.W. Speiser, D.M. Styne, V.M. Montori, "Prevention and treatment of pediatric obesity: an Endocrine Society clinical practice guideline based on expert opinion," *J Clin Endocrinol Metab* 93 (2008) 4576-4599.

43. "Comorbidity," *Dorland's Illustrated Medical Dictionary*, 30th ed: 397.

44. G.P. August, S. Caprio, I. Fennoy, M. Freemark, F.R. Kaufman, R.H. Lustig, J.H. Silverstein, P.W. Speiser, D.M. Styne, V.M. Montori, "Prevention and treatment of pediatric obesity: an Endocrine Society clinical practice guideline based on expert opinion," *J Clin Endocrinol Metab* 93 (2008) 4576-4599.

45. K.A. Schutzer, B.S. Graves, "Barriers and motivation to exercise in older adults," *Prev Med* 39 (2004) 1056-1061.

46. *"2008 physicalactivity guidelines for Americans,"* (Washington, DC: US Department of Health and Human Services, 2008) 32.

47. E.M. Phillips, J.C. Schneider, G.R. Mercer, "Motivating elders to initiate and maintain exercise," *Arch Phys Med Rehab* 85 (2004) S52-S57.

48. T.N. Frimel, D.R. Sinacore, D.T. Villareal, "Exercise attenuates the weight-loss induced reduction in muscle mass in frail obese older adults," *Med Sci Sports Exer* 40 (2008) 1213-1219.

49. K. Shah, A. Stufflebam, T.N. Hilton, D.R. Sinacore, S. Klein, D.T. Villareal, "Diet and exercise interventions reduce intrahepatic fat content and improve insulin sensitivity in older adults," *Obesity* 126 (2009) 1-7.

50. D.T. Villareal, M. Banks, D.R. Sinacore, C. Siener, S. Klein, "Effect of weight loss and exercise on frailty in obese older adults," *Arch Intern Med* 166 (2006) 860-866.

51. R. Pendola, S. Gen, "BMI, auto use, and the urban environment in San Francisco," *Health Place* 13 (2007) 551-556.

52. E.M. Phillips, J.C. Schneider, G.R. Mercer, "Motivating elders to initiate and maintain exercise," *Arch Phys Med Rehab* 85 (2004) S52-S57.

53. K.A. Schutzewr, B.S. Graves, "Barriers and motivations to exercise in older adults," *Prev Med* 39 (2004) 1056-1061.

54. G. Dubnov, A. Brzezinski, E.M. Berry, "Weight control and the management of obesity after menopause: the role of physical activity," *Maturitas* 44 (2003) 89-101.

55. M.T. Railey, "Patterns of obesity and African-American women," *J Nat Med Assoc* 92 (2000) 481-484.

56. *"Ace personal trainer manual-American Council on Exercise,"* 3rd ed (San Diego, CA: *American Council on Exercise*, 2003) 366.

57. University of Michigan News Service, *"Pregnant women who exercise should listen to their bodies,"* http://www.ns.umich.edu/htdocs/releases/story.php?id=1271

58. A. Prentice, "Nutrition and pregnancy," *Women's Health Med* 1 (2004) 22-24.

59. V. Tsagareli, M. Noakes, R.J. Norman, "Effect of a very-low calorie diet on in vitro fertilization outcomes," *Fertil Steril* 86 (2006) 227-229.

60. A.K. Sebert-Kuhlmenn, P.M. Dietz, C. Galavotti, L.J. England, "Weight-management interventions for pregnant or postpartum women," *Am J Prev Med* 34 (2008) 523-5528.

61. N. Ochsenbein-Kolble, M. Roos, T. Gasser, R. Zimmermann, "Cross-sectional study of weight gain and increase in BMI throughout pregnancy," *Euro J Obstet Gynecol Rep Bio* 130 (2007) 180-186.

62. F. Galtier, I. Raingeard, E. Renard, P. Boulot, J. Bringer, "Optimizing the outcome of pregnancy in obese women: from pregestational to long-term management," *Diab Metab* 34 (2008) 19-25.

63. K.J. Calfas, B.H. Marcus, "Postpartum weight retention: a mother's weight to bear?" *Am J Prev Med* 32 (2007) 356-357.

64. A. Prentice, "Nutrition and pregnancy," *Women's Health Med* 1 (2004) 22-24.

65. F. Galtier, I. Raingeard, E. Renard, P. Boulot, J. Bringer, "Optimizing the outcome of pregnancy in obese women: from pregestational to long-term management," *Diab Metab* 34 (2008) 19-25.

66. A. Merlino, L. Laffineuse, M. Collin, B. Mercer, "Impact of weight loss between pregnancies on recurrent preterm birth," *Am J Obstet Gynecol* 195 (2006) 818-821.

67. A.K. Sebert-Kuhlmenn, P.M. Dietz, C. Galavotti, L.J. England, "Weight-management interventions for pregnant and postpartum women," *Am J Prev Med* 34 (2008) 523-528.

68. *"Lifestyle and weight management consultant manual-American Council on Exercise,"* (San Diego, CA: *American Council on Exercise*, 2005) 261.

69. A. Merlino, L. Laffineuse, M. Collin, B. Mercer, "Impact of weight loss between pregnancies on recurrent preterm birth," *Am J Obstet Gynecol* 195 (2006) 818-821.

70.   D. Duncombe, E.H. Wertheim, J. Skouteris, S.J. Paxton, L. Kelly, "Factors related to exercise over the course of pregnancy including women's beliefs about the safety of exercise during pregnancy," *Midwifery* 25 (2009) 4300438.

71.   D.S. Downs, H.A. Hausenblas, "Women's exercise beliefs and behaviors during their pregnancy and postpartum," *J Midwifery Womens Health* 49 (2004) 138-144.

72.   Ibid.

73.   *"2008 physicalactivity guidelines for Americans,"* (Washington, DC: US Department of Health and Human Services, 2008) 41.

74.   S. Phelan, "Pregnancy: a teachable moment for weight control and obesity prevention," *Am J Obstet Gynecol* 210 (2009) 1.e1-1.e8.

75.   T.W. Wang, B.S. Apgar, *"Exercise during pregnancy,"* (An American Academy of Family Physicians Study), http://www.aafp.org/afp/980415ap/wang.html

76.   American Pregnancy Association, *"Top recommended exercises,"* http://www.americanpregnancy. org/pregnancyhealth/toprecommendedexercises.html

77.   *"Ace personal trainer manual-American Council on Exercise,"* 3rd ed (San Diego, CA: *American Council on Exercise,* 2003) 366.

78.   T.W. Wang, B.S. Apgar, *"Exercise during pregnancy,"* (An American Academy of Family Physicians Study), http://www.aafp.org/afp/980415ap/wang.html

79.   American Pregnancy Association, *"Top recommended exercises,"* http://www.americanpregnancy. org/pregnancyhealth/toprecommendedexercises.html

80.   *"Ace personal trainer manual-American Council on Exercise,"* 3rd ed (San Diego, CA: *American Council on Exercise,* 2003) 366.

81.   *"Lifestyle and weight management consultant manual-American Council on Exercise,"* (San Diego, CA: *American Council on Exercise,* 2005) 262.

82.   S. Yeo, *"Pregnant women who exercise should listen to their bodies,"* (University of Michigan News Service 1996), http://www.ns.umich.edu/htdocs/releases/story.php?id=1271

83.   *"Fitness for two,"* (March of Dimes 1996). www.marchofdimes.com/professionals/14332_1150. asp

84.   T. Ostbye, K.M. Krause, C.A. Lovelady, M.C. Morey, L.A. Bastian, B.L. Peterson, G.K. Swamy, R.J.N. Brouwer, C.M. McBride, "Active mother's postpartum: a randomized controlled weight-loss intervention trial," *Am J Prev Med* 37 (2009) 173-180.

85.   S. Gennaro, W. Fehder, "Health behaviors in postpartum women," *Fam Community Health* 22 (2000) 16-26

86.   K.J. Calfas, B.H. Marcus, "Postpartum weight retention: a mother's weight to bear?" *Am J Prev Med* 32 (2007) 356-357.

87.   M. Maddah, B. Nikooyeh, "Weight retention from early pregnancy to three years postpartum: a study in Iranian women," *Midwifery* (2008) 1-7.

88.   H. Nuss, J. Freeland-Graves, K. Clarke, D. Klohe-Lehman, T.J. Milani, "Greater nutrition knowledge is associated with lower 1-year postpartum weight retention in low-income women," *J Am Diet Assoc* 107 (2007) 1801-1806.

89.   F.M. Kramer, A.J. Stunkard, K.A. Marshall, S. McKinney, J. Liebschutz, "Breast-feeding reduces maternal lower-body fat," *J Am Diet Assoc* 93 (1993) 429-433.

90.   "Position of the American Dietetic Association: promoting and supporting breast-feeding," *J Am Diet Assoc* 105 (2005) 810-818.

91.   D.A. Krummel, "Postpartum weight control: a vicious cycle," *J Am Diet Assoc* 107 (2007) 37-40.

92. C.M. Devine, C.F. Bove, C.M. Olson, "Continuity and change in women's weight orientations and lifestyle practices through pregnancy and the postpartum period: the influence of life course trajectories and transitional events," *Soc Sci Metab* 50 (2000) 567-582.

93. T.B. VanItallie, "Sleep and energy balance: interactive homeostatic systems," *Metab Clin Exper* 55 (2006) S30-S35.

94. *"Why do we need so much sleep,"* (msnbc.com), http://www.msnbc.msn.com/id/3076707/

95. N.L. Rogers, M.P. Szuba, J.P. Staab, D.L. Evans, D.F. Dinges, "Neuroimmunologic aspects of sleep and sleep loss" *Sem Clin Neuropsychiatry* 6 (2001) 295-307.

96. R. Klatz, R. Goldman, *"Stopping the clock: longevity for the new millennium,"* 2nd ed, (North Bergen, NJ: *Basic Health Publications, Inc.*, 2002) 305.

97. *"Why do we need so much sleep,"* (msnbc.com), http://www.msnbc.msn.com/id/3076707/

98. H.R. Colten, B.M. Altevogt editors, committee on sleep medicine and research board on health sciences policy, *"Sleep disorders and sleep deprivation: an unmet public health problem,"* (Washington, DC: The National Academies Press 2006) 20.

99. Ibid., 21.

100. K.G. Berge, *"Sleep guidelines: how many hours of sleep are enough?"* (MayoClinic.com reprints), http://www.mayoclinic.com/health/how-many-hours-of-sleep-are-enough/AN01487

101. P.C. Zee, *"The normal duration of daily sleep for different age groups,"* (Medscape Family Medicine), http://cme.medscape.com/viewarticle/511229

102. K.G. Berge, *"Sleep guidelines: how many hours of sleep are enough?"* (MayoClinic.com reprints), http://www.mayoclinic.com/health/how-many-hours-of-sleep-are-enough/AN01487

103. Ibid.

104. E.C. Hanlon, M.E. Andrzejewski, B.K. Harder, A.E. Kelley, R.M. Benca, "The effect of REM sleep deprivation on motivation for food reward," *Behav Brain Res* 163 (2005) 58-69.

105. Ibid.

106. K.L. Knutson, "Sex differences in the association between sleep and body mass index in adolescents," *J Ped* 147 (2005) 830-934.

107. C.S. Berkey, H.R.H. Rockett, G.A. Colditz, "weight gain in older adolescent females: the Internet sleep coffee and alcohol," *J Ped* 153 (2008) 635-639.

108. K.L. Knutson, K. Spiegel, P. Penev, E. Van Cauter, "The metabolic consequences of sleep deprivation," *Sleep Med Rev* 11 (2007) 163-178.

109. E. Van Cauter, K. Spiegel, E. Tasali, R. Leproult, "Metabolic consequences of sleep and sleep loss," *Sleep Med* 9 (2008) S23-S28.

110. N.S. Marshall, N. Glozier, R.R. Grunstein, "Is sleep duration related to obesity? A critical review of the epidemiological evidence," *Sleep Med Rev* 12 (2008) 289-298.

111. F. Jiang, S. Zhu, C. Yan, X. Jin, H. Bandla, X. Shen, "Sleep and obesity in preschool children," *J Ped* 154 (2009) 814-818.

112. J. Horne, "Short sleep is a questionable risk factor for obesity and related disorders: statistical versus clinical significance," *Bio Psych* 77 (2008) 266-276.

113. K.A. Stamatakis, R.C. Brownson, "Sleep duration and obesity-related risk factors in the rural Midwest," *Prev Med* 46 (2008) 439-444.

114. S. Stranges, F.P. Cappuccio, N-B Kandala, M.A. Miller, F.M. Taggart, M. Kumari, J.E. Ferrie, M.J. Shipley, E.J. Brunner, M.G. Marmot, "Cross-sectional versus prospective associations of sleep duration with changes in relative weight and body fat distribution: the Whitehall II study," *Am J Epidemiol* 167 (2007) 321-329.

115. J.E. Gangwisch, D. Malaspina, B. Boden-Albala, S.B. Heymsfield, "Inadequate sleep as a risk factor for obesity: an analysis of the NHANES I," *Sleep* 28 (2005) 1289-1296.

116. Z. Xiaozhe, " A clinical survey of acupuncture slimming," *J Trad Chin Med* 28 (2008) 139-147.

117. K.K. Khoo, "Acupuncture treatment for obesity: a randomized controlled trial," *Medical Acupuncture* 17 (2006).

118. M.T. Cabyoglu, N. Ergene, "The treatment of obesity by acupuncture," *Inter J Neuroscience* 116 (2006) 165-175.

119. Z-J Zhang, H-Y Chen, K-C Yip, R. Ng, V.T. Wong. "The effectiveness and safety of acupuncture therapy in depressive disorders: systematic review and meta-analysis," *J Affect Disord* (2009) 1-13.

120. W-F Yeung, K-F Chung, Y-K Leung, S-P Zhang, A.C.K. Law, "Traditional needle acupuncture treatment for insomnia: a systematic review of randomized controlled trials," *Sleep Med* 10 (2009) 694-704.

121. *"Massage therapy: an introduction"* (National Center for Complementary and Alternative Medicine), http://nccam.nih.gov/health/massage/

122. *"Massage information center research in massage: Glossary of research terminology"* (American Massage Therapy Association), http://www.amtamassage.org/infocenter/research_glossery-of-research-terminology.html

123. T. Field, M. Diego, M. Hernandez-Reif, "Massage therapy research," *Dev Rev* 27 (2007) 75-89.

124. G.W. Bell, "Aquatic sports massage therapy," *Clin Sports Med* 18 (1999) 427-435.

125. M.L. Hannuksela, S. Ellahham, "Benefits and risks of sauna bathing," *Am J Med* 110 (2001) 118-126.

126. M. Hutchison, *"Mega brain power: transform your life with mind machines and brain nutrients,"* (NY, NY: *Hyperion*, 1994) 316.

127. Ibid., 329.

9   The Last Resort - A Hidden Trap Awaits

In the case of the morbidly obese, their excess body weight is usually life threatening, in which case weight reduction is imperative. Many of these individuals have repeatedly attempted to lose weight using conventional techniques but have become disillusioned and frustrated by their lack of success. This chapter was written specifically for those people. I consider the therapies that follow to be extreme, (i.e. the last resort), and they are not intended for people attempting to lose a few pounds so that they might look better at an upcoming class reunion. The reason that I consider these therapies a last resort is because of the far-reaching negative health consequences associated with them. I am certain that because of the potential for fast, easy weight loss associated with some of the following techniques, many people will be tempted to make use of them, instead of making the lifestyle changes outlined in this book. As the chapter title suggests, *a hidden trap awaits* those people, who for whatever reason choose to embrace the following therapies. Read on and you will see why I believe these therapies could lead the unwary down a very slippery slope.

Prescription Drugs

Because of the huge worldwide obesity epidemic and the amount of money that could be made from an easy obesity solution, the use of prescription and over-the-counter drugs, for weight loss, has drawn a lot of attention in recent years. Many anti-obesity drugs were originally developed for the treatment of psychiatric diseases,[1] therefore they work on the nervous system rather than on digestion. As a result many of the side effects relate to anxiety, nervousness

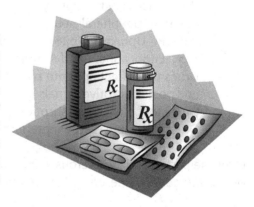

and depression. Wouldn't it be great if: (1) we could lose weight by simply taking a pill, and (2) such a pill had no side effects? Yes it would but, as you will see in the following pages, such a belief borders on pure fantasy. Developing such a drug is an extremely complicated process, because it involves a sensitive and dynamic interplay between the brain and gut. For example, peptides are a class of compounds that yield two or more amino acids,[2] and researchers have claimed that they are the main components the body uses to communicate the status of energy balance between the brain and the gut, and because of the complexity of the peripheral-neural circuitry the search for useful weight loss drugs is extremely complicated.[3] Others have shown that while there is substantial redundancy in this neural circuitry, which operates to maintain nutritional homeostasis, it is this redundancy that thwarts drug interventions.[4] In reality, "pharmacologic approaches may be helpful for some severely obese people, but will not be applicable for prevention of moderate obesity for the whole population."[5]

Let's look at one basic fact that you must understand. **All drugs have unwanted side effects**. Sometimes the side effects are known and sometimes they are unknown. Anyone who tries to convince you otherwise either doesn't know any better or is in a total state of denial. In fact Moore goes further when he says that, "there is no such thing as a safe drug."[6] Consider this! The primary function of your liver is to remove everything from your body that is biologically incompatible, (e.g. pathogens, chemicals, toxins) and this includes every chemical pharmaceutical product on the earth. Most likely you have noticed that the majority of the drug commercials on television tell you that you cannot take their product if you have liver disease. What these advertisers are really trying to convey is that if you take their product it will put a stress on your liver and for those with liver disease that stress may be life threatening. For the rest of us it is just potentially liver damaging. Furthermore, I maintain that if you don't already have liver disease but take enough of these liver-stressing chemicals, for a long enough period of time, you certainly increase the possibility of developing it.

Fundamentally there are a number of different types of anti-obesity drugs that are either currently undergoing clinical development or have in the past. They fall into the following categories:

- Drugs that affect appetite and energy regulation by influencing or controlling the brain/gut peripheral-neural circuitry, and these include:
  - Re-Uptake Inhibitors (e.g. Sibutramine),
  - Endocannabinoid Antagonists (e.g. Rimonabant),
- Drugs that affect appetite by regulating feeding behavior, which include both pre and post-absorptive signals,
- Drugs that block fat absorption (e.g. Orlistat),
- Drugs that increase the metabolism.[7]

Over the past decade numerous weight-loss drugs have been brought to market and because of the dangerous side effects, discovered after their introduction, all but a few have been removed. Some of those that have been banned from use as weight-loss drugs were initially developed for other purposes, (e.g. Bupropion - used as a depression treatment, Topiramate and Zonisamide - used as seizure treatments, and Metformin - used as a diabetes treatment).[8] Of those that remain only two, Orlistat and Sibutramine, enjoy sustained popularity, probably because they are the only ones that may be used for up to one year. It does puzzle me as to what good they might be if you can't take them for more than a year, because it's a fairly sure bet that once you stop taking them, in the absence of the appropriate lifestyle changes, you will regain the weight you have already lost. In addition, the fact that they are still legally available should not imply that they are by any means safe; wait until you see the list of related side effects. Let's take a more detailed look at some of the most well known drugs available in the US today, for the treatment of adult obesity.

Drug Name - **Orlistat**

How it works -   Orlistat, first approved in 1998 by the FDA as a gastric and pancreatic lipase inhibitor,[9] is the most popular weight-loss drug in the US today. It is the only drug in this list that is a fat inhibitor, which means that it "reduces the body's ability to absorb dietary fat by...blocking the enzyme lipase, which is responsible for breaking down dietary fat."[10] Bray showed that orilstat blocks up to 30 percent of dietary fat.[11] As the body passes this unabsorbed fat through the digestive system, it also passes a lot of unabsorbed nutrition through with it. In 2007 the FDA approved a watered-down version of orlistat, under the trade name of alli, to be sold over the counter to adults over the age of 18.[12] Once a person loses weight and progresses into the weight maintenance phase, a reasonable lifestyle modification program is as effective as the use of orlistat in helping maintain a stabilized weight.[13]

Max Usage -   one year

Side Effects -   Cramping, diarrhea, leakage of an oily stool,[14] decreased absorption of fat-soluble vitamins,[15] increased oxidative stress,[16] interference with the absorption of many drugs (e.g. warfarin, amiodarone, ciclosporin, thyroxine), hepatitis and liver failure.[17]

Drug Name - **Sibutramine**

How it works -   Sibutramine, first approved in 1997 by the FDA as an antidepressant,[18] works as an appetite suppressant, which causes its user to feel full, thereby reducing food consumption.[19]

Max Usage -   one year

Side Effects -   Increased blood pressure, increased heart rate,[20] (note this drug "should be used cautiously or avoided in the presence of vascular diseases, which are more prevalent in obese patients),"[21] constipation[22] and depression.[23]

Drug Name - **Phentermine**

How it works -   Phentermine is an appetite suppressant, which along with sibutramine are the most popular appetite suppressants in the US.[24] Phentermine is typically prescribed for use in conjunction with a very low calorie diet (i.e. usually less than 800 calories/day).[25] If you are going to eat such a starvation diet, which I would never recommend, you should lose weight without the phentermine.

Max Usage -   12 weeks

Side Effects -   Increased blood pressure, increased heart rate, sleeplessness, nervousness,[26] dry mouth, agitation, insomnia, nausea, diarrhea, and constipation.[27]

Drug Name - **Diethylpropion**

How it works -   Diethylpropion is an appetite suppressant.

Max Usage -   12 weeks

Side Effects -   Dizziness, headache, sleeplessness, nervousness,[28] increased blood pressure, blurred vision, insomnia, dry mouth, unpleasant taste, nausea and constipation.[29]

Drug Name - **Phendimetrazine**

How it works -   Phendimetrazine is an appetite suppressant.

Max Usage -   12 weeks

Side Effects -   Sleeplessness, nervousness,[30] restlessness, insomnia, agitation, increased heart rate, increased blood pressure, dry mouth, nausea, abdominal pain, constipation, diarrhea and increased urination frequency.[31]

One drug with a good side effect is orlistat, which has been shown to have a cholesterol-lowering effect, not seen in other weight-loss drugs.[32] Of course this would be significant to most people attempting to lose weight since overweight individuals frequently have high cholesterol.

Research raises a couple of additional questions:

- Short-term obesity management is more effective using pharmaceutical intervention than a diet and exercise regime,
- Sibutramine used alone is more effective than orlistat used alone,
- Orlistat and sibutramine taken together is a more effective weight-loss strategy than the use of orlistat alone, but the combination is no more effective than sibutramine taken by itself,
- The safety of orlistat and sibutramine or a combination of the two remains unclear.[33]

I realize that research studies have to be of limited scope but often times that limited scope becomes very misleading. The scope of the above mentioned research, conducted by Kaya et al, has been limited so much that it concerns me, for several reasons.

- Researchers, including Kaya, define short-term obesity intervention, as up to 12 weeks and long-term intervention from 12 weeks to one year. As noted above, the 12-week time frame matches the maximum length of time that three of the five drugs can be used. It is great that Kaya found short-term benefits, but after 12 weeks then what? What happens when you have to cycle off the drugs? If you are obese and trying to lose weight you will surely not reach your goal in 12 weeks, so who cares about what this, or any other, study claims they found in 12 weeks. It would be best to refrain from focusing on either a short-term or long-term obesity intervention and gear you're thinking for a timeframe well beyond one year. The real question is how will you reach your weight loss goal and how will you carry that success into the future?

  Kaya also talked about how they think pharmaceutical intervention is superior to a program of diet and exercise, but failed to consider how all three might complement each another. Most drug researchers today agree that the best drug induced weight-loss results are achieved when medication is used in conjunction with an integrated program of diet, exercise, and behavioral therapy.[34] I do realize that Kaya did not have the benefit of this research, since it was reported a year later, but I merely present this evidence for the benefit of you, my reader.

- While Kaya suggested that sibutramine was found to be a more effective weight-loss drug than orlistat, again later research data has shown that the drug selection process would be better if it included consideration of the patient's personality traits. For example, "patients with personality traits that imply order and consciousness may do better with orlistat, while those patients with little control over their eating habits may respond better to the satiety-enhancing properties of sibutramine."[35]

- If as Kaya suggests the safety of both orlistat and sibutramine remains unclear, why would anyone want to take them in combination? It strikes me as illogical to think that two drugs of questionable safety might become any safer if taken in combination.

Finally, there is one more drug that you need to know about. Its name is rimonabant. Rimonabant was the first selective CB_1 receptor blocker to be approved for use anywhere in the world, and it originally had the dual purpose of: (1) treating obesity, and (2) aiding in smoking cessation.[36] This drug was the darling of 18 EU countries,[37] where legal use began in 2006,[38] and was not only touted by many as the best weight-loss drug in existence, but was widely regarded as a shoe-in for US FDA approval. In 2007 rimonabant was presented to the FDA for approval,[39] but despite its popularity it wasn't without its problems. Although rimonabant has the opposite effects of another well-known CB_1 receptor influencing drug marijuana, its central nervous system altering characteristics raised serious questions.

Among the unfavorable side effects of rimonabant are: nausea, dizziness, diarrhea, insomnia,[40] upper respiratory tract infection, nasopharyngitis, influenza, arthralgia, anxiety, viral gastroenteritis, depressed mood, fatigue,[41] and suicidal thoughts.[42] Researchers raised additional concerns: (1) since the sensitive hormonal signaling system involved plays a major role in energy homeostasis rimonabant might inadvertently upset the balance,[43] and (2) rimonabant could possibly affect a number of systems unrelated to feeding.[44] Later in 2007 a committee advising the FDA voted not to recommend rimonabant for approval because of concerns over a variety of psychiatric side effects including, anxiety, depression, insomnia, panic attacks and suicidal thoughts.[45] Subsequently the manufacturer of rimonabant (Sanofi-Aventis) withdrew its request for FDA approval. In a 2008 press release, the European Medicines Agency recommended the suspension of Sanofi-Aventis' marketing authorization for rimonabant, throughout the entire EU, stating that rimonabant's benefits no longer outweigh its risks.[46] Finally, in 2009 Sanofi-Aventis voluntarily withdrew its EU marketing authorization.[47]

All of this makes me wonder about the validity of the drug approval process. How can a drug like this get to market in the first place and over a short three year period have more than 700,000 people use it,[48] only then to have all these safety issues come to light? I think I know who the real test monkeys are!

Children's Issues with Prescription Drugs

Treating childhood obesity with drugs is far different than treating adult obesity with the same drugs. These drugs can be taken by an adult but are often not tolerated well by a child's more sensitive system and/or they may be downright unsafe for a child. In fact, there are no weight loss drugs currently approved by the FDA for use in children under 12 years old. Orlistat may be prescribed for children over 12, sibutramine may be prescribed for children over 16 and a reduced strength over-the-counter version of orlistat called alli may be purchased and used by children over 18.[49] Furthermore, even if orlistat and sibutramine could be prescribed for more than one year, it is hard to visualize a person beginning in childhood and continuing to take weight loss drugs for their entire lifetime, in order to control obesity.[50]

So what if you've made your best effort to improve your lifestyle by incorporating exercise, nutritional improvement and psychological counseling. You know that your hormone levels are where they should be for your age, and perhaps you have even coupled all that with drug therapy. However you have lost little or no weight and you realize that obesity is killing you. Bariatric surgery still remains an option. But before we explore that option, understand that the health risks associated with bariatric surgery cannot be overstated. Let's take a further look.

Bariatric Surgery

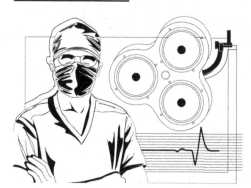

Bariatric surgery is the process of surgically altering the digestive system for the purpose of limiting the amount of food that can be eaten.[51] Not only does bariatric surgery restrict food intake but it also interferes with the body's absorption of nutrients.[52] I envision this to be a major problem, one that we typically think of as malnutrition. I seriously doubt that obese people were born with an oversized stomach that requires this kind of procedure, and I just can't give up the thought that the problem might lie elsewhere.

When you look at the list of surgery risks and complications listed below notice that protein, vitamin and mineral deficiency is listed. It gets worse, "if the malnutrition is not addressed promptly, diseases such as pellagra, beri beri and kwashiorkor may occur along with permanent damage to the nervous system."[53] Here are the two basic approaches to bariatric surgery:

- **Gastric Bypass Surgery** - is the process of surgically reducing the size and functional volume of the stomach and bypassing part of the small intestine, which leads to fewer calories being absorbed.[54] Gastric bypass surgery is the most common bariatric surgery performed in the United States, and is only recommended for people with a BMI greater than 40, or a BMI greater than 35 accompanied by serious weight related health risk factors, that might be improved by weight loss.[55] "Current evidence, although predominantly observational, consistently demonstrates greater weight loss and improvements in obesity-related conditions with...gastric bypass compared with laparoscopic adjustable gastric banding,"[56] which is discussed below. One of the positive impacts of gastric bypass surgery is that patients appear to produce less of the appetite-stimulating hormone Ghrelin, which may explain why their appetites are markedly suppressed after surgery.

The Western Pennsylvania Hospital claims that, "the risks and complications of surgical treatment of obesity are most often due to the patient's obesity related health problems."[57] In order to help alleviate this situation the hospital encourages their patients to improve their health status prior to surgery, and among the improvements suggested is that they want their patients to lose weight.[58] One obvious question is, if the patient could lose weight why would they need the surgery? In any event, here are some of the surgery risks and complications experienced by Western Pennsylvania Hospital:

- Death,
- Pulmonary embolism (i.e. the closure of the pulmonary artery or one of its branches),
- Gastrointestinal tract leakage,
- Bowel obstruction,
- Excessive scar tissue where the stomach pouch connects to the bowel,
- Internal bleeding, at the site of the surgery,
- Ulcers,
- Gallstones,
- Infections,
- Protein, vitamin and mineral deficiency,
- Failure of weight loss,
- Weight gain,
- Too much weight loss,
- Chronic symptoms of nausea, vomiting and abdominal pain,
- Depression,
- Hypoglycemia,
- Kidney failure,
- Kidney stones.[59]

Some claim these two should be added:
- Anxiety,
- Body image dissatisfaction.[60]

- **Laparoscopic Adjustable Gastric Banding** - is the process of reducing the size of the stomach by placing a small band around the stomach's entrance to restrict the volume of incoming food.[61] Use of the laparoscopic band is the preferred approach in Australia and Europe.[62] Laparoscopic banding is often preferred over gastric bypass surgery because: (1) it is minimally invasive,[63] (2) results in a shorter hospital stay,[64] (3) is totally reversible,[65] and (4) is performed from outside the abdomen by the insertion of a laparoscope through small incisions, which makes it a much simpler procedure than the more invasive open abdominal gastric bypass surgery.[66] The early US experience reported a high complication rate and poor weight loss results using the lap band, however more recent data is more encouraging.[67] Although the amount of weight lost may not be as great or occur as fast as it does with gastric bypass surgery, it still is clinically meaningful and rarely associated with life-threatening complications.[68]

Here are some of the surgery risks and complications experienced by the University of California, San Diego Medical Center:

- o Band leakage,
- o Reflux or vomiting,
- o Erosion of the band into the stomach,
- o Difficulty swallowing,
- o Enlargement of the stomach pouch,
- o Band slippage,
- o Dehydration,
- o No weight loss,
- o Blockage of the stomach outlet,
- o Bloating,
- o Nausea,
- o Constipation,
- o Ulceration,
- o Weight regain,
- o Gastritis,
- o Death.[69]

One final thought if you're considering bariatric surgery. There are a number of physicians who are minimizing the invasiveness of typical gastric bypass surgery by utilizing a laparoscopic technique. Morbidly obese patients may receive the benefits of full-blown gastric bypass surgery without the necessity of such an invasive procedure,[70] and this procedure has spread to Asia where it is rapidly becoming the preferred bariatric surgery.[71]

Children's Issues with Bariatric Surgery

If a child between the ages of 2-18 years old has a BMI between the 85th and 95th percentile for their age and gender, steps should be taken to improve that situation. If on the other hand their BMI is over the 95th percentile for their age and gender or their BMI is greater than 30, whichever is the smaller number, they are obese and their weight must be reduced.[72] To determine your child's BMI, BMI data tables and calculators have been developed that will give you that information. Go online and Google BMI calculator to find many of them. To determine what percentile your child's BMI falls in compared to other children, you may need to consult a professional, (e.g. doctor, school nurse) or you may be also able to find that information on the Internet. In any event these are some of the parameters that your doctor will use to help determine if and what corrective action needs to be taken to help your child lose weight.

The possibility of subjecting a child to bariatric surgery presents some unique challenges. There are five specific challenges that need to be included in any successful childhood weight management plan:

- Involve the whole family in a healthy lifestyle,
- Monitor and adjust the program to avoid malnutrition,
- Minimize overly strict or unpalatable food choices or schedules,
- Work to improve the possibilities for success in school, work, social and family relationships,
- Since the child's entire lifetime is ahead of him/her, maintain vigilance for new and emerging obesity treatments.[73]

If all avenues have been explored unsuccessfully and the child continues to gain weight beyond what is normal for his/her age and gender, bariatric surgery may be considered, but it must be regarded as the last resort. Between 1996 and 2003 slightly over 2700 adolescent bariatric surgeries were performed, with this surgery occurring with increasing frequency each year from 1996 to 2003 and culminating in a total of 771 procedures in 2003.[74] Although juvenile bariatric surgery is not a wildly popular idea in the US, even though it is more widely accepted elsewhere, (e.g. Australia),[75] it is gaining more acclaim in the US as one tool in the arsenal for reducing the risks associated with morbid obesity in adolescents,[76] and for improving health related quality of life.[77]

If you choose bariatric surgery for your child, there are ethical considerations that should be a basic part of the operating system of the pediatric hospital that will be caring for him/her. One suggestion is that there should be:

- "Sufficient oversight of clinical and research activities,
- Provision of adequate resources for comprehensive pre-and postoperative care,
- Administrative leadership that keeps abreast of the short and long-term clinical outcomes."[78]

It is imperative that you the parent understand the heavy burden that you bear in protecting your child's interests, should you decide on a weight loss plan of action as severe as bariatric surgery.

Liposuction

Since the goal of this book is health enhancing weight loss rather than fat removal for cosmetic purposes, I have only included the following discussion of liposuction to provide you with a basic understanding of the topic, not to promote its use. Liposuction is a popular cosmetic surgery,[79] most often performed by a plastic surgeon,[80] resulting in the removal of localized fat deposits,[81] from just under the skin.[82] "In 2006, liposuction was the most common cosmetic surgery performed in the United States."[83] Good candidates for liposuction are people who generally:

- Are average or only slightly above average in body weight,
- Are in good health,
- Have small fat concentrations that don't respond well to diet or exercise,[84]
- Have fat deposits that are out of proportion to the rest of the body, and are located in body areas with minimal amounts of excess skin.[85]

Like other surgeries liposuction is not risk-free. Here are some of the risks listed by the US National Library of Medicine in conjunction with the National Institute of Health (NIH):

- Shock (usually when not enough fluid is replaced during the surgery),
- Fluid overload,
- Infections,
- Bleeding and blood clots,
- Fat embolism (i.e. tiny globules of fat in the bloodstream that block blood flow),
- Nerve, skin, tissue, organ damage or burns from the heat of the instruments used,
- Uneven fat removal resulting in a lumpy look,
- Drug reactions,
- Scarring.[86]

Should liposuction be of interest to you, consult your physician for more details.

Summary

The topic of extreme weight loss measures rarely arises without the discussion being accompanied by the necessity of concurrent lifestyle changes. Some research has made this point very clear by saying, "a lifestyle-based weight loss program that includes dietary changes, increased physical activity, and behavioral therapy is the cornerstone of treatment for overweight and obesity. Pharmacotherapy may be added if lifestyle interventions alone are insufficient. For morbidly obese individuals, bariatric surgery may be an appropriate option when combined with long-term lifestyle modifications."[87] In plain words drug therapy or bariatric surgery should not be attempted until all possible lifestyle changes have been proven ineffective.

The basic rules for the use of prescription weight loss medications are that:

- They should only be used by patients who are at increased medical risk because of their weight,
- They should not be used for the purpose of cosmetic weight loss,
- They should only be used after extensive lifestyle interventions have been exhausted,[88]
- From a safety standpoint, obesity treatment products need special consideration before their use because, "few other diseases have such a poor pharmaceutical safety record,"[89] and this poor safety record is frequently expressed as unacceptable side effects.[90]

The most extreme obesity treatment is obviously bariatric surgery. Since this group of procedures is fraught with so many negatives it must be selected as the treatment of choice with the utmost of caution. Researchers claim that bariatric surgery is neither practical nor desirable as a treatment for obesity, since this intervention has not produced consistently effective long-term weight loss.[91] Not only does it result in unsatisfactory weight loss, it has been shown to have no beneficial effect on mortality.[92] Another major drawback to bariatric surgery is that the patient frequently suffers from nutritional malabsorption also know as malnutrition.[93] To me bariatric surgery makes about as much sense as deciding that you can save gas by putting less in your car's tank. For those that do turn to bariatric surgery, one great way to ensure you get adequate nutrition is by juicing. Buy a juicer, juice a lot of vegetables, (with a limited amount of fruit sprinkled in) and consume at least 12-24 ounces of juice per day.

The biggest difficulty with drugs and surgery for the obese is in trying to apply these tools to children and adolescents. These techniques rarely work the same on a child as they do on an adult. In some cases the side effects may be very severe. In other cases some of these techniques are illegal to use on a child. Not only is the utmost caution suggested in choosing one of these techniques for a child, but also the physician selection process becomes even more important. These techniques should only be applied to an adult as a last resort, and to a child as a life saving measure.

Endnotes

1. R.A.H. Adan, L.J.M.J. Vanderschuren, S.E. la Fleur, "Anti-obesity drugs and neural circuits of feeding," *Trends Pharma Sci* 29 (2008) 208-217.
2. "Peptide," *Dorland's Illustrated Medical Dictionary*, 30th ed: 1396.
3. H. Mendieta-Zeron, M. Lopez, C. Dieguez, "Gastrointestinal peptides controlling body weight homeostasis," *Gen Compar Endocrinol* 155 (2008) 481-495.
4. E. Valassi, M. Scacchi, F. Cavagnini, "Neuroendocrine control of food intake," *Nutri Metab Cardio Dis* 18 (2008) 158-168.

5. S.C. Grundy, "Multifactorial causation of obesity: implications for prevention," *Am J Clin Nutr* 67 (1998) 563S-572S.

6. T,J. Moore, *"Prescription for Disaster,"* (NY, NY: *Simon & Schuster,* 1998) 21.

7. J.C.G. Halford, "Obesity drugs in clinical development," *Cur Opin Invest Drugs* 7 (2006) 312-318.

8. Weight-Control Information Network - The National Institute of Diabetes and Digestive and Kidney Diseases (NIDDK) in conjunction with the National Institute of Health, *"Prescription medications for the treatment of obesity,"* http://win.niddk.nih.gov/Publications/prescription.htm

9. R.S. Padwal, S.R. Majumdar, "Drug treatments for obesity: orlistat, sibutramine, and rimonabant," *Lancet* 369 (2007) 71-77.

10. Weight-Control Information Network - The National Institute of Diabetes and Digestive and Kidney Diseases (NIDDK) in conjunction with the National Institute of Health, *"Prescription medications for the treatment of obesity,"* http://win.niddk.nih.gov/Publications/prescription.htm

11. G.A. Bray, "A concise review on the therapeutics of obesity," *Nutrition* 16 (2000) 953-960.

12. Weight-Control Information Network - The National Institute of Diabetes and Digestive and Kidney Diseases (NIDDK) in conjunction with the National Institute of Health, *"Prescription medications for the treatment of obesity,"* http://win.niddk.nih.gov/Publications/prescription.htm

13. J. Woo, M.M.M. Sea, P. Tong, G.T.C. Ko, Z. Lee, J. Chan, F.C.C. Chow, "Effectiveness of the lifestyle modification programme in weight maintenance in obese subjects after cessation of treatment with orlistat," *J Eval Clin Prac* 13 (2007) 853-859.

14. Weight-Control Information Network - The National Institute of Diabetes and Digestive and Kidney Diseases (NIDDK) in conjunction with the National Institute of Health, *"Prescription medications for the treatment of obesity,"* http://win.niddk.nih.gov/Publications/prescription.htm

15. G.A Bray, D.H. Ryan, "Drug treatment of the overweight patient," *Gastroenterology* 132 (2007) 2239-2252.

16. O. Ozcelik, Y. Ozkan, F. Karatas, H. Kelestimur, "Exercise training as an adjunct to orlistat therapy reduces oxidative stress in obese subjects," *Tohoku J Exp Med* 206 (2005) 313-318.

17. T.D. Filippatos, C.S. Derdemezis, I.F. Gazi, E.I. Nakou, D.P. Mikhailidis, M.E. Elisaf, "Orlistat associated adverse effects and drug interactions: a critical review," *Drug Safety* 31 (2008) 53-65.

18. R.S. Padwal, S.R. Majumdar, "Drug treatments for obesity: orlistat, sibutramine, and rimonabant," *Lancet* 369 (2007) 71-77.

19. Weight-Control Information Network - The National Institute of Diabetes and Digestive and Kidney Diseases (NIDDK) in conjunction with the National Institute of Health, *"Prescription medications for the treatment of obesity,"* http://win.niddk.nih.gov/Publications/prescription.htm

20. Ibid.

21. W.Y.S. Leung, G.N. Thomas, J.C.N. Chan, B. Tomlinson, "Weight management and current options in pharmacotherapy: orlistat and sibutramine," *Clin Ther* 25 (2003) 58-80.

22. A. Avenell, T.J. Brown, M.A. McGee, M.K. Campbell, A.M. Grant, J. Broom, R.T. Jung, W.C.S. Smith, "What interventions should we add to weight reducing diets in adults with obesity? A

systematic review of randomized controlled trials of adding drug therapy, exercise, behavior therapy or combinations of these interventions," *J Human Nutr Diet* 17 (2004) 293-316.

23. K. Elfhag, S. Rossner, B. Barkeling, P. Rooth," Sibutramine treatment in obesity: initial eating behavior in relation to weight loss results and changes in mood," *Pharmacol Res* 51 (2005) 159-163.

24. Weight-Control Information Network - The National Institute of Diabetes and Digestive and Kidney Diseases (NIDDK) in conjunction with the National Institute of Health, "*Prescription medications for the treatment of obesity*," http://win.niddk.nih.gov/Publications/prescription.htm

25. Z. Li, K. Hong, I. Yip, S. Huerta, S. Bowerman, J. Walker, H. Wang, R. Elashoff, V. Liang, D. Heber, "Body weight loss with phentermine alone versus phentermine and fenfluramine with very-low-calorie diet in an outpatient obesity management program: a retrospective study," *Curr Ther Res* 64 (2003) 447-460.

26. Weight-Control Information Network - The National Institute of Diabetes and Digestive and Kidney Diseases (NIDDK) in conjunction with the National Institute of Health, "*Prescription medications for the treatment of obesity*," http://win.niddk.nih.gov/Publications/prescription.htm

27. S.B. Moyers, "Medications as adjunct therapy for weight loss: approved and off-label agents in use," *J Am Diet Assn* 105 (2005) 948-959.

28. Weight-Control Information Network - The National Institute of Diabetes and Digestive and Kidney Diseases (NIDDK) in conjunction with the National Institute of Health, "*Prescription medications for the treatment of obesity*," http://win.niddk.nih.gov/Publications/prescription.htm

29. S.B. Moyers, "Medications as adjunct therapy for weight loss: approved and off-label agents in use," *J Am Diet Assn* 105 (2005) 948-959.

30. Weight-Control Information Network - The National Institute of Diabetes and Digestive and Kidney Diseases (NIDDK) in conjunction with the National Institute of Health, "*Prescription medications for the treatment of obesity*," http://win.niddk.nih.gov/Publications/prescription.htm

31. S.B. Moyers, "Medications as adjunct therapy for weight loss: approved and off-label agents in use," *J Am Diet Assn* 105 (2005) 948-959.

32. E. Mannucci, I. Dicembrini, F. Rotella, C.M. Rotella, "Orlistat and sibutramine beyond weight loss," *Nutr Metab Cardio Dis* 18 (2008) 342-348.

33. A. Kaya, N. Aydin, P. Topsever, M. Filiz, A. Ozurk, A. Dagar, E. Kilinc, C. Ekmekcioglu, "Efficacy of sibutramine, orlistat and combination therapy on short-term weight management in obese patients," *Biomed Pharmacotherapy* 58 (2004) 582-587.

34. T.A. Wadden, R.I. Berkowitz, L.G. Womble, D.B. Sarwer, S. Phelan, R.K. Cato, L.A. Hesson, S.Y. Osei, R. Kaplan, A.J. Stunkard, "Randomized trial of lifestyle modification and pharmacotherapy for obesity," *New England J Med* 353 (2005) 2111-2120.

35. G. Wittert, I. Caterson, N. Finer, "The clinical effectiveness of weight loss drugs," *Obes Res Clin Prac* 1 (2007) 1-5.

36. R.S. Padwal, S.R. Majumdar, "Drug treatments for obesity: orlistat, sibutramine, and rimonabant," *Lancet* 369 (2007) 71-77.

37. Press Release Sanofi Aventis, "Sanofi-aventis is complying with the EMEA's recommendation to temporarily suspend the marketing authorisation of Acomplia in obese and overweight

patients," http://www.acomplia.com/acl/cx/medias/D934A348-65E0-4115-AED6-89578F366C13.pdf

38. European Medicines Agency (Press Release), *"The European Medicines Agency recommends suspension of the marketing authorisation of Acomplia (Rimonabant),"* http://www.ema.europe.eu/humandocs/PDF's/EPAR/acomplia/53777708en.pdf

39. Weight-Control Information Network - The National Institute of Diabetes and Digestive and Kidney Diseases (NIDDK) in conjunction with the National Institute of Health, *"Prescription medications for the treatment of obesity,"* http://win.niddk.nih.gov/Publications/prescription.htm

40. R.S. Padwal, S.R. Majumdar, "Drug treatments for obesity: orlistat, sibutramine, and rimonabant," *Lancet* 369 (2007) 71-77.

41. G.A Bray, D.H. Ryan, "Drug treatment of the overweight patient," *Gastroenterology* 132 (2007) 2239-2252.

42. BBC News, *"Suicide risk fears over diet pill,"* http://news.bbc.co.uk/2/hi/health/6755665.stm

43. I. Matias, L. Cristino, V. Di Marzo, "Endocannabinoids: some like it fat (and sweet too)," J *Neuroendocrinol* 20 (2008) 100-109.

44. J.C.G. Halford, "Obesity drugs in clinical development," *Cur Opin Invest Drugs* 7 (2006) 312-318.

45. BBC News, *"Suicide risk fears over diet pill,"* http://news.bbc.co.uk/2/hi/health/6755665.stm

46. Press Release - European Medicines Agency, *"The European Medicines Agency recommends suspension of the marketing authorisation of Acomplia (Rimonabant),"* http://www.ema.europe.eu/humandocs/PDFs/EPAR/acomplia/53777708en.pdf

47. Press Release Sanofi Aventis, "Sanofi-aventis is complying with the EMEA's recommendation to temporarily suspend the marketing authorisation of Acomplia in obese and overweight patients," http://www.acomplia.com/acl/cx/medias/D934A348-65E0-4115-AED6-89578F366C13.pdf

48. Ibid.

49. MayoClinic.com, *"Childhood Obesity; Treatments and Drugs,"* http://www.mayoclinic.com/health/childhood-obesity/DS00698/DSECTION=treatments-and-drugs

50. H.R. Berthoud, C. Morrison, "The brain, appetite and obesity," *Annual Rev Psych* 59 (2008) 55-92.

51. MayoClinic.com, *"Gastric Bypass Surgery,"* http://www.mayoclinic.com/health/gastric-bypass/my00825

52. Weight-Control Information Network - The National Institute of Diabetes and Digestive and Kidney Diseases (NIDDK) in conjunction with the National Institute of Health, *"Bariatric Surgery for Severe Obesity,"* http://win.niddk.nih.gov/publications/gastric.htm

53. Ibid.

54. WebMD, *"Weight Loss Surgery Health Center - Gastric Bypass,"* http://www.webmd.com/diet/weight-loss-surgery/gastric-bypass

55. MayoClinic.com, *"Gastric Bypass Surgery,"* http://www.mayoclinic.com/health/gastric-bypass/MY00825/DSECTION=why-its-done

56. J.A. Tice, L. Karliner, J. Walsh, A.J. Petersen, M.D. Feldman, "Gastric banding or bypass? a systematic review comparing the two most popular bariatric procedures," *Am J Med* 121 (2008) 885-893.

57. Bariatric surgery at the Western Pennsylvania Hospital, *"Risks and Complications of Gastric Bypass Surgery,"* http://www.bariatricsurgerypittsburgh.com/surgery/risks.html

58.   Ibid.

59.   Ibid.

60.   T.A. Wadden, M.L. Butryn, D.B. Sarwer, A.N. Fabricatore, C.E. Crerand, P.E. Lipschutz, L. Faulconbridge, S.E. Raper, N.N. Williams, "Comparison of psychosocial status in treatment-seeking women with class III versus class I-II obesity," *Obesity* 12 (2006) 90S-98S.

61.   Weight-Control Information Network - The National Institute of Diabetes and Digestive and Kidney Diseases (NIDDK) in conjunction with the National Institute of Health, "*Bariatric Surgery for Severe Obesity,*" http://win.niddk.nih.gov/publications/gastric.htm

62.   J.A. Tice, L. Karliner, J. Walsh, A.J. Petersen, M.D. Feldman, "Gastric banding or bypass? a systematic review comparing the two most popular bariatric procedures," *Am J Med* 121 (2008) 885-893.

63.   W-J Lee, W. Wang, P-L Wei, M-T Huang, "Weight loss and improvement of obesity-related illness following laparoscopic adjustable gastric banding procedure for morbidly obese patients in Taiwan," *J Formos Med Assn* 105 (2006) 887-894.

64.   J.D. Evans, M.H. Scott, A.S. Brown, J. Rogers, "Laparoscopic adjustable gastric banding for the treatment of morbid obesity," *Am J Surgery* 184 (2002) 97-102.

65.   L. Meyer, S. Rohr, J. Becker, A. Pradignac, C. Meyer, J.L. Schlienger, C. Simon, "Retrospective study of laparoscopic adjustable silicone gastric banding for the treatment of morbid obesity: results and complications in 127 patients," *Diabetes Metab* 30 (2004) 53-60.

66.   J.W. Allen, M.G. Coleman, G.A. Fielding, "Lessons learned from laparoscopic gastric banding for morbid obesity," *Am J Surgery* 182 (2001) 10-14.

67.   J.A. Holloway, G.A. Forney, D.E. Gould, "The lap-band is an effective tool for weight loss even in the United States," *Am J Surgery* 188 (2004) 659-662.

68.   H. Spivak, M.F. Hewitt, A. Onn, E.E. Half, "Weight loss and improvement of obesity-related illness in 500 U.S. patients following laparoscopic adjustable gastric banding procedure," *Am J Surgery* 189 (2005) 27-32.

69.   University of California, San Diego Medical Center, Center for the Treatment of Obesity, "*Gastric Band Surgery - Risks,*" http://health.ucsd.edu/specialties/lapband/about/risks.htm

70.   L. Biertho, R. Steffen, T. Ricklin, F.F. Horber, A. Pomp, W.B. Inabnet, D. Herron, M. Gagner, "Laparoscopic gastric bypass versus laparoscopic adjustable gastric banding: a comparative study of 1200 cases," *J Am Coll Surgeons* 197 (2003) 536-547.

71.   W-J Lee, "Surgical treatment of obesity: an Asian perspective," *Tzu Chi Med J* 19 (2007) 200-206.

72.   S.E. Barlow and the expert committee, "Expert committee recommendations regarding the prevention, assessment, and treatment of child and adolescent overweight and obesity: summary report" *Pediatrics* 120 (2007) S164-S192.

73.   A.F. Browne, T. Inge, " How young for bariatric surgery in children," *Seminars Ped Surgery* 18 (2009) 176-185.

74.   W.S. Tsai, T.H. Inge, R.S. Burd, "Bariatric surgery and adolescents: recent national trends in use and in-hospital outcome," *Arch Ped Adolescent Med* 161 (2007) 217-221.

75.   J.B. Dixon, K. Jones, M. Dixon, "Medical versus surgical interventions for the metabolic complications of obesity in children," *Seminars Ped Surgery* 18 (2009) 168-175.

76.   E.P. Nadler, S. Reddy, A. Isenalumhe, H.A. Youn, V. Peck, C.J. Ren, G.A. Fielding, "laparoscopic adjustable gastric banding for morbidly obese adolescents affects android fat loss, resolution of comorbidities, and improved metabolic status," *J Am Coll Surgeons* 209 (2009) 638-644.

77. T.J. Loux, R.N. Haricharan, R.H. Clements, R.L. Kolotkin, S.E. Bledsoe, B. Haynes, T. Leath, C.M. Harmon, "Health-related quality of life before and after bariatric surgery in adolescents," *J Ped Surgery* 43 (2008) 1275-1279.

78. D.A. Caniano, "Ethical issues in pediatric bariatric surgery," *Seminars Ped Surgery* 18 (2009) 186-192.

79. Medline Plus, *"Liposuction,"* http://www.nlm.nih.gov/medlineplus/ency/article/002985.htm

80. The American Society for Aesthetic Plastic Surgery, *"Liposuction (Lipoplasty),"* http://www.surgery.org/consumers/procedures/body/liposuction

81. "Liposuction," *Dorland's Illustrated Medical Dictionary*, 30th ed: 1058.

82. *"Lifestyle and weight management consultant manual-American Council on Exercise,"* (San Diego, CA: *American Council on Exercise*, 2005) 176.

83. M.W. Mann, M.D. Palm, R.D. Sengelmann, "New advances in liposuction technology," *Seminars Cutan Med Surgery* 27 (2008) 72-82.

84. WebMD, *"Cosmetic Procedures and Liposuction,"* http://www.webmd.com/skin-beauty/guide/cosmetic-procedure-liposuction

85. The American Society for Aesthetic Plastic Surgery, *"Liposuction (Lipoplasty),"* http://www.surgery.org/consumers/procedures/body/liposuction

86. Medline Plus, *"Liposuction,"* http://www.nlm.nih.gov/medlineplus/ency/article/002985.htm

87. C.P. Cannon, A. Kumar, "Treatment of overweight and obesity: lifestyle, pharmacologic, and surgical options," *Clin Cornerstone* 9 (2009) 55-71.

88. Weight-Control Information Network - The National Institute of Diabetes and Digestive and Kidney Diseases (NIDDK) in conjunction with the National Institute of Health, *"Bariatric Surgery for Severe Obesity,"* http://win.niddk.nih.gov/publications/gastric.htm

89. E.G. Jackson, "Eating order: a 13-week trust model class for dieting casualties," *J Nutr Ed Behav* 40 (2008) 43-48.

90. D. Cooke, S. Bloom, "The obesity pipeline: current strategies in the development of anti-obesity drugs," *Nat Rev Drug Discovery* 5 (2006) 919-931.

91. R.S. Padwal, S.R. Majumdar, "Drug treatments for obesity: orlistat, sibutramine, and rimonabant," *Lancet* 369 (2007) 71-77.

92. A.J. Walley, A.I.F. Blakemore, P. Froguel, "Genetics of obesity and the prediction of risk for health," *Hum Mole Gen* 15 (2006) R124-R130.

93. S.P. Davison, M.W. Clemens. "Safety first: precautions for the massive weight loss patient," *Clin Plastic Surgery* 35 (2008) 173-183.

10   Summary - What Action to Take Now

You obviously took time to read this book because you have an interest in the subject of weight loss. I also addressed health because the two are inseparable. By now you realize that:

- "Obesity alone is not a disease,"[1]
- By itself weight loss is seldom the complete solution for treating chronic medical conditions,[2]
- The loss of excess body weight can play an important role in the prevention and elimination of many diseases.

Living a long, healthy and happy life seems to be a common interest throughout mankind. Here are four weight related factors that have been estimated to add years to your life, if you control them properly. One important thing to notice is that they are additive.[3]

Adding Years to Your Life	
Factor	**Live More Years**
Maintain Normal Weight	+11.0
Remain Non-Diabetic	+6.6
Maintain Normal Blood Pressure	+3.7
Exercise Regularly	+2.4[4]
Sub Total Potential	**23.7 yrs**

Here's one additional non-weight related factor worth considering:

Factor	Live More Years
Non-Smokers Add Years of Life (Men +13.2 & Women +14.5)	
Average Men & Women	+13.8[5]
Grand Total Potential	**37.5 yrs**

We also know that people who try to lose weight often thwart their own effort because they do not use the correct combination of caloric restriction and exercise,[6] coupled with the behavioral and hormonal considerations that they need in order to be successful.

Now we will precisely distill the knowledge you have gained from the previous chapters into one simple, cohesive set of tactics that will allow you to: (1) effectively construct your own personal weight loss plan, and (2) successfully implement it.

Remember the Basic Rules

There are a number of considerations in any weight loss effort but I believe the following two are paramount:

- **There is No Single Answer** - Many would have you believe that if you eat a certain diet, engage in a certain exercise regime, take certain drugs or have your intestinal system surgically revamped, you will lose weight, look good and live happily ever after. It is true that any one of these may give you a quick, short-term result, but over time all suffer the same fatal flaw, their benefits simply aren't sustainable. Even if they were, any single approach is so lopsided that it becomes unhealthy. The answer lies in incorporating a sensible, personalized, never-ending, balanced lifestyle that will work for you. For that lifestyle to be optimal, during its development it must consider all of the following:

  o Your personal genetics,
  o Proper food planning,
  o Appropriate exercise,
  o Any behavioral modifications needed,
  o Personal support you might require (e.g. family, friends, support group),
  o Your hormone profile,
  o Possible last resort measures like drugs or surgery.

Losing weight is like the US trying to break its dependency on foreign oil. There are many possible approaches. Any one by itself is nothing more than a band-aid on a wound that really requires stitches, but several logically selected choices taken in the aggregate will get a more satisfactory result.

• **Control Calorie Intake / Output** - The hallmark of losing weight is the act of burning more calories than you consume! Once you reach your desired weight you must balance your caloric intake with the amount of calories than you burn, in order to remain at that weight. Put another way you must remain vigilant with regard to the difference between the total number of calories in the food you eat, compared to the total number of calories your body is burning during your daily activities. As you already know I am not an advocate of counting calories, one simple way to control caloric intake is by following my Rule of Thirds (identified in chapter 3). The secret lies in eating the right foods and eating them in the right quantities. Scientists have shown that chocolate doesn't make your clothes shrink.

Evaluate Your Readiness for Change

A critical component of success in any weight loss program is to ensure that you are ready to make the changes necessary. Many times in life circumstances beyond your control can present a roadblock to even the best-laid weight-loss plan. Here are some examples:

• Generally during a pregnancy your doctor will not let you undertake a severely restrictive food plan or an aggressive new exercise regime.

• If you are suffering from a major emotional upheaval in your life (e.g. a death in the family, a divorce, a job loss) you may not be emotionally prepared to undertake the rigors of a weight-loss program.

You must recognize these impediments and deal with them appropriately.

If you are working with an experienced lifestyle and weight management coach he/she should conduct an in-depth assessment of your readiness for change. In doing so they may inquire into your: (1) personal history, (2) dieting history, (3) exercise history, (4) psychological history, (5) psychosocial history, (6) health and medical history, and (7) they may examine your current eating and exercise patterns.[7] If you are working alone or in a small group, complete the *Self-Evaluation of Readiness for Weight Loss* portion of the *Weight Loss Plan*, discussed below and proceed as directed. The first key factor to recognize is that not everyone is prepared to plow headlong into a weight-loss program without first correcting some long-standing issues, that could easily derail such an effort. The second important factor and the one most critical to you is to understand that if you are the person I am talking about, you must recognize the problem, face it head on, and get the help you need.

Here is an example of what I mean. As discussed in chapter 5, if you are 50, 75, 100 or more pounds overweight, it may be a mistake to start a weight loss program without first understanding your true psychological condition. Dealing with that situation rationally and honestly will enable you to take more deliberate and effective steps toward resolving your weight problem.

Goal Setting

Goal setting is an absolutely critical part of any successful weight management program, and most authorities agree that it is vital to not only target specific weight loss objectives, but those targets must precisely focus on the long term behavior changes that are needed in order to accomplish those objectives.[8] For example, it is not enough to think that you would like to lose 10, 20, 30, or more pounds, but the plan must pinpoint exactly which areas of your life pressure must be brought to bear. Looking down the road towards the end result is wonderful, but make sure to focus on the incremental steps required to remove the barriers that stand in the way of achieving that result. Examples might be to: (1) reduce the fat intake in your diet, (2) reduce the total calories you consume, (3) begin an exercise program.

There are a number of barriers that can inhibit successful obesity management strategies. Among them are: (1) a failure to recognize obesity as a chronic condition, (2) a low socioeconomic status, (3) time constraints, (4) intimate saboteurs, and (5) a wide range of health challenges including mental health dysfunction, sleep deprivation, chronic pain, and musculoskeletal, cardiovascular, respiratory, digestive and endocrine disorders.[9] A failure to identify and address any of these barriers can cause you to experience a continuing sense of failure and frustration, which often undermines an already potentially low self-esteem and negative sense of self-efficacy.[10]

- **Set Achievable Goals**
  As mentioned in an earlier chapter, the hallmark of any reachable goal is that it must be: (1) specific, (2) measurable, (3) achievable, (4) realistic/relevant, and (5) time bound. Frequently in the realm of weight loss specific goals that can be measured over a defined period of time are relatively easy to establish. The much bigger issue becomes how realistic is the goal? "One of the biggest challenges in the clinical management of obese patients is addressing the significant disparity between the actual and expected weight losses."[11] Successful weight-loss interventions focus on modest weight losses, which include improvements in body image and eating behaviors and result in healthier psychological and eating behavioral characteristics.[12] It has been claimed many times by numerous professionals that a ten percent weight loss is a success,[13] however I am inclined to argue that a ten

percent weight loss may prove excessive for some people and woefully inadequate for many others. Strategy rich goals should be:

- o   The result of an honest appraisal of what a realistic body weight is for you, based on your age, sex, gender, ethnicity, etc., and not on what you might consider your ideal body weight to be,

- o   Based on an incremental approach, where small measurable steps can be achieved on the way to the final overriding goal. Be sure to incorporate as many small improvement steps as possible because the satisfaction of accomplishing those incremental goals will motivate you to continue the process.

- **Implement the Changes Needed**
Once the plan is developed it does you no good if it isn't implemented. You must proceed to implement the plan immediately before you lose interest or become distracted. At this point implementation of necessary changes should have been adequately considered and should contain well-defined, measurable outcomes. Be careful not to try and force yourself to implement extraneous elements that were not originally incorporated in the plan, because all that will do is introduce useless stress that well distract you from execution of the real plan.

- **Develop a Strong Support System**
Social support, given to you by your family, friends, coworkers and/or others, results from your knowing that you are part of a community of people who love and care for you and value what you think and do. For support to be effective you must understand it and believe it to be supportive. Those that you select for support will be critical to your success. You must use great care to surround yourself with people you can count on to be a positive influence, while carefully avoiding the negative forces in your life. Many people you might think would willingly support your effort may for whatever reason find it in their own personal interest to sabotage you. For example, it might be natural to assume that family members would want to support your weight loss effort. However, if they also have a weight problem, as you become more successful they may feel weak, unmotivated or lazy, if other people are constantly making comparisons between the two of you. It might be wise to select your supporting cast from people who you can easily distance yourself from should true, effective support fail to materialize.

- **Monitor Your Progress**
Once you develop your plan and begin to work it, it becomes important to monitor your progress. Monitoring your progress is akin to driving to a neighboring town that is 50 miles away, with the knowledge that it will take you about 50 minutes to

get there. You will most likely check your progress by periodically looking at your car's odometer and clock. Likewise you must keep a close eye on your weight-loss progress, which can be done by utilizing such simple measures as: (1) employing my <u>Belt Hole Rule</u>, (2) looking in the bathroom mirror, and (3) weighing yourself occasionally.

As you will see in the last section of this chapter an important part of evaluating your progress is keeping ongoing records. Through the review of accurate historical data you will understand where you were and how far you've come. If you try to rely on your memory alone you may fool yourself into thinking you are making better progress than you really are, or you may have made more progress than you can recall. Either situation can prove detrimental to your effort.

Equally important to monitoring your progress is making midcourse adjustments to your plan, when you discover you are not making satisfactory progress. Even the very best plans must be flexible enough to allow for adjustment as changes in circumstances dictate. Never be reluctant to change a plan that isn't working.

Finally, your monitoring may periodically reveal that forward progress has stopped or that you have actually taken a step backward. Lapses are certain to occur in almost every weight-loss program, and should be viewed as an expected part of the process of developing a healthy new lifestyle.[14] Whatever you do don't let a lapse or even a series of lapses permanently derail your overall program. Lapses can serve as signals you may need additional professional help. Use a lapse as a learning tool, not an excuse to beat yourself up or abandon the program.

- **Maintain, Maintain, Maintain**
  Once you have reached your target bodyweight the game shifts from one of weight loss to one of weight maintenance. The good news is that you should find the weight maintenance phase to be easier than the weight-loss phase. You have been in a struggle, perhaps for an extended period of time, to reach this desirable and rewarding goal, but now the struggle becomes less intense. While the weight maintenance phase could be thought of as a holding pattern, all too often those who have lost weight use the success of goal achievement as an endpoint where they stop doing the things that got them there, and return to their previously unhealthy lifestyle. Along with that original lifestyle comes the return of the weight that was lost, often accompanied by additional weight.

By the maintenance phase you will have learned new habits that worked for you in the weight-loss phase, and now for you to be successful going forward you must continue to employ many of them, to whatever extent is necessary to maintain your body weight. These new habits have at a minimum incorporated changes in diet and exercise[15] that must become a part of your long-term strategy. I realize that may sound intimidating, unexciting, time-consuming, demanding and not very glamorous, but keep in mind that everything of value in life is a trade off, the process of giving up one thing to get another.

Several factors predict success with weight maintenance. Among them are:

o   Maintaining ongoing contact with weight management professionals,
o   Exercise adherence,
o   Extent of body weight monitoring,[16] since frequent self-weighing is part of a group of behaviors associated with dietary restraint, decreases in disinhibition, and decreases in depressive symptoms.[17]

Because of the potential monotony of the weight maintenance phase, this phase becomes more mentally challenging than was the weight-loss phase. I believe those who construct little self-serving games out of the various aspects of weight maintenance have the most success. For example, I make use of a rowing machine several times a week where I row for a half hour at a time. My goal is to warm up for five to ten minutes at which point I am working at my target rate of 80 percent VO_{2max}. From that point I continue until I have reached the 30 minute mark, at which time I cool down for two or three minutes and stop. Before I reach the end of the session I am tired, sweating heavily, and finding that hard little seat that I am sitting on to be increasingly annoying, so it goes without saying that I seldom find this event to be some kind of euphoric intoxication.

Here is what I do: I visualize myself leading the pack in a prestigious rowing race. To win I simply have to continue my tempo for the duration in order to stay ahead of the pack, which I do every time. Sure it's a game of mental gymnastics, but it works effectively for me and similar mental games can work for you as well. My hope is that you too can create ways of visualizing yourself as the successful winner that you were created to be. In the long run you will never be a bigger winner than you are when you shed those excess pounds, improve your health and remain strong, mobile and active, well into old age.

Putting it all Together - Proceeding From Here

As we reach the end of this book the most important information is yet to come. One of the biggest limitations of most weight-loss interventions today is they: (1) remain one dimensional, (2) lack individualization, (3) present few options for participants, and (4) generally cannot easily be adapted to the personal characteristics of the individual.[18] Your personal weight loss plan cries out for input that only you can provide. Any weight loss plan that lacks your input and is not completely customized to meet your individual needs should be shunned, because it will make your struggle much more difficult and will not achieve the result you want.

Because of this reality, I have developed a series of simple tools that will help you construct and activate your own personalized plan. The tools are comprised of the following:

- Three flowcharted plans identified as the *Week 1 Plan*, the *Week 2 & 3 Plan*, and the *Week 4 & Beyond Plan*. Notice that these plans are in a simple flowcharted format, instead of written paragraphs. The reason flowcharts were used is that you will find them easier to understand. As you look at them you will see each one contains three different shaped boxes, which have the following meaning:

  o   A rectangle signifies a simple step in the process,
  o   A diamond signifies a decision point where a question is asked, frequently resulting in a yes or no answer,
  o   A rectangular shaped box with a squiggly line on the bottom signifies the creation of a record or the completion of a form.

You will also find two additional forms that will be an integral part of your planning and execution. They are:

  o   A *Calorie Consumption Diary*,
  o   A *Weight Loss Plan*.

You will work back-and-forth between the three Weekly Plans, the Calorie Consumption Record and the Weight Loss Plan, as directed in the Weekly Plans. Let's take a look at how that will work.

The Planning Phase

Objective #1 - Determine Readiness for Weight Loss
Steps to Take
1.   Review boxes 1-3 on <u>Week 1 Plan</u>
2.   Complete p1 of <u>Weight Loss Plan</u>
3.   Determine your readiness to proceed. If you are not ready to proceed, make necessary adjustments and re-evaluate your readiness. If you are ready to proceed, move to objective #2

Objective #2 - Gather Personal Foundational Data
Steps to Take
1. Review boxes 4-6 on <u>Week 1 Plan</u>
2. Complete top 1/2 of p2 of <u>Weight Loss Plan</u>
3. Move to objective #3

Objective #3 - Determine Need for Psychological Counseling
Steps to Take
1. Review boxes 7-11 on <u>Week 1 Plan</u>
2. Begin preparing bottom 1/2 of p2 <u>Weight Loss Plan</u>
3. Move to objective #4

Objective #4 - Gather Trend Data Regarding Eating Habits
Steps to Take
1. Review box 12 on <u>Week 1 Plan</u>
2. Document everything that you eat and drink, for the next seven - ten days on the <u>Calorie Consumption Diary</u>
3. Move to objective #5

Objective #5 – Determine Possible Need for Physical Exam
Steps to Take
1. Review boxes 13-15 on <u>Week 1 Plan</u>
2. Begin preparing top 1/3 of page 3 of <u>Weight Loss Plan</u>
3. Move to objective #6

Week 1 Plan

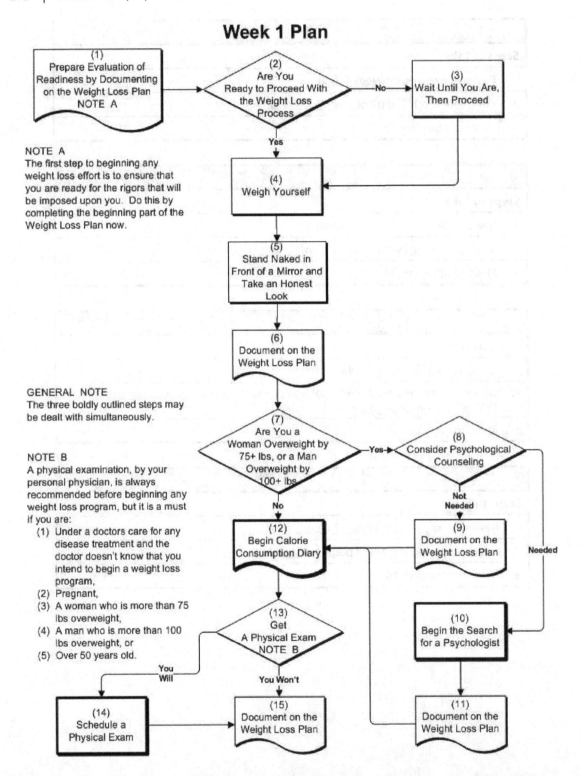

NOTE A
The first step to beginning any weight loss effort is to ensure that you are ready for the rigors that will be imposed upon you. Do this by completing the beginning part of the Weight Loss Plan now.

GENERAL NOTE
The three boldly outlined steps may be dealt with simultaneously.

NOTE B
A physical examination, by your personal physician, is always recommended before beginning any weight loss program, but it is a must if you are:
(1) Under a doctors care for any disease treatment and the doctor doesn't know that you intend to begin a weight loss program,
(2) Pregnant,
(3) A woman who is more than 75 lbs overweight,
(4) A man who is more than 100 lbs overweight, or
(5) Over 50 years old.

Weight Loss Plan

Name _____ Age _____ Date _____

On Each Line Circle Your Yes or No Answer to the Question

Self-Evaluation of Readiness for Weight Loss

<u>Personal History</u>

Are Your Parents Overweight	Yes	No
Are Your Siblings Overweight	Yes	No
Were You Overweight as a Child	Yes	No

<u>Health and Medical History</u>

Do You Have Any of the Following

High Blood Pressure	Yes	No
High Cholesterol	Yes	No
Stroke	Yes	No
Cardiovascular Disease	Yes	No
Heart Disease	Yes	No
Diabetes	Yes	No
Arthritis	Yes	No
Alzheimer's / Parkinson's	Yes	No
Autoimmune Disease	Yes	No

Note: If You Circled Any of the Spotted Yes Boxes, Get Your Doctor's Approval Before Proceeding

<u>Dieting History</u>

Have You Dieted Before		Yes	No		
If Yes - How Many Diets	1	2	3	4	5+
Most Pounds Lost on Any Diet	0 - 5	5 to 10	10 to 20	20 to 40	40+
Are You Currently on a Diet		Yes	No		

<u>Exercise History</u>

Have You Exercised Regularly Before		Yes	No		
If Yes - Was it in a Fitness Center		Yes	No		
Did You Work With a Personal Trainer		Yes	No		
How Many Months of Help Did You Get	0 to 1	1 to 2	2 to 4	4 to 6	6+
Are You Currently Exercising Regularly		Yes	No		

<u>Current Eating Pattern</u>

Do You Have Anorexia or Bulimia	Yes	No
Do You Eat 25% of Your Food After Dinner	Yes	No
Do You Eat When You Are Under Stress	Yes	No
Do You Binge Eat	Yes	No

How Many Shaded Boxes Did You Circle _____

Key   0 to 8 - You Should be OK to Proceed
9 to 12 - You Are Urged to Consider Psychological Counseling
13 to 16 - You Are Strongly Urged to Obtain Psychological Counseling

Additional Data and Observations

Actual Body Weight (in Lbs.) _____

Reasonable Body Weight _____

How Overweight are You _____

What Did You See in the Mirror

Explain _____

_____

_____

_____

What Do You Want to See

Explain _____

_____

_____

_____

Psychological Counseling

Do You Need Psychological Counseling   Yes   No

If No
Explain _____

_____

_____

_____

                                                          Select
                                                          One

If Yes:

Psychologists Considered _____ ☐

_____ ☐

_____ ☐

Counseling Scheduled to Begin   Date _____

Physical Exam

<u>Do You Need a Physical Exam</u>   Yes   No

If No
Explain   _____

     _____

     _____

     If Yes: Exam Scheduled For   Date   _____

Personal Trainer

<u>Do You Need a Personal Trainer</u>   Yes   No

If No
Explain   _____

     _____

     _____

                                                      Select
                                                      One
     If Yes:
          Trainers Considered   _____   ☐

                              _____   ☐

                              _____   ☐

          Exercise Scheduled to Begin   Date   _____

Note: Do Not Begin Exercising Without a Doctor's Approval to Proceed

Nutritionist

<u>Do You Need a Nutritionist</u>   Yes   No

If No
Explain   _____

     _____

     _____

                                                      Select
                                                      One
     If Yes:
          Nutritionists Considered   _____   ☐

                              _____   ☐

                              _____   ☐

          Counseling Scheduled to Begin   Date   _____

Goal Setting & Monitoring

Date Goal Set _____

Goal Setting Guidelines

1. A Reasonable Weight Loss Goal is No More than 5% - 10% of Total Bodyweight
   (Once the Goal is Reached, a New or Different One Can be Set)
2. Maximum Effective Weight Loss is 1 - 2 Pounds Per Week
3. 95% of the Time, Dieting Alone Results in Failure

Goal	Bodyweight Goal	Pounds _____	Date _____

How Frequently Will You Monitor Your Progress _____

When Will You Set New / Different Goals   Date _____

What Dietary Changes Will You Make

Explain   _____

_____

_____

What Exercise Changes Will You Make

Explain   _____

_____

_____

What Stress Reduction Changes Will You Make

Explain   _____

_____

_____

Monitoring - How Are You Doing

Result   _____   Date _____

Result   _____   Date _____

Result   _____   Date _____

Result   _____   Date _____

Result   _____   Date _____

Calorie Consumption Diary

Name _____

Date	Item Consumed (Includes Both Food and Drinks)	How Much	When
____	_____	____	____
____	_____	____	____
____	_____	____	____
____	_____	____	____
____	_____	____	____
____	_____	____	____
____	_____	____	____
____	_____	____	____
____	_____	____	____
____	_____	____	____
____	_____	____	____
____	_____	____	____
____	_____	____	____
____	_____	____	____
____	_____	____	____
____	_____	____	____
____	_____	____	____
____	_____	____	____
____	_____	____	____
____	_____	____	____
____	_____	____	____
____	_____	____	____
____	_____	____	____
____	_____	____	____
____	_____	____	____

Comments _____

_____

Objective #6 – Determine Possible Need for Personal Trainer
Steps to Take
1. Review boxes 1 – 3 on <u>Week 2 & 3 Plan</u>
2. Begin preparing center 1/3 of page 3 of <u>Weight Loss Plan</u>
3. Move to objective #7

Objective #7 – Evaluate Your Current Diet
Steps to Take
1. Review boxes 4 – 7 on <u>Week 2 & 3 Plan</u>
2. Review your <u>Calorie Consumption Record</u> to see if you can determine detrimental trends. Proceed to make adjustments by removing excess fats, sugar, etc.)
3. Move to objective #8

Objective #8 – Determine Possible Need for a Nutritionist
Steps to Take
1. Review boxes 8 – 10 on <u>Week 2 & 3 Plan</u>
2. Begin preparing bottom 1/3 of page 3 of <u>Weight Loss Plan</u>
3. Move to objective #9

Objective #9 – Begin Using <u>Rule of Thirds</u>
Steps to Take
1. Review boxes 11 – 13 on <u>Week 2 & 3 Plan</u>
2. Begin following <u>Rule of Thirds</u> when you eat
3. Move to objective #10

Week 2 & 3 Plan

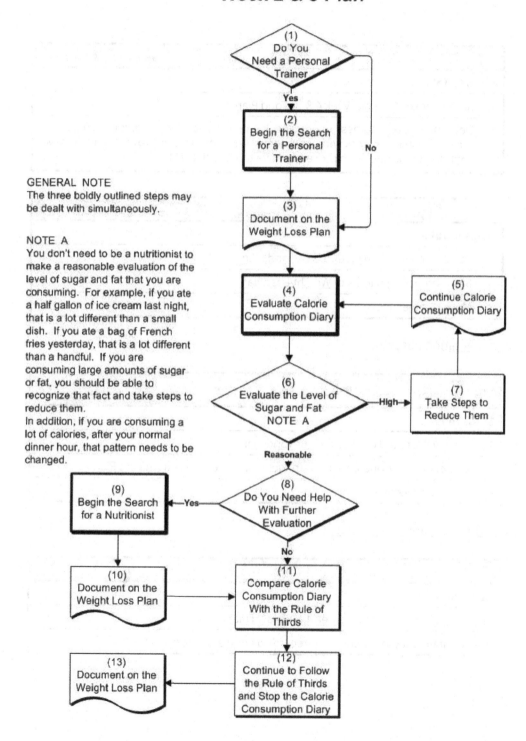

GENERAL NOTE
The three boldly outlined steps may be dealt with simultaneously.

NOTE A
You don't need to be a nutritionist to make a reasonable evaluation of the level of sugar and fat that you are consuming. For example, if you ate a half gallon of ice cream last night, that is a lot different than a small dish. If you ate a bag of French fries yesterday, that is a lot different than a handful. If you are consuming large amounts of sugar or fat, you should be able to recognize that fact and take steps to reduce them.
In addition, if you are consuming a lot of calories, after your normal dinner hour, that pattern needs to be changed.

(1) Do You Need a Personal Trainer

(2) Begin the Search for a Personal Trainer

(3) Document on the Weight Loss Plan

(4) Evaluate Calorie Consumption Diary

(5) Continue Calorie Consumption Diary

(6) Evaluate the Level of Sugar and Fat NOTE A

(7) Take Steps to Reduce Them

(8) Do You Need Help With Further Evaluation

(9) Begin the Search for a Nutritionist

(10) Document on the Weight Loss Plan

(11) Compare Calorie Consumption Diary With the Rule of Thirds

(12) Continue to Follow the Rule of Thirds and Stop the Calorie Consumption Diary

(13) Document on the Weight Loss Plan

Objective #10 – Ensure Doctors Approval of Your Program
Steps to Take
1. Review boxes 1 – 2 on <u>Week 4 & Beyond Plan</u>
2 Determine your readiness to proceed. If you don't have your doctor's approval to proceed, you must work with your doctor until you have approval. If you do have your doctor's approval to proceed, move to objective #11

Objective #11 - Establish Specific Goals
Steps to Take
1. Review boxes 3-4 on <u>Week 4 & Beyond Plan</u>
2. Begin preparing page 4 of <u>Weight Loss Plan</u>
3. Move to objective #12

The Implementation Phase

Objective #12 - Determine Psychologist, Personal Trainer and/or Nutritionist, if Required, and Implement Plan
Steps to Take
1. Review boxes 5-9 on <u>Week 4 & Beyond Plan</u>
2. Complete appropriate sections (pages 2 and 3) of the <u>Weight Loss Plan</u>
3. Move to objective #13

The Execution and Monitoring Phase

Objective #13 - Work Plan and Monitor Your Results
Steps to Take
1. Review boxes 10-11 on <u>Week 4 & Beyond Plan</u>
2. Maintain ongoing monitoring records p4 of <u>Weight Loss Plan</u>

Week 4 & Beyond Plan

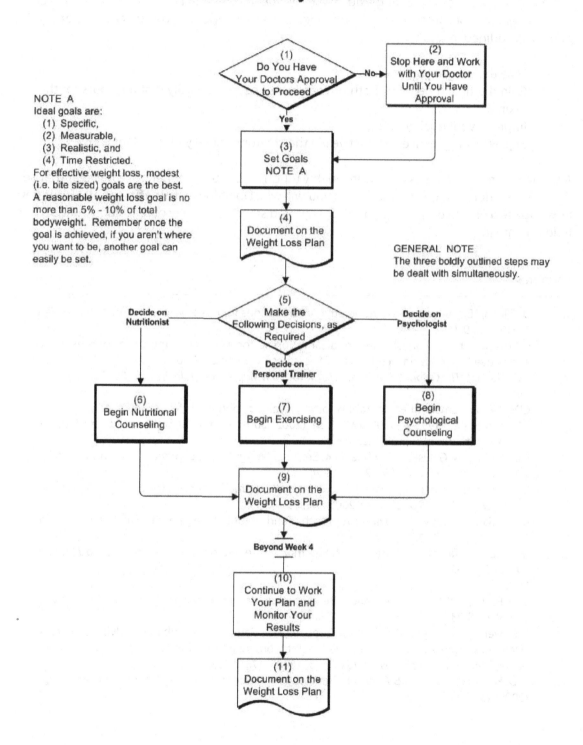

NOTE A
Ideal goals are:
(1) Specific,
(2) Measurable,
(3) Realistic, and
(4) Time Restricted.
For effective weight loss, modest (i.e. bite sized) goals are the best. A reasonable weight loss goal is no more than 5% - 10% of total bodyweight. Remember once the goal is achieved, if you aren't where you want to be, another goal can easily be set.

GENERAL NOTE
The three boldly outlined steps may be dealt with simultaneously.

(1) Do You Have Your Doctors Approval to Proceed

(2) Stop Here and Work with Your Doctor Until You Have Approval

No

Yes

(3) Set Goals NOTE A

(4) Document on the Weight Loss Plan

(5) Make the Following Decisions, as Required

Decide on Nutritionist

Decide on Psychologist

Decide on Personal Trainer

(6) Begin Nutritional Counseling

(7) Begin Exercising

(8) Begin Psychological Counseling

(9) Document on the Weight Loss Plan

Beyond Week 4

(10) Continue to Work Your Plan and Monitor Your Results

(11) Document on the Weight Loss Plan

By now you have a good idea of the personal benefits you can achieve by losing excess body weight. You also have at your fingertips the tools, techniques and knowledge that you need to make weight loss become a reality in your life. I sincerely hope that you successfully apply the principles outlined in this book to:

- Lose the weight you desire,
- Gain the health benefits, both physically and psychologically that are yours for the taking,
- Improve your quality of life,
- Enjoy the long, active, productive life the creator originally planned for you.

Although there will be times that are invariably tough, and you'll experience setbacks and lapses, if you remain determined and motivated you will win. Don't forget **this effort is all about you, and your success**, so don't let anybody or anything stand in the way of reaching your goal and holding onto it.

Endnotes

1. D. Ciliska, "Evaluation of two nondieting interventions for obese women," *West J Nursing Res* 20 (1998) 119-135.
2. P. Ernsberger, R.J. Koletsky, "Biomedical rationale for a wellness approach to obesity: an alternative to a focus on weight loss," *J Soc Issues* 55 (1999) 221-260.
3. S.G. Aldana, "*The Culprit & the Cure*," (Mapleton, UT: *Maple Mountain Press*, 2005) 6.
4. Ibid.
5. CDC, "Annual smoking-attributable mortality, years of potential life lost and economic costs---United States, 1995—1999" MMWR 51 (2002) 300-303, also http://www.cdc.gov/mmwr/preview/mmwrhtml/mm5114a2.htm
6. E.C. Weiss, D.A. Galuska, L.K. Khna, M.K. Serdula, "Weight-control practices among US adults, 2001-2001," *Am J Prev Med* 31 (2006) 18-24.
7. "*Lifestyle and weight management consultant manual-American Council on Exercise*," (San Diego, CA: *American Council on Exercise*, 2005) 50.
8. K.L-M Liao, "cognitive-behavioral approaches and weight management: an overview," *J Royal Society Prom Health* 120 (2000) 27-30.
9. M. Mauro, V. Taylor, S. Wharton, A.M. Sharma, "Barriers to obesity treatment," *Euro J Int Med* 19 (2008) 173-180.
10. Ibid.
11. G.D. Foster, A.P. Makris, B.A. Bailer, "Behavioral treatment of obesity," *Am J Clin Nutr* 82supp (2005) 230S-235S.
12. V. Provencher, C. Begin, M-P Gagnon-Girouard, H.C. Gagnon, A. Tremblay, S. Bolvin, S. Lemieux, "Defined weight expectations in overweight women: anthropometrical, psychological and eating behavioral correlates," *Intl J Obes* 31 (2007) 1731-1738.
13. G.D. Foster, A.P. Makris, B.A. Bailer, "Behavioral treatment of obesity," *Am J Clin Nutr* 82supp (2005) 230S-235S.

14. *"Lifestyle and weight management consultant manual-American Council on Exercise,"* (San Diego, CA: *American Council on Exercise*, 2005) 60.

15. S. Ziebland, J. Robertson, J. Jay, A. Neil, "Body image and weight change in middle age: a qualitative study," *Intl J Obes* 26 (2002) 1083-1091.

16. *"Lifestyle and weight management consultant manual-American Council on Exercise,"* (San Diego, CA: *American Council on Exercise*, 2005) 114.

17. R.R. Wing, D.F. Tate, A.A. Gorin, H.A. Raynor, J.L. Fava, J. MacHan, "Stop regain: are there negative effects of daily weighing," *J Counsult Clin Psych* 75 (2007) 652-656.

18. P.J. Teixeira, S.B. Going, L.B. Houtkooper, E.C. Cussler, C.J. Martin, L.L. Metcalfe, N.R. Finkenthal, R.M. Blew, L.B. Sardinha, T.G. Lohman, "Weight loss readiness in middle-aged women: psychosocial predictors of success for behavioral weight reduction," *J Behav Med* 25 (2002) 499-523.

Appendix

How to Find Help

It is important to be able to find the help you need, in addition to the list of professionals you may already know. Here are some helpful suggestions.

<u>Medical Doctors</u>

Since an understanding of hormone function and balance may be critical to your success you may want to find a medical doctor who is either board-certified in:

- Endocrinology, or
- Anti-Aging.

If you have exhausted all other possibilities and bariatric surgery is the only remaining option you will need help in finding a qualified and experienced surgeon.

The following methods will work equally well for any of the three medical specialties mentioned:

- Get a referral from your primary care physician.
- Get a recommendation from a friend or relative. Most of the time you will still need a referral from a primary care physician, in order to get an appointment with the specialist.
- Search the Yellow Pages in your local telephone book.
- Search the Internet. In the Google Search Window enter the words *Find a Local Doctor*. Dozens of web sites will appear, leaving you with many good options. In most cases you will be able to enter your zip code or city name and find someone close-by. Again, you may need to have your primary care physician refer you to the specialist of your choice.

- Local, state or federal medical directories. If you have access to one of these hard copy directories, you will find them to work much like your local Yellow Pages.
- American Medical Association
  515 N. State Street
  Chicago, IL 60654
  800-621-8335
  http://www.ama-assn.org/ama/pub/patients/patients.shtml

Psychologists

Here are some ways to find a psychologist:

- Get a recommendation from a friend or relative.
- Search the Yellow Pages in your local telephone book.
- Search the Internet. In the Google Search Window enter the words *Find a Local Psychologist*. Dozens of web sites will appear, leaving you with many good options. In most cases you will be able to enter your zip code or city name and find someone in your local area.
- American Psychological Association
  750 First Street NE
  Washington, DC 20002-4242
  800-374-2721
  http://www.apa.org/topics/obesity/index.aspx

Nutritionists

Here are some ways to find a nutritionist:

- Get a referral from your primary care physician.
- Get a recommendation from a friend, relative or exercise professional.
- Search the Yellow Pages in your local telephone book.
- Search the Internet. In the Google Search Window enter the words *Find a Local Nutritionist*. Dozens of web sites will appear, leaving you with many good options. In most cases you will be able to enter your zip code or city name and find someone in your local area.
- International and American Associations of Clinical Nutritionists
  15280 Addison Road, Suite 130
  Addison, TX 75001
  972-407-9089
  http://www.iaacn.org/
- The Nutritionists Directory
  http://nutritionists.healthprofs.com/cam/

<u>Personal Trainers</u>

Here are some ways to find a personal trainer:

- Get a recommendation from a friend or relative.
- Search the Yellow Pages in your local telephone book.
- Search the Internet. In the Google Search Window enter the words *Find a Local Personal Trainer*. Dozens of web sites will appear, leaving you with many good options. In most cases you will be able to enter your zip code or city name and find someone in your local area.
- National Federation of Professional Trainers
  PO Box 4579
  Lafayette, IN 47903
  800-729-6378
- American Council on Exercise
  4851 Paramount Drive
  San Diego, CA 92123
  888-825-3636
  http://www.acefitness.org
- National Strength and Condition Association
  1885 Bob Johnson Drive
  Colorado Springs, CO 80906
  800-815-6826
  http://www.nsca-lift.org

Index

A

absence of protection model 4
accelerated starvation in pregnancy 227
action planning 193
acupuncture 235
adenosine triphosphate 4
adipogenesis 16
adiponectin 162
adjustment disorder 114
adult-onset diabetes 77
aerobic 84
aerobic capacity 80, 84
aerobic exercise 75, 77, 80, 82, 84, 85, 86, 88
Aldana, S.G. 70
altered fats 26, 45, 57, 58
Alzheimers disease xxvii
American Council on Exercise ix, 287
American Heart Association 57
American Pregnancy Association 229
anaerobic 84
anaerobic exercise 84, 85, 93
anaerobic metabolism 5
anaerobic threshold 84
anorexia athletica 121
anorexia nervosa 121, 122
anti-obesity drugs 245
arterial elasticity 75
atherosclerosis xxix, 82
Atkins diet 28, 59
auditory visual stimulation devices 237
autoimmune disease 77, 82

B

Ballantine, R. 44
bariatric surgery 251
basal metabolic rate 10

behavioral contract 132
behavioral cue 185
behavioral factors xxix, 18
behavior Initiation 133
behavior maintenance 134
Bennett, B 222
Bennett, W. 6
beta oxidation 54, 71
binge eating disorder syndrome 123
binge eating/purging type 121
bio-available hormones 166
bioelectric impedance 9
bio-identical, hormones 166
blood test 165
body composition 7, 15, 43, 72, 77, 90, 156
body image dissatisfaction 105, 106, 252
body mass index (BMI) 5, 8, 162
body type 7
bone density 79, 80, 81, 157, 230
bone mass 79, 80, 81
bone mineral density 79, 80, 157
brain atrophy xxx
bulimia nervosa 122
Burrows, M. 81
Bush, R.A. 81

C

calorie 17, 26, 32, 50, 58, 72, 74, 109, 113, 223, 227, 233, 248
cancer 75
Capsaicin 33
carbohydrates 25, 28, 29, 36, 40, 42, 54, 57, 113, 116, 163
cardiovascular disease xxvii, 70, 73, 74, 156, 158
Center for Disease Control (CDC)

235
Central Michigan University ix
central resistance model 4
Chantre, P. 55
cholesterol xxvii, 5, 29, 40, 46, 55, 58, 83, 134, 155, 248
chromosomes 14, 15
chronic stress 111
civilization syndrome 111
Cleveland Clinic 82
clinical depression 114
clustering of risk factors xxviii
cognitive behavioral therapy 123, 124
cognitive decline xxvii
cognitive restructuring 112, 132
comfort foods 113
co-morbid 78
complete protein 43
complex carbohydrates 42
conflictual family relationships 106
coping planning 193
coronary artery calcification xxix
corticotropin-releasing hormone (CRH) 164
cortisol 112, 163
cost-benefit analysis 185
c-reactive protein 117
creatine phosphate 84
Cushing Syndrome 112
cynical hostility 116
cytokines 117, 154

D

deadly quartet xxvii
dehydroepiandrosterone (DHEA) 163
dementia 79
depressed mood 114
depression xxvii, 43, 79, 111,

114, 134, 166, 195, 236
diabetes 76
diabetes mellitus 76
diet 26
dietary fiber 29, 57
diethylpropion 248
disability limitation 220
discipline xxii, 177, 182, 204
disuse atrophy 80
DNA 14, 19, 77
dopamine 109
drug 16, 25, 30, 37, 41, 77, 122, 224, 245
dysmetabolic syndrome xxvii

E

eating disorders 118
ectomorphic 7
ego depletion 183
empty calories 49
endocannabinoid system 110
endocrine system 154
endomorphic 7
endorphins 73
endothelial cells 74
entropy xxii, 3
environmental cues 132
environmental factors 8, 16, 137
Erasmus, U. 44
erectile dysfunction xxvii
essential amino acids 43
essential fats 28, 30, 40, 41
essential fatty acids 41
estrogen 157
European Medicines Agency 250
exercise 69

F

false hope 192
fantasy realization theory 188
fasting glucose xxvii, xxviii
fat xx, xxv, xxviii, 5, 13, 25, 28, 34, 40, 49, 57, 70, 111, 121, 130, 156, 160, 246, 255

fat balance 71
fat free mass 9
fat gene 14
fat oxidation 54, 71, 93
fatty degeneration 40
fight or flight response 112
financial incentives 133
Fishbach, A. 179
fitting the norms of appearance perspective 115
five why 194
Food and Drug Administration (FDA) 235
food label 57
Frawley, D. 53
free testosterone 156

G

gastric bypass surgery 251
gene 15
General Motors Institute ix
genetic viii, xxv, 5, 13, 94
glucocorticoid therapy 81
glucose 76
glucose tolerance xxix, 77, 89
glycemic index 26, 29, 42
glycemic load 28, 59
goal achievement 190
goal maintenance 190
goal orientation 187
goal representations 185
goal setting 132, 186
goal setting theory 187
gray matter 108
green tea 33, 55
grehlin 160
group support 199
growth hormone 158
Gurin, J. 6

H

health action process approach 188
health at every size approach 134
health belief model 130

health locus of control 131
health risk factors xxviii, 71, 158, 251
heart disease 74
heart rate recovery 75
high blood pressure xxvii
Hind, K. 81
Holmes, S. 31
hoodia 56
hoodia gordonii 56
hormone replacement therapy 166
hormones 153
hormone substitution therapy 166
Horne, J. 233
Hubert, M. 39
hydrogenated 38, 45
hydrostatic weighing 9
hyperthyroidism 155
hypogonadism 157
hypothalamic-pituitary-adrenal (HPA) axis 111
hypothyroidism 155

I

incomplete protein 43
infant development 227
inflammation 49, 73, 82, 117, 166
insoluble fiber 57
Institute of Medicine xxxi
insulin 76
insulin-dependent diabetes 77
insulin resistance xxvii, xxviii, 76, 108, 155, 158, 162
insulin resistance syndrome xxvii
International Agency for Research on Cancer 75
interpersonal therapy 125
interpersonal vulnerability 106
inverse dose response 72

J

jolly fat hypothesis 116

juicing 256
juvenile-onset diabetes 77

K

Kaiser Family Foundation 222
Koo, M. 179
Kretschmer, E. 116
kwashiorkor 31, 251

L

laparoscopic adjustable gastric
 banding 252
lapses 133, 268
Latham, G.P. 187
law of stimulus-response 177
Layman, D.K. 43
lean body mass 8, 9, 157, 158
lean muscle mass 7, 10, 32, 35,
 70, 72, 80, 86, 87
learning goal orientation 187
left ventricular hypertrophy 74
leptin 160
light/sound machine 237
lipid metabolism 16, 164
liposuction 255
Locke, E.A. 178, 187
low calorie diet 27, 248
low self-esteem 33, 106, 115,
 118, 122, 128

M

Macdonald, A. 193
macronutrients 25
major depression 114
major depressive disorder 114
marasmus 31
March of Dimes 229
marijuana 110
massage therapy 236
maternal morbidity 227
maximum oxygen consumption
 84
maximum oxygen uptake 84
meal skipping 34
medical nutrition therapy 37

melatonin 163
mental contrasting 183
mesomorphic 7
metabolic rate 10, 35, 87, 155,
 225
metabolic syndrome xxvii, 162
metabolism 10
metformin 157
mind machines 237
mind technology 110
mitochondria 4, 71
modified fats 46
monoamine-oxidase inhibitors
 117
mortality xxvii, xxix, 73, 75, 117,
 122, 227, 232, 256
motivation xxii, 16, 109, 130,
 178, 188, 195, 203, 227

N

National Institute of Health (NIH)
 235, 255
National School Lunch Program
 223
natural foods 38
negative caloric balance 59
neurovegetative symptoms 124
Nielsen Company 222
night eating/drinking syndrome
 126
night eating syndrome 125
nocturnal sleep related eating
 disorder 126
nocturnal snacking 126
nonessential amino acids 43
nonessential fats 40
non-insulin-dependent diabetes
 77
nutrients 25
nutrition facts 57

O

obesity xvii, xix, xxv, 4, 8, 71, 76,
 83, 94, 110, 114, 154, 227,
 235, 245, 249, 263, 286
omega-3 26, 40, 41

omega-6 26, 41, 44
optimism 193
orlistat 247
Ornish diet 59
osteoporosis xxvii, 80
outcome expectancies 191
over active thyroid 155
overweight xix, xxv, 8, 13, 26,
 38, 72, 86, 131, 155, 190,
 200, 223, 248

P

Palfai, T. 193
parathyroid hormone 164
partially hydrogenated 45
perceived health risk 191
perfectionism 193
performance goal orientation
 187
Perricone, N. 82
personal identity 201
phendimetrazine 248
phentermine 248
physical activity 69
plurimetabolic syndrome xxvii
portion control 60
portion distortion 60
preterm birth 227
progesterone 157
protein 10, 25, 28, 43, 57, 81,
 158

R

rate of perceived exertion 229
reflected self-appraisal
 perspective 115
repair and restoration theory
 231
resting energy expenditure 158
resting metabolic rate 10, 32, 35
restrained eating 113
restraint pathway 106
restricting type 121
rimonabant 250
runner's high 73

S

saliva test 165
Sanofi-Aventis 250
sarcopenia xxvii
sauna 236
schema 194
secretagogues 159
selective serotonin reuptake
     inhibitors 117, 126
self-control 183
self-defeating behavior 184
self determination theory 188
self-directed dieting 31
self-discipline 182
self-efficacy 131
self-efficacy appraisals 185
self-help groups 199
self-monitoring 132
self-regulation 182
set point theory xxii, 6
sex hormone binding globulin
     156
Sheldon, W. 7
sibutramine 247
simple carbohydrates 42
skin fold measurements 9
sleep apnea xxvii
SlimFast 55
Snyder, C.R. 188
social cognitive theory 188
social comparison theory 127
social identity 201
social reinforcement 106
social support 133, 199
soluble fiber 57
somatic cells 15
somatotype 7
Sothern, M.S. 222
steam room 236
stress 111, 135
stress hormone 112, 163
stress management 133
Stunkard, A.J. 125
support systems xxii
syndrome X xxvii
synthetic hormones 166

systolic blood pressure xxviii, 5

T

testosterone 156
theory of compensation 206
theory of planned behavior 178
theory of social network
     substitution 206
theory of the reasoned action
     178
thermic effect of activity 33
thermic effect of food 32
thermogenesis 32, 34
thermogenic response 54
Thomas M. Cooley Law School
     ix
thrifty gene 13
thyroid - hyperthyroid 155
thyroid - hyperthyroidism 155
thyroid - hypothyroid 155
thyroid - hypothyroidism 155
thyrotropin 155
thyroxine 155
total testosterone 156
Toyota Motor Corporation 194
transdiagnostic theory 120
trans fats 26, 45, 54, 57, 60
transtheoretical model 130
tri-cyclic antidepressants 117
triglycerides xxvii, 5, 75, 89, 110,
     161
tri-iodothyronine 155
Trinity College of Natural Health
     ix
trust model 34
type 1 diabetes 77
type 2 diabetes 77

U

under active thyroid 155
unipolar depression 114
University of California 80, 253
US Centers for Disease Control
     and Prevention 71
US Department of Agriculture
     (USDA) 47, 69, 223

US Department of Health and
     Human Services 228
US Department of Health and
     Human Services physical
     activity guidelines for
     Americans 222
US National Library of Medicine
     255

V

vegan diet 28, 30
vegetarian diet 28, 30
very low calorie diet 29
visceral adipose tissue xxix
visceral fat 111, 114, 115, 154,
     156, 163
visceral fat rebound 89
visceral obesity 111
VO2max 84
VO2peak 84

W

waist circumference 9
waist to hip ratio 8
Weight Watchers diet 59
Western Pennsylvania Hospital
     252
white matter 108

Z

Zone diet 59